Primary Care Medically Underserved

Editors

VINCENT MORELLI
ROGER J. ZOOROB
JOEL J. HEIDELBAUGH

PHYSICIAN ASSISTANT CLINICS

www.physicianassistant.theclinics.com

Consulting Editor
JAMES A. VAN RHEE

January 2019 • Volume 4 • Number 1

ELSEVIER

1600 John F. Kennedy Boulevard • Suite 1800 • Philadelphia, Pennsylvania, 19103-2899

http://www.theclinics.com

PHYSICIAN ASSISTANT CLINICS Volume 4, Number 1
January 2019 ISSN 2405-7991, ISBN-13: 978-0-323-65487-6

Editor: Jessica McCool
Developmental Editor: Casey Potter

Physician Assistant Clinics (ISSN: 2405–7991) is published quarterly by Elsevier Inc., 360 Park Avenue South, New York, NY 10010-1710. Months of issue are January, April, July, and October. Periodicals postage paid at New York, NY and additional mailing offices. Subscription prices are $150.00 per year (US individuals), $205.00 (US institutions), $100.00 (US students), $150.00 (Canadian individuals), $257.00 (Canadian institutions), $100.00 (Canadian students), $150.00 (international individuals), $257.00 (international institutions), and $100.00 (international students). Foreign air speed delivery is included in all *Clinics* subscription prices. All prices are subject to change without notice. POSTMASTER: Send address changes to *Physician Assistant Clinics*, Elsevier Periodicals Customer Service, 11830 Westline Industrial Drive, St. Louis, MO 63146. Customer Service Health Sciences Division, Subscription Customer Service, 3251 Riverport Lane, Maryland Heights, MO 63043. **Customer Service: 1-800-654-2452 (U.S. and Canada); 314-447-8871 (outside U.S. and Canada). Fax: 314-447-8029. E-mail: journalscustomerservice-usa@elsevier.com (for print support); journalsonlinesupport-usa@elsevier.com (for online support).**

Reprints. For copies of 100 or more, of articles in this publication, please contact the Commercial Reprints Department, Elsevier Inc., 360 Park Avenue South, New York, NY 10010-1710. Tel. 212-633-3874; Fax: 212-633-3820; E-mail: reprints@elsevier.com.

Physician Assistant Clinics is covered in *EMBASE/Excerpta Medica and ESCI.*

PROGRAM OBJECTIVE

The goal of the *Physician Assistant Clinics* is to keep practicing physician assistants up to date with current clinical practice by providing timely articles reviewing the state of the art in patient care.

TARGET AUDIENCE

Physician Assistants and other healthcare professionals.

LEARNING OBJECTIVES

Upon completion of this activity, participants will be able to:

1. Review environmental justice and climate change in underserved communities.
2. Discuss issues in underserved populations such as diet and obesity, exercise and sports, and infectious disease.
3. Recognize medical care issues for undocumented immigrants and for the homeless.

ACCREDITATION

The Elsevier Office of Continuing Medical Education (EOCME) is accredited by the Accreditation Council for Continuing Medical Education (ACCME) to provide continuing medical education for physicians.

The EOCME designates this enduring material for a maximum of 15 *AMA PRA Category 1 Credit*(s) ™. Physicians should claim only the credit commensurate with the extent of their participation in the activity.

All other health care professionals requesting continuing education credit for this enduring material will be issued a certificate of participation.

DISCLOSURE OF CONFLICTS OF INTEREST

The EOCME assesses conflict of interest with its instructors, faculty, planners, and other individuals who are in a position to control the content of CME activities. All relevant conflicts of interest that are identified are thoroughly vetted by EOCME for fair balance, scientific objectivity, and patient care recommendations. EOCME is committed to providing its learners with CME activities that promote improvements or quality in healthcare and not a specific proprietary business or a commercial interest.

The planning committee, staff, authors and editors listed below have identified no financial relationships or relationships to products or devices they or their spouse/life partner have with commercial interest related to the content of this CME activity:

Teresa L. Beck, MD, FAAFP; Jonathan A. Becker, MD; Daniel L. Bedney, MD; Juliana Berenyi, DO; Ramon Cancino, MD, MSc; Arie (Eric) Dadush, MD; Lauren deCaporale-Ryan, PhD; Konstantinos E. Deligiannidio, MD, MPH, FAAFP; Neerav Desai, MD; Mathew Devine, DO; Omotayo Fawibe, MD; Luz M. Fernandez, MD; Sheryl B. Fleisch, MD; Sandra J. Gonzalez, PhD; Samuel Neil Grief, MD, FCFP; Michael Hayden, MD; Queen Henry-Okafor, PhD, FNP-BC; Paul Hutchinson, PhD; Casey Potter; Medhat Kalliny, MD, PhD; Alison Kemp; Alicia Ann Kowalchuk, DO; Thien-Kim Le, MD; Robert S. Levine, MD; Magdalene Lim, PsyD; Jessica McCool; Judith Green McKenzie, MD, MPH; Maria C. Mejia de Grubb, MD, MPH; John Paul Miller, MD; Vincent Morelli, MD; Charles P. Mouton, MD, MS; Robertson Nash, PhD, ACNP, BC; Stephanie L. Neary, MPA, MMS, PA-C; Oluwadamilola O. Olaku, MD, MPH; Arunkumar Rangarajan; Brian C. Reed, MD; Mary Elizabeth Romano, MD, MPH; Megha K. Shah, MD, MSc; Mary Showstark, MS, PA-C; Mohamad A. Sidani, MD, MS; Janet H. Southerland, DDS, PhD, MPH; Jeffrey Steinbauer, MD; Emmanuel A. Taylor, MSc, DrPH; Carol Ziegler, DNP, APRN, NP-C, RD; Roger J. Zoorob, MD, MPH.

The planning committee, staff, authors and editors listed below have identified financial relationships or relationships to products or devices they or their spouse/life partner have with commercial interest related to the content of this CME activity:

James A. Van Rhee, MS, PA-C: receives royalties and/or holds patents from Kaplan, Inc.

UNAPPROVED/OFF-LABEL USE DISCLOSURE

The EOCME requires CME faculty to disclose to the participants:

1. When products or procedures being discussed are off-label, unlabelled, experimental, and/or investigational (not US Food and Drug Administration [FDA] approved); and
2. Any limitations on the information presented, such as data that are preliminary or that represent ongoing research, interim analyses, and/or unsupported opinions. Faculty may discuss information about pharmaceutical agents that is outside of FDA-approved labelling. This information is intended solely for CME and is not intended to promote off-label use of these medications. If you have any questions, contact the medical affairs department of the manufacturer for the most recent prescribing information.

TO ENROLL

The CME program is available to all *Physician Assistant Clinics* subscribers at no additional fee. To subscribe to the *Physician Assistant Clinics*, call customer service at 1-800-654-2452 or sign up online at www.physicianassistant.theclinics.com/.

METHOD OF PARTICIPATION

In order to claim credit, participants must complete the following:
1. Complete enrolment as indicated above.
2. Read the activity.
3. Complete the CME Test and Evaluation. Participants must achieve a score of 70% on the test. All CME Tests and Evaluations must be completed online.

CME INQUIRIES/SPECIAL NEEDS

For all CME inquiries or special needs, please contact elsevierCME@elsevier.com.

Contributors

CONSULTING EDITOR

JAMES A. VAN RHEE, MS, PA-C
Associate Professor, Program Director, Yale School of Medicine, Yale Physician Assistant Online Program, New Haven, Connecticut

EDITORS

VINCENT MORELLI, MD
Department of Family and Community Medicine, Meharry Medical College, Nashville, Tennessee

ROGER J. ZOOROB, MD, MPH
Professor and Chair, Department of Family and Community Medicine, Baylor College of Medicine, Houston, Texas

JOEL J. HEIDELBAUGH, MD, FAAFP, FACG
Clinical Associate Professor, Departments of Family Medicine and Urology, Clerkship Director, Department of Family Medicine, University of Michigan Medical School, Ann Arbor, Michigan; Ypsilanti Health Center, Ypsilanti, Michigan

AUTHORS

TERESA L. BECK, MD, FAAFP
Assistant Professor, Program Director, Emory Family Medicine Residency Program, Department of Family and Preventive Medicine, Emory School of Medicine, Atlanta, Georgia

JONATHAN A. BECKER, MD
Associate Professor, Department of Family and Geriatric Medicine, University of Louisville, Louisville, Kentucky

DANIEL L. BEDNEY, MD
Resident, Department of Family and Community Medicine, Meharry Medical College, Nashville, Tennessee

JULIANA BERENYI, DO
University of Rochester Family Medicine Resident, Rochester, New York

RAMON CANCINO, MD, MSc
Chief Medical Officer, Mattapan Community Health Center, Assistant Professor of Family Medicine and Community Health Sciences, Boston University School of Medicine, Boston, Massachusetts

ARIE (ERIC) DADUSH, MD
Resident, Department of Family and Community Medicine, Meharry Medical College, Nashville, Tennessee

LAUREN DECAPORALE-RYAN, PhD
Assistant Professor, Departments of Psychiatry, Medicine, and Surgery, University of Rochester Medical Center, Rochester, New York

KONSTANTINOS E. DELIGIANNIDIS, MD, MPH, FAAFP
Director, House Calls Education Program, Northwell Health Solutions, New Hyde Park, New York

NEERAV DESAI, MD
Assistant Professor, Division of Adolescent Medicine & Young Adult Health, Monroe Carell Jr. Children's Hospital at Vanderbilt, Vanderbilt University Medical Center, Nashville, Tennessee

MATHEW DEVINE, DO
Associate Medical Director, Highland Family Medicine; Assistant Professor, Department of Family Medicine, Associate Medical Director, Accountable Health Partners, Rochester, New York

OMOTAYO FAWIBE, MD
Occupational Medicine Resident, Department of Family and Community Medicine, Meharry Medical College, Nashville, Tennessee

LUZ M. FERNANDEZ, MD
Assistant Professor, Department of Family and Geriatric Medicine, University of Louisville, Louisville, Kentucky

SHERYL B. FLEISCH, MD
Assistant Professor of Psychiatry and Medical Director, Homeless Health Services at Vanderbilt, Vanderbilt Street Psychiatry, Vanderbilt University School of Medicine, Nashville, Tennessee

SANDRA J. GONZALEZ, PhD
Instructor, Department of Family and Community Medicine, Baylor College of Medicine, Houston, Texas

SAMUEL NEIL GRIEF, MD, FCFP
Associate Professor, Department of Family Medicine, University of Illinois at Chicago, Chicago, Illinois

MICHAEL HAYDEN, MD
Department of Internal Medicine, School of Medicine, Meharry Medical College, Nashville, Tennessee

QUEEN HENRY-OKAFOR, PhD, FNP-BC
Family Nurse Practitioner Program, Assistant Professor, Vanderbilt University School of Nursing, Nashville, Tennessee

PAUL HUTCHINSON, PhD
Associate Professor, Global Community Health Sciences, Tulane University School of Public Health and Tropical Medicine, New Orleans, Louisiana

MEDHAT KALLINY, MD, PhD
Assistant Professor, Department of Family and Community Medicine, Meharry Medical College, Nashville, Tennessee

ALICIA ANN KOWALCHUK, DO
Assistant Professor, Department of Family and Community Medicine, Baylor College of Medicine, Houston, Texas

THIEN-KIM LE, MD
Department of Family and Preventive Medicine, PGY2 Resident, Emory School of Medicine, Atlanta, Georgia

ROBERT S. LEVINE, MD
Department of Family and Community Medicine, Professor, Baylor College of Medicine, Houston, Texas

MAGDALENE LIM, PsyD
Psychology Fellow, Departments of Psychiatry and Medicine, University of Rochester Medical Center, Rochester, New York

JUDITH GREEN McKENZIE, MD, MPH
Division of Occupational Medicine, Associate Professor, Department of Emergency Medicine, Hospital of the University of Pennsylvania, Philadelphia, Pennsylvania

MARIA C. MEJIA de GRUBB, MD, MPH
Department of Family and Community Medicine, Assistant Professor, Baylor College of Medicine, Houston, Texas

JOHN PAUL MILLER, MD
Program Director, Bakersfield Memorial Family Medicine Residency Program; Assistant Clinical Professor, Department of Family Medicine, University of California Irvine School of Medicine, Bakersfield, California

VINCENT MORELLI, MD
Department of Family and Community Medicine, Meharry Medical College, Nashville, Tennessee

CHARLES P. MOUTON, MD, MS
Department of Family and Community Medicine, School of Medicine, Meharry Medical College, Nashville, Tennessee

ROBERTSON NASH, PhD, ACNP, BC
Assistant in Medicine, Vanderbilt Comprehensive Care Clinic, Vanderbilt Health at One Hundred Oaks, Nashville, Tennessee

STEPHANIE L. NEARY, MPA, MMS, PA-C
Instructor, Yale University Physician Assistant Online Program, New Haven, Connecticut

OLUWADAMILOLA O. OLAKU, MD, MPH
Office of Cancer Complementary and Alternative Medicine, National Cancer Institute, Bethesda, Maryland; Kelly Services, Rockville, Maryland

BRIAN C. REED, MD
Department of Family and Community Medicine, Associate Professor, Baylor College of Medicine, Houston, Texas

MARY ELIZABETH ROMANO, MD, MPH
Assistant Professor, Division of Adolescent Medicine & Young Adult Health, Monroe Carell Jr. Children's Hospital at Vanderbilt, Vanderbilt University Medical Center, Nashville, Tennessee

MEGHA K. SHAH, MD, MSc
Department of Family and Preventive Medicine, Assistant Professor, Emory School of Medicine, Atlanta, Georgia

MARY SHOWSTARK, MS, PA-C
Instructor, Physician Assistant Online Program, Yale University, New Haven, Connecticut

MOHAMAD A. SIDANI, MD, MS
Department of Family and Community Medicine, Professor, Baylor College of Medicine, Houston, Texas

JANET H. SOUTHERLAND, DDS, PhD, MPH
Department of Oral and Maxillofacial Surgery, School of Dentistry, Meharry Medical College, Nashville, Tennessee

JEFFREY STEINBAUER, MD
Department of Family and Community Medicine, Professor, Baylor College of Medicine, Houston, Texas

EMMANUEL A. TAYLOR, MSc, DrPH
Center to Reduce Cancer Health Disparities, National Cancer Institute, Rockville, Maryland

CAROL ZIEGLER, DNP, APRN, NP-C, RD
Assistant Professor, Vanderbilt University School of Nursing, Family Nurse Practitioner and Instructor, Department of Family and Community Medicine, Meharry Medical College, Nashville, Tennessee

ROGER J. ZOOROB, MD, MPH
Professor and Chair, Department of Family and Community Medicine, Baylor College of Medicine, Houston, Texas

Contents

> This article addresses the scope of the problem primary care physicians
> face when caring for the underserved, both nationally and internationally.
> It touches on the statistics used to define medically underserved commu-
> nities, the pervasiveness of poverty, and how primary care physician short-
> ages may soon reach a crisis point. The definitions of socioeconomic
> status, allostatic load, and structural violence are also reviewed.

> Rural populations have different demographics and health issues
> compared to their metropolitan counterparts, including higher mortalities
> from ischemic heart disease, chronic obstructive pulmonary disease, un-
> intentional injuries, motor vehicle accidents, and suicide. Rural primary
> care physicians (PCPs) have a unique position in counseling, preventing,
> and treating common issues that are specific to rural populations, such
> as motor vehicle accidents, unintentional injuries, pesticide poisoning,
> occupational respiratory illnesses, and mental illness. They are also in a
> unique position to address prevention and social determinants of health.
> Rural PCPs can use multiple strategies to improve access to medical care.

> Inner-city patient populations are high-risk for poor outcomes, including
> increased risk of mortality. Barriers to delivering high-quality primary
> care to inner-city patients include lack of access, poor distribution of pri-
> mary care providers (PCPs), competing demands, and financial restraints.

Health care issues prevalent in this population include obesity, diabetes, cancer screening, asthma, infectious diseases, and obstetric and prenatal care. Population health management and quality improvement (QI) activities must target disparities in care. Partnering with patients and focusing on social determinants of health and medical care are key areas in which to focus to improve overall health outcomes in this population.

The number of undocumented immigrants (UIs) varies worldwide, and most reside in the United States. With more than 12 million UIs in the United States, addressing the health care needs of this population presents unique challenges and opportunities. Most UIs are uninsured and rely on the safety-net health system for their care. Because of young age, this population is often considered to be healthier than the overall US population, but they have specific health conditions and risks. Adequate coverage is lacking; however, there are examples of how to better address the health care needs of UIs.

Children and adolescents in underserved populations have health care risks that are different from those of the adult population. Providers need to be aware of these needs and the available resources. Providers should work with school and community organizations to provide timely and appropriate preventive health care and screen for medical and mental health problems that occur more commonly in these high-risk patient populations.

The purpose of this article is to review women's health issues that affect underserved populations. Certain groups have a lack of health care resources or inability to access resources. Individuals encounter barriers to accessing health care due to socioeconomic status, transportation, intimate partner issues, and distrust of the health care system. These factors lead to health care disparities and a lack of appropriate care or quality care as it pertains to breast cancer screening, cervical cancer screening, and obtaining contraceptive care. Identifying available resources in response to community-based needs assessment is among the tools available to combat these inequalities.

Homeless persons die significantly younger than their housed counterparts. In many cases, relatively straightforward primary care issues escalate into life-threatening, expensive emergencies. Poor health outcomes driven by negative interactions between comorbid symptoms meet the definition of a health syndemic in this population. Successful primary care of patients struggling with homelessness may result in long-term lifesaving measures along with decreased expenditure to hospital systems. This primary prevention requires patience, creativity, and acknowledgment that the source of many confounders may lay outside the control of these patients.

Sleep disorders and occupational hazards, injuries, and illnesses impact an individual's overall health. In the United States, substantial racial, ethnic, and socioeconomic disparities exist in sleep and occupational health. Primary care physicians working in underserved communities should be aware of this disparity and target these higher-risk populations for focused evaluation and intervention.

Infectious disease has a major impact on the health outcomes of underserved populations and is reported at significantly higher rates among these populations compared with the general population. Overcoming barriers and obstacles to health care access is key to addressing the disparity regarding the prevalence of infectious disease. Enhancing cultural competency and educating practitioners about underserved populations' basic health needs; optimizing health insurance for the underserved; increasing community resources; and improving access to comprehensive, continuous, compassionate, and coordinated health care are strategies for diminishing the burden of infectious disease in underserved populations.

The US population has a subset of those that are underserved who are in need of primary care and also suffer from mental health disorders. In this article, categories of underserved populations are described. Each section defines the population being presented, identifies the mental health problems each is likely to encounter, explores the barriers that prevent access to care, and identifies potential methods to minimize such barriers. The ways in which psychiatric issues vary in underserved settings compared with the general population are differentiated. Recommendations are offered for primary care physicians to support improved recognition and management of psychosocial stressors and psychiatric illness among the underserved.

Substance use affects people of all ages, cultures, and socioeconomic levels. Most underserved populations have lower rates of substance use than the general population in a given society, excluding tobacco use. The impact of substance use is more severe, however, in the underserved, with higher rates of incarceration, job loss, morbidity, and mortality. Innovative solutions are being developed to address these differences. Working together, underserved patients with substance use problems can be helped on their journeys toward health and wholeness.

The goal of this article is to inform new directions for addressing inequalities associated with obesity by reviewing current issues about diet and obesity among socioeconomically vulnerable and underserved populations. It highlights recent interventions in selected high-risk populations, as well as gaps in the knowledge base. It identifies future directions in policy and programmatic interventions to expand the role of primary care providers, with an emphasis on those aimed at preventing obesity and promoting healthy weight.

Primary care providers can make a strong argument for exercise promotion in underserved communities. The benefits are vitally important in adolescent physical, cognitive, and psychological development as well as in adult disease prevention and treatment. In counseling such patients, we should take into account a patient's readiness for change and the barriers to exercise.

Underserved communities suffer from environmental inequities. Gases lead to hypoxia and respiratory compromise, ozone to increased respiratory illnesses and decreased mental acuity, and mercury to prenatal cognitive disabilities and antisocial behaviors. Lead toxicity is associated with developmental delays. Cadmium is linked with cancer. The smaller sizes of air pollution particulate matter are pathogenic and are associated with cardiovascular and pulmonary disease and nervous system disorders. Bisphenol A is being studied for possible links to cancer and pregnancy risks. Physicians should be aware of these dangers, especially in underserved communities and populations. Investigating possible environmental risks and education are key.

Climate change is the greatest global health threat of the twenty-first century, yet it is not widely understood as a health hazard by primary care providers in the United States. Aside from increasing displacement of populations and acute trauma resulting from increasing frequency of natural disasters, the impact of climate change on temperature stress, vectorborne illnesses, cardiovascular and respiratory illnesses, and mental health is significant, with disproportionate impact on underserved and marginalized populations. Primary care providers must be aware of the impact of climate change on the health of their patients and advocate for adaptation and mitigation policies for the populations they serve.

rates of diseases accompanying poverty and hunger. There has been a shift away from the infectious diseases so deadly in developing nations toward first-world conditions. This article presents health care statistics across age groups and geographic areas to help the primary care physician understand these changes. There is a special focus on underserved populations. New technologies in health and health care spending internationally are addressed, emphasizing universal health care. The article concludes with recommendations for the future.

PHYSICIAN ASSISTANT CLINICS

SERIES OF RELATED INTEREST

Medical Clinics
https://www.medical.theclinics.com/
Primary Care: Clinics in Office Practice
http://www.primarycare.theclinics.com/

THE CLINICS ARE AVAILABLE ONLINE!
Access your subscription at:
www.theclinics.com

Foreword

The Underserved

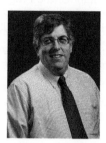

James A. Van Rhee, MS, PA-C
Consulting Editor

There have been many articles over the years regarding the care that physician assistants provide to patients in underserved areas. In 2009, Everett and colleagues identified characteristics and outcomes of patients who use physician assistants as a usual source of care. They noted that physician assistants are acting as primary care providers to underserved patients with a range of disease severity with no difference in outcomes when compared with physicians.[1] Henry and colleagues completed a literature review looking at the role of physician assistants in rural care. The review noted that physician assistants possess the broad range of skills and knowledge necessary to meet the health care needs of the underserved rural population.[2] Because this topic is so relevant to physician assistants today, we are reprinting a number of articles from *Primary Care: Clinics in Office Practice*. The articles have been divided into three areas:

- Medically underserved areas: these articles look at primary care issues in rural populations and inner-city America.
- Medically underserved populations: these articles look at medical care for undocumented immigrants, homeless patients, and pediatric, women's, and geriatric issues in underserved populations.
- Specific medical issues faced by the underserved: the focus of these articles is on cardiovascular, infectious disease, cancer, psychological, substance abuse, and obesity in the underserved population.

This issue of *Physician Assistant Clinics* not only provides the reader with the current issues related to care of underserved populations but also provides the reader with the knowledge needed to care for the wide variety of medical problems common to the underserved population. Neary and Showstark in their articles suggest ways that physician assistants can get involved in providing care to the underserved at both the

Physician Assist Clin 4 (2019) xvii–xviii
https://doi.org/10.1016/j.cpha.2018.10.001
2405-7991/19/© 2018 Published by Elsevier Inc.

physicianassistant.theclinics.com

domestic and the international levels and provide examples of their experiences. Our next issue will provide you with a review of the latest in Critical Care Medicine.

James A. Van Rhee, MS, PA-C
Yale School of Medicine
Yale Physician Assistant Online Program
100 Church Street South, Suite A230
New Haven, CT 06519, USA

E-mail address:
james.vanrhee@yale.edu

Website:
https://www.paonline.yale.edu

REFERENCES

1. Everett CM, Schumacher JR, Wright A, et al. Physician assistants and nurse practitioners as a usual source of care. J Rural Health 2009;25:407–14.
2. Henry LR, Hooker RS, Yates KL. The role of physician assistants in rural health care: a systematic review of the literature. J Rural Health 2011;27:220–9.

Preface

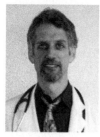 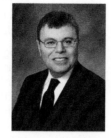

Vincent Morelli, MD   Roger J. Zoorob, MD, MPH
Editors

As primary care physicians on the frontlines of the world's health care delivery system, most of us are tasked daily with providing care for the underserved: the homeless, the aged, the undocumented, the uninsured. Such populations experience unique exposure risks and face significant barriers to care. Our medical training, though excellent in many aspects, fails to adequately spotlight these populations and discuss their unique medical needs. We hope that this publication will help overcome this deficiency and offer the primary care physician a new perspective when caring for these segments of our population.

Also, as we have researched and written for this issue, we have realized how important our social policies are in affecting the health of our citizens. We hope that policy-makers will take the time to consider the information contained in this issue when setting future health care policies.

Finally, we are honored to serve as guest editors for this issue of *Physician Assistant Clinics*, and we feel privileged to have worked with such a distinguished group of collaborators. Many thanks to our contributing authors, who have worked diligently to make their articles scholarly and clinically relevant. We also thank the Departments of Family and Community Medicine at Meharry Medical College and Baylor College of Medicine for providing us with the support needed to complete this project. Finally, thanks to our editors at Elsevier, without whose help this project would never have been accomplished.

Physician Assist Clin 4 (2019) xix–xx
https://doi.org/10.1016/j.cpha.2018.08.013
2405-7991/19/© 2018 Published by Elsevier Inc.

Vincent Morelli, MD
Department of Family and
Community Medicine
Meharry Medical College
1005 Dr D.B. Todd Boulevard
Nashville, TN 37208, USA

Roger J. Zoorob, MD, MPH
Family and Community Medicine
Baylor College of Medicine
3701 Kirby Drive, Suite 600
Houston, TX 77098, USA

E-mail addresses:
morellivincent@yahoo.com (V. Morelli)
roger.zoorob@bcm.edu (R.J. Zoorob)

Editorial

Serving the Underserved Internationally

INTRODUCTION

Underserved communities exist both domestically and internationally. Underserved populations internationally suffer from unclean water, lack of medical providers, or access to care. Although every country has underserved populations, every country has their own interpretation of what this means.[1] Over four million people worldwide lack access to quality health services, in large part because of a huge shortage, imbalanced skill mix, and uneven geographical distribution of health workers.[2]

In the World Health Report 2017, it was estimated that approximately one-half of the global population lives in rural areas. Of the 43.5 million health workers in the world, it is estimated that 20.7 million are nurses and midwives, yet 50% of World Health Organization (WHO) Member States report to have less than 3 nursing and midwifery personnel per 1000 population (about 25% report to have less than 1 per 1000), according to the 2017 Global Health Observatory. Over 45% of WHO Member States report to have less than 1 physician per 1000 population[3] (Appendix 1).

The United Nations (UN) World Populations Prospects lists the 10 countries with the largest populations and projects population growth over time (**Table 1.**).[4] This, of course, leads to increasing numbers of underserved and medical disparities, thus increasing the health care burden (**Fig. 1**).

Working as a Physician Assistant (PA) abroad, I have had the opportunity to work with the underserved internationally. I have had a wide range of opportunities. These vary from setting up clinics in remote locations, to sponsoring local villages, to performing medical needs assessments, to working in disaster zones, and to remotely assisting in evacuation. In all of these situations, the goal is to help create sustainability, educate, and work toward improving safety.

Many underserved populations would never call themselves underserved. In many remote areas, such as when I was working in Nepal after the earthquake in 2015, the village I was helicoptered into to provide medical care pulled together and rebuilt their community. They supported each other; they sought out others in other remote villages to let them know that we were on the ground providing medical assistance for those in need. This area in the Ganesh mountain chain was a four-day walk to Kathmandu with strenuous changes in altitude. Villagers relied on each other to provide care, to bandage, and to emotionally support each other after the trauma and losses they sustained. When working abroad in times of disaster, sometimes you are only able to provide temporary care; however, there are plenty of opportunities for education, which we hope lasts a lifetime. There is also the psychological component, whereby people here now know they are not alone.

Previously, there has been much discussion as to whether PAs should be working internationally in countries that do not recognize the profession. There is the question of medical liability. What do you do if something goes wrong? Will a PA be blamed

Physician Assist Clin 4 (2019) xxi–xxxix
https://doi.org/10.1016/j.cpha.2018.08.015

Table 1
UN predicted populations

	Ten Countries with the Largest Populations, 2017 and 2050			
Rank	Country	2017 Population (Millions)	Country	2050 Population (Millions)
1	China	1410	India	1659
2	India	1339	China	1364
3	United States of America	324	Nigeria	411
4	Indonesia	264	United States of America	390
5	Brazil	209	Indonesia	322
6	Pakistan	197	Pakistan	307
7	Nigeria	191	Brazil	233
8	Bangladesh	165	Bangladesh	202
9	Russian Federation	144	Dem. Rep. of the Congo	197
10	Mexico	129	Ethiopia	191

Among the ten most populous countries of the world today, one is in Africa (Nigeria), five are in Asia (Bangladesh, China, India, Indonesia, and Pakistan), two are in Latin America (Brazil and Mexico), one is in Northern America (United States of America), and one is in Europe (the Russian Federation). Amongst these, Nigeria's population, currently the seventh largest in the world, is growing the most rapidly and is projected to surpass that of the United States shortly before 2050. In 2050, the populations in six of the ten largest countries are expected to exceed 300 million: China, India, Indonesia, Nigeria, Pakistan, and United States of America (in alphabetical order).

From United Nations. World Populations Prospects 2017 Revision. Available at: https://esa.un.org/unpd/wpp/Publications/Files/WPP2017_DataBooklet.pdf. Accessed June 6, 2018.

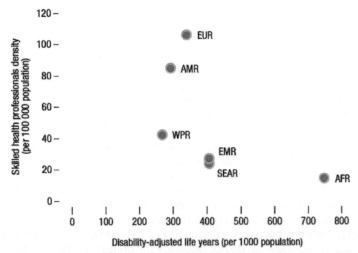

Fig. 1. Regional health workforce density, 2005–2015, and estimated total burden of disease, 2010. AFR, Africa; AMR, Americas; EMR, Eastern Mediterranean; EUR, Europe; SEAR, South-East Asia; WPR, Western Pacific. (*From* United Nations. World Populations Prospects 2017 Revision. Available at: https://esa.un.org/unpd/wpp/Publications/Files/WPP2017_DataBooklet.pdf. Accessed June 6, 2018. ©2017 United Nations. *Reprinted* with the permission of the United Nations.)

publicly and it may look bad for the profession? Will people understand what a Physician Assistant is? What type of liability insurance does one carry? Will people sue you if they don't know/understand the care that you are providing them, and what if that care is not able to be obtained? There are many criticisms to this; however, if one is trained, has a supervising MD in some capacity, then why would we do people a disservice by not providing care, when we are fully capable and they are more than willing to accept it?

HISTORY OF ADVANCED PRACTICE PROVIDERS GLOBALLY

Advanced practice providers similar to PAs have worked throughout history taking care of the underserved. Feldshers in Russia, barefoot doctors in China, and military corpsman were some of the first "midlevel" providers.[5]

PAs are present in Australia, India, the Netherlands, Liberia, New Zealand, Germany, Saudi Arabia, Afghanistan, Israel, Ireland, and Canada. Physician associates work in the United Kingdom, medical associates in Ghana, and clinical associates in South Africa.[6] More and more countries are becoming accustomed to the advanced practice provider.

In the past several years, increasing conflicts have arisen, and as many as 20 people are forcibly displaced every minute as a result of conflict or persecution. Many displaced persons end up in refugee camps and are totally dependent on humanitarian aid. They fall susceptible to disease, physical and sexual abuse, and human trafficking.[7] Advanced practice providers can and have played a huge role in providing care to these camps and internationally filling the gap.

American Academy of Physician Assistants and the Physician Assistant's Scope Internationally

The American Academy of Physician Assistants (AAPA) in 2016 has reaffirmed their guidelines for an international standard for a code of conduct for PAs practicing internationally (**Box 1**). While PAs should only provide care in their scope of practice, PAs may be called upon to play many other roles.[8,9] These roles include logistical support and aiding in communication to receiving hospitals, local governances, other nongovernmental organizations (NGOs), and other global entities, such as the UN and the WHO to report statistics to.

The PA may be assisting in setting up the clinic, anything from setting up a basic tent and tarp to a Western Shelter, scoping out and drawing the site for a helicopter pad, to working with incident command structures (**Fig. 2**).[10–12]

The PA may be a part of the medical team, where the PA functions in their typical role as a medical provider, or as the safety officer, or one of the safety officer's assistants. The safety officer handles everything from unsafe work environments to personal protection equipment (PPE), ensures adequate sanitation and safety in food preparations, and listens in on tactical options being considered.[12] The safety officer (see **Fig. 2**) may also ensure that risk management addresses safety, occupational health, and environmental health at all levels.[12,13]

The PA may handle everything from medical care to digging latrines, and ensuring safe water sources.

Licensure

Licensure for PAs practicing abroad with the underserved is a common question. In situations such as disaster, this may be waived, or you are working with an MD on your disaster team that supervises you. A PA should contact the Ministry of Health

Box 1

American Academy of Physician Assistants guidelines for Physician Assistants working internationally

AAPA: Guidelines for PAs Working Internationally: HP-3700.3.0 International [Adopted 2001, reaffirmed 2006, amended 2011, reaffirmed 2016]

1. PAs should establish and maintain the appropriate physician-PA team

2. PAs should accurately represent their skills, training, professional credentials, identity, or service both directly and indirectly

3. PAs should provide only those services for which they are qualified via their education and/ or experiences, and in accordance with all pertinent legal and regulatory processes

4. PAs should respect the culture, values, beliefs, and expectations of the patients, local health care providers, and the local health care systems

5. PAs should be aware of the role of the traditional healer and support a patient's decision to utilize such care

6. PAs should take responsibility for being familiar with, and adhering to, the customs, laws, and regulations of the country where they will be providing services

7. When applicable, PAs should identify and train local personnel who can assume the role of providing care and continuing the education process

8. PA students require the same supervision abroad as they do domestically

9. PAs should provide the best standards of care and strive to maintain quality abroad

10. Sustainable programs that integrate local providers and supplies should be the goal

11. PAs should assign medical tasks to nonmedical volunteers only when they have the competency and supervision needed for the tasks for which they are assigned

From AAPA. American Academy of Physician Assistants Policy Manual. 2016. Available at: https://www.aapa.org/wp-content/uploads/2017/02/International-Policy.pdf. Accessed June 6, 2018.

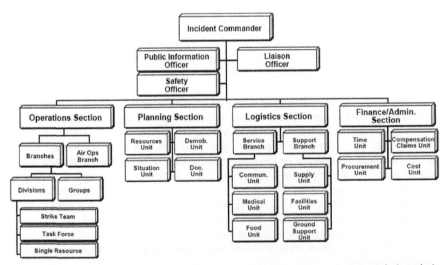

Fig. 2. Incident command structure: Federal Emergency Management Agency. Admin, administrator; Commun, communications; Demob, demobilization; Doc, documentation; Ops, operations. (*From* Federal Emergency Management Agency—Federal Emergency Management Agency (May 2008). Incident Command System Training Review Material. Available at: http://www.training.fema.gov/EMIWeb/IS/ICSResource/assets/reviewMaterials.pdf. Accessed June 6, 2018.)

in the country or discuss options with the organization they are working with. The PA may also establish a relationship with a provider in the host country or their supervising physician in their established practice. Section HP-3700.3.1 of AAPA's policy manual states that PAs must establish the appropriate physician-PA team.[9] There are no established laws for PAs practicing in underserved areas internationally.[14,15] It is recommended to bring photocopies of your licenses, passport, and vaccines as local government and NGO agencies, hospitals, and land border control may wish to keep a copy.

Liability

When working with the underserved, will they sue? When working in a US hospital Emergency Department in an underserved area, we had a woman who would constantly visit and threaten to sue; she even would phone the Chief Medical Officer of the hospital and tell them of her care that she didn't approve of. When working internationally with the underserved, it feels like there will be less of a chance to be sued; however, one should not take that chance.

Liability for a PA comes into question here, as is it the PA's personal coverage or the doctor or organization that they are working with? Will the liability insurance policy even cover you internationally? It is recommended that PAs look into their own personal coverage. Checking with the Ministry of Health in that country or a local consulate is also recommended. In times of a disaster, this may be waived.

Certain countries, such as Tahiti, require you to work under the supervision of a French Polynesian trained doctor, no matter their specialty. This holds true for physicians as well as PAs.

PAs should also keep in mind that Good Samaritan laws do not provide either authorization to practice or, in most cases, liability protection when they are working in disaster relief situations.[15] Certain countries honor the Good Samaritan law, such as Tahiti, Australia, and the Philippines; however, Australia has multiple different states, and one should check specifically before providing care.[16] Some of these countries will honor a medical mission under the law; however, one should always make sure to check with the above agencies first and have it in writing.

MEDICATIONS

One of the other big factors to address when working in an underserved area is that medicines may not be readily available. A provider may not be familiar with the local medications either. Medical providers cannot haul large amounts of medications in without being given the proper permissions.

When working in Indonesia, I met with the local consulate to receive permission to bring in the medications that were necessary. Upon entering the country, Indonesia has a sign that says death penalty for bringing in drugs (**Fig. 3**). In Fiji, one must contact the Ministry for approval; however, customs still have the right to search you and may detain your goods. In previous trips to underserved areas, I have a full itemized list of what is being brought in; I have the consulate review and stamp their seal of approval. It is not always easy to get appointments with consulates nor are they always readily accessible in smaller towns.

Pill bottles should always be labeled, and a provider should always carry their medical license and copies of it in case of being detained at customs. In Japan, Vicks and Sudafed are illegal due to containing pseudoephedrine. In Costa Rica, you may only bring in enough meds for the length of your stay with a doctor's note. In Hong Kong and Greece, codeine is illegal. Tramadol may get you imprisoned in Egypt.

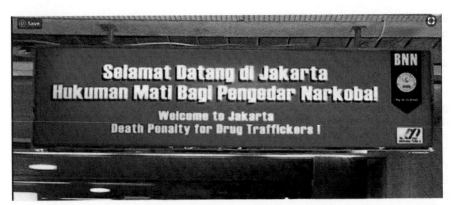

Fig. 3. Sign in Indonesia. (*From* Wikimedia Commons. Available at: https://commons.wikimedia.org/wiki/File:2011-08-06_Drug_sign_in_Soekarno_Hatta_Airport.jpg.   Accessed June 6, 2018.)

Drug resistance in an underserved area should also be noted. If a provider enters the country and tries to prescribe a resistant antibiotic, they are not of service and are adding to the crisis.

PAs should also be aware of drug dosages. When administering medications in Tahiti, the measurements were not the same. In a comparison, between Japan, Europe, and the United States, multiple differences in approved dosing for drugs exist.[17,18]

A provider must also understand that what you might wish to give a patient is a nonsteroidal anti-inflammatory drug, but they may want an herbal lotion or an ointment instead.

DONATIONS

Many developing countries are increasingly dependent on donor assistance to meet the equipment needs of their health care systems.[19,20] A provider must think before bringing in supplies to another country. Will the community know how to use the supplies? Are they reusable? Will harm occur to them if they run out?

The WHO has donation guidelines. These guidelines include that the health care equipment donation should benefit the recipient to the maximum extent possible; a donation should be given with the respect and wishes of the recipient and governing/administrative policies. There should be no double standard of care—if the item is unacceptable in the donor's country, then it is also unacceptable in the receiving country. And, last, there should be effective communication between the donor and the recipient, with all donations resulting from a need expressed by the recipient. Donations (solicited) should never be sent unannounced.[21]

There are also certain organizations that will help you transport medical supplies into different countries or provide you with prepackaged travel packs.

In Haiti, after the 2010 earthquake, drugs and supplies were shipped in containers. There were tons of containers at the airport and all over the tarmacs. There was no one to empty them, nor did anyone know where they were best suited. Bringing in all of the supplies does not mean that the community knows what to do with them.

While working in a remote island in the Philippines, we taught over 100 people basic life support. We purchased two automated external defibrillators and gave one to the clinic and one to the Coast Guard and trained them how to use them. While you can tell people what to do, that does not mean they know how to do it. Teaching and demonstrating how to perform certain tasks and how to use drugs/supplies and where they could be best utilized are key.

RESOURCE UTILIZATION

One of the most important things working in underserved environments is to understand resource utilization. One must work with what is given to them. They must understand how to triage who needs what. There is not an unlimited supply. You can't just call central supply and have something delivered to you within the hour.

One may reuse c-collars; sterilization may vary, and clinics may soak needles and sutures in Chlorhexidine for 14 days before reusing them. In Malawi, the hospital would send people to the pharmacy to buy clean needles to ensure that they were given them.

Providers who are accustomed to working in a hospital will need to think outside of the box. They will need to set up their own water filtration systems, such as the ones from Waves4Water; they will need to use old bottles to collect rain water to help with delivery of babies, irrigate wounds, and utilize during surgery. In Haiti, the surgeon and I couldn't close the abdomen due to abdominal compartment syndrome and we didn't have Vac-packs or even an operating table, so we utilized a take on the Bogota bag, by cutting empty saline bags and sewing them to the skin and sterile wet towels on top of, all while operating on a table with a wood plank as our bed (**Fig. 4**D). We also ran out of Foley catheter bags, so we used gloves instead (**Fig. 4**B). In Nepal, we created a walking boot out of an extra Sharps box (**Fig. 4**C). In Africa, an intracranial pressure (ICP) monitor was created with tubing and cardboard (**Fig. 4**A).

PERSONAL PACKING

What do you pack for yourself? A provider going to work abroad with the underserved should take what you can carry and no more than that. You will need to be able to take care of yourself. In Nepal, we had to allot for weight on the helicopters that were flying into treacherous areas with high wind gusts. Several helicopters had crashed in that region within the week. We also had to be prepared to hike steep elevation gains with our gear on our back. You cannot rely on having someone carry your bags. The US federal government recommends MOUSE, an acronym which means: mobile, organized, utility, safety and self, and environment. This means you must be able to move with your gear, know where stuff is in your bag, have appropriate tools such as work gloves, duct tape, and a travel shovel with you. Safety should include N95 and PPE. Self includes meals ready to eat (MREs), eyeshades, earplugs, raingear, water filtration, hand hygiene kits, first-aid kit, and personal medications. Environment means one should have sturdy boots and clothing that suits the 3W's: wicking, warmth, weather.[22] I have included a pack list (Appendix 2). I also recommend carrying a wire saw, which can cut anything from a piece of paper to tree limbs for firewood, and can be use for limb amputation. I also recommend packing your happy foods (remember that chocolate melts); a mixture of goji berries, cacao, and goldenberries is a great superfood that packs well in a Ziplock bag. One should also remember cash/local currency, as many locations will not have access to ATMs.

EVACUATION

Working in Haiti after the earthquake as a PA, I communicated with the military hospital ship, the SS Comfort, as well as worked with hospitals along the US east coast

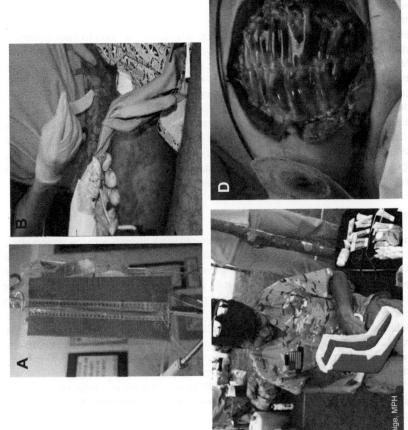

R. Kurashige, MPH

Fig. 4. Resource utilization. (*A*) ICP monitor. (*B*) Catheter bags made with gloves. (*C*) Walking boot made from Sharps box. (*D*) Saline bag "Bogota bag." (*From* Wikipedia. Available at: https://en.wikipedia.org/wiki/Bogota_bag#/media/File:Bogota_bag.png. Accessed June 6, 2018.)

transporting patients out that needed emergency care. In underserved areas, one typically works with the resources that they are given; however, there are those few times when one can really make a difference and organize a patient to be evacuated. In Nepal, we got report that a pregnant woman who we saw the day before was seizing. We were able to organize a helicopter and deliver mother and baby safely in Kathmandu. The local midwife was not present, and we were able to arrange transport, so we did. This does not always happen.

You must be sensitive that you are separating families as well as working with agencies to allow noncitizens right of entry into the country for medical care.

Evacuation insurance for yourself should be also be purchased. What happens if you break your leg or become ill? Make sure you and your family have a plan of action and make sure someone knows where you are at. GPS satellite devices such as SPOT can send out messages to those you designate on your list to let them know you are safe. SPOT also has tracking so those at home can see where you are located on a map when you ping the device.

One thing you will find is that written record is very common in underserved areas. Normally, this is quite difficult; however, after a disaster, this becomes very difficult. Families from other locations do not know if the person is alive or not. Patients in Haiti after the earthquake did not have any records of who they were. I went through over 400 patients creating a medical record system so that people would know who they were. This also becomes very difficult as these patients don't have records of owning their homes, bank records, or identification/passports to be evacuated. It is advisable that when working in an underserved area that you counsel your patients to have backup records.

CULTURAL BARRIERS

Overcoming cultural barriers is another factor one must take into consideration. Providers may need to use translators. They may have to use other words as words might not exist in the patient's language. One must be considerate as eye contact, touch, and gestures vary from culture to culture. Expressions of pain may differ. Patients may speak in tongues when in pain. While working in Africa, patients postoperation did not have a patient-controlled analgesia pump for pain. They did not take pain medicine. Attitudes toward pain may be very stoic.

Every culture has its own way of responding to important life events, such as birth, puberty, childbearing, illness, disease, and death. Cultural norms affect the way people react when they face the stresses of crises, disasters, ill health, detention, and uncertain futures.[22] In Nepal after the earthquake that destroyed their village and killed their loved ones in front of their very eyes, they sat in circles and played music and hand-clapping games and sang together. It was their way of coping. It was what they knew how to do (**Fig. 5**).

Foods are part of every culture. Patients may eat hot, spicy, kosher, vegetarian, and meals different than you are accustomed to. They may not want to stop eating certain foods that you recommend not to eat, or they may believe certain foods may cure them. In many cultures, refusing food offered to you is a sign of disrespect.

One should pay attention to religious beliefs, appropriate dress, cultures that are male dominant, and attitudes toward menstruation. Many women are not allowed to live in their homes when it is that time of month.

Many cultures believe that when inflicted with disease it is due to some causality. Deuteronomy 28:20-22 states that, because of various transgressions, God strikes people with diseases, fever, and inflammation.[23]

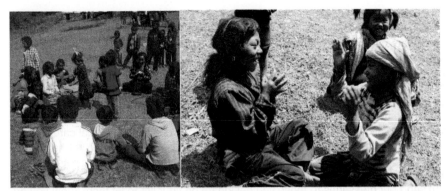

Fig. 5. Children in remote village in Ganesh Mountain Chain. (*Courtesy of* Mary Showstark, MS, PA-C, New Haven, CT.)

Death rituals are also carried out differently. Mourning and burials may differ from what one normally sees. In India, the men line up in the street; there are so many gathering in this procession carrying the casket, and it is so festive that you might think it is a party. Some cultures have burials, some cremations, and some funeral pyres. When training to work on Ebola, we learned that burial rites involve bathing the deceased. This can lead to the spread of infection. This is not something that we are used to in the Western world.

According to WHO, about 70% to 80% of the population in some West African countries depend on traditional medicine.[24] This exists in many different cultures, not just West Africa. One must be nonjudgmental and have openness to shamans, and other practitioners of traditional medicine, who may be known as "mediums," "witch doctors," "spiritual healers," "prophets," "medicine man/woman," "healers," "Txiv Neeb," "Sorcerers," "Dukun," and "Babaylan."

Culturally, one may encounter rituals for Pachamama, also known as Mother Earth, Anito in the Philippines, which refers to ancestor spirits, nature spirits, and deities. Many people practice plant medicine, only wishing to have herbal pills and ointments. In South America, ayahuasca is a hallucinogenic herbal plant that is used as traditional medicine and cultural psychiatry.[25]

Communicating with patients may be quite difficult not just due to the language barriers; patients may not know exactly what is going on with them. After the earthquake in Nepal, patients were all complaining of dizziness; while there is some sense of disequilibrium after an earthquake,[26] many were experiencing episodes of posttraumatic shock and unable to communicate it otherwise.

The Spirit Catches You and You Fall Down is a book about Hmongs that immigrated to the United States. A doctor in the book states: "The language barrier was the most obvious problem, but not the most important. The biggest problem was the cultural barrier. There is a tremendous difference between dealing with the Hmong and dealing with anyone else. An infinite difference."[27]

BURNOUT AND WELL-BEING

Provider burnout and stress is something that is very common when working with the underserved populations. Sometimes we feel as if we are providing them everything, and it feels so hopeful; however, there are times when workers share a common feeling that there is so much work that needs to be done and so little time in which to do it.[28]

Besides the never-ending work, there are many hardships that the provider faces. It is not easy living with people 24/7 in harsh, crowded conditions, possibly listening to military helicopters circling, sharing the same squatter hole, eating MREs day after day (**Fig. 6**).

What happens when you get out on the field or to the underserved area and it's not what you expected? How do you cope? Can you leave? What if there is perceived danger? In Nicaragua, we have evacuated efforts at a clinic due to the local protests becoming violent over the country's 2018 social security program.

How do you take care of your emotional well-being? In Africa, patients were being dropped off daily who were beaten with Sjamboks, a heavy whip made of rhino or hippo's hide; virgins wore red bows in their hair and were being raped because culturally there were stories that having sex with a virgin would cure AIDS/HIV. The president at the time told the media that by simply taking a shower one will be cured of HIV/AIDS. How do you cope with seeing this day after day? How do you counsel these patients? How do you educate and change public opinion?

First, by taking care of yourself, by making sure you are well fed, well hydrated, and well rested, and by making sure that you have moments for yourself. I bring my own food, as I stated; that gives me a feeling of home. I also make sure I have my air mattress and my pillow that compress and weigh less than one pound. I make sure I have at least ten minutes alone whether that is in my tent or behind the squatter hole. Recognizing burnout in yourself is just as important as recognizing it in others. Maslach and Leiter[29] define burnout as a prolonged response to stressors on the job that encompass overwhelming exhaustion, feelings of cynicism and detachment from the job, and a sense of ineffectiveness and a lack of accomplishment. This can occur rapidly when one is away from home, living in scarce conditions, and one feels there is an overwhelming amount of people to help.

One also has to make sure they are fit, that they have proper shoes—not new ones, and are capable of hiking to remote areas to help the underserved. This is your responsibility. Most organizations will ask you your fitness level, but it is very important that you identify your fitness level. This is because this can hinder the whole team, or you can start to draw resources out of the area because you become ill. We have had many providers who have needed IVs due to lack of hydration and self-care and even those who have had to be sent home.

In the Disaster Management Assistance Teams (DMAT) fitness (note, not IMSURT [International Medical/Surgical Response Teams]), of the 57 DMATs identified, 31 had publicly available Web sites. Of these, six publish fitness requirements, and one team requires a self-administered fitness assessment. By mitigating the risk of illness or injury to disaster responders, the likelihood of mission success and provider wellness can be increased.[30]

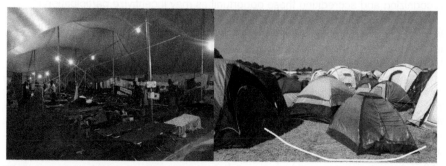

Fig. 6. Crowded conditions in the field.

INNOVATIVE PLANS AND THE FUTURE

In 2015, an estimated 303,000 women worldwide died due to maternal causes. Almost all of these deaths (99%) occurred in low- and middle-income countries, with almost two-thirds (64%) occurring in the WHO African Region.[31]

More than 90% of the world's population was living in places where air quality fell below WHO standards.[31] In India, air pollution is so bad that green projects have been initiated whereby plants are being placed on the sides of every building, and advertisements state to protect your children with PPEs as the air pollution is worse than smoking. Utilization of social media and advertising for educational purposes are on the rise.

The WHO 2030 plans have sustainable development goals (SDGs) for underserved areas. These plans include everything from water to sanitation, poverty, unhealthy food consumption, air pollution, food insecurity, malaria/HIV/AIDS/TB prevention, injuries and violence, disease outbreaks, reproductive health, and hazardous and unsafe work environments to name a few. There are over 50 SDG indicators that have been agreed upon to monitor health outcomes (**Table 2**).[31,32] The UN General Assembly stresses they, too, will make efforts and measures to identify those who are seeking international protection as refugees into the United States.[33]

Innovative ideas by corporate companies are taking shape in the global health world. One thing is for sure, Coca-Cola was in the most remote regions of Africa when I lived there. The *Cola Road* film documents how using the extra space in the Coke crates was able to deliver oral rehydration salts, zinc to treat diarrhea, and a bar of soap to the most remote villages.

By utilizing The Coca-Coca Company's business, route-to-market strategy, Project Last Mile is helping by getting medical supplies the "last mile" to remote communities in Africa. Since the initiative launched in 2010, Tanzania's Medical Stores Department reports that it has been able to improve medicine availability by 20% to 30% in some regions where new processes have been rolled out.[34] There are many possibilities for global corporations to aid in global health.

One of the biggest challenges is retention of health care workers in rural communities. This relies on policymakers, budgets, and the ability to create training programs. Implementations such as education and financial incentives, recruitment and retention strategies, and overall impact need to be assessed[35] (**Table 3**). The WHO Global Strategy on HRH: Workforce 2030 encourages countries to adopt a diverse, sustainable skills mix, harnessing the potential of community-based and midlevel health workers in interprofessional primary care teams. The goal is to have universal health coverage and accomplish the health SDG targets.[36]

In-service training for current health care workers seems to be underrecognized by existing professional development and continuing education programs. Formally recognizing and accrediting these opportunities may incentivize participation.[37]

Utilization of educational online platforms is also a useful way to keep providers with up-to-date materials. Massive open online courses (MOOC), such as Coursera, MIT-Harvard edX, Khan Academy partnered with Stanford School of Medicine, and Udacity, have been changing the way the world receives education.[38] There is the story of the 15-year-old from Mongolia who enrolled in an MOOC from MIT and was one out of 300 who received a perfect score out of 140,000 people who took it and then went on to get accepted at MIT. When interviewed, he said "for the underprivileged people, the learning more is almost like a punishment because it reminds you more about the resource restrictions." He suggested colleges and institutions make learning spaces in developing countries to help students put their knowledge to use.[39]

Table 2
Examples of opportunities for leveraging intersectoral action to improve health and achieve multiple other SDG targets

Exposure	Key Health Outcomes	Intersectoral Action: Examples of Key Actions Beyond the Health Sector	SDG Targets
Inadequate water, sanitation and hygiene	Diarrhoeal diseases, protein-energy malnutrition, intestinal nematode infections, schistosomiasis s, hepatitis A and E, typhoid and poliomyelitis	Actions by water, sanitation, and education sectors to improve management, affordability, and use of appropriate technologies, while empowering communities	1.4; 4.1; 6.1; 6.2; 16.7
Poverty and food insecurity	Under-five child deaths, stunting and wasting	Social welfare cash transfer programmes for better child nutrition and improved use of preventive health services	1.1; 1.2; 1.3; 2.1; 2.2; 10.4
Air pollution	Cardiovascular diseases (CVDs), chronic obstructive pulmonary disease (COPD), respiratory infections and lung cancer	Health-promoting urban design and transport systems resulting in multiple health and environmental co-benefits	7.1; 7.2; 9.1; 11.2; 11.6; 13.1
Substandard and unsafe housing, and unsafe communities	Asthma, CVDs, injuries and violence deaths	Implementation of housing standards and urban design that promote health	1.4; 5.2; 7.1; 7.2; 9.1; 11.1; 11.6; 12.6; 16.1
Hazardous, unsafe and unhealthy work environments	COPD, CVDs, lung cancer, leukaemia, hearing loss, back pain, injuries, depression	Labour sector promotion of occupational standards and workers' rights to protect worker health and safety across different industries (including the informal economy)	8.5; 8.8; 12.6; 13.1; 16.10
Exposure to carcinogens through unsafe chemicals and foods	Cancers, neurological disorders	Sound management of chemicals and food across the food industry, agriculture sector, and different areas of industrial production	6.3; 12.3; 12.4
Unhealthy food consumption and lack of physical activity	Obesity, CVDs, diabetes, cancers and dental caries	Improving product standards, public spaces, and using information and financial incentives, involving the education, agriculture, trade, transport, and urban planning sectors	2.2; 2.3; 4.1; 9.1; 12.6
Inadequate child care and learning environments	Suboptimal cognitive, socia and physical development	Specific early child development programmes designed by the health and other sectors, with supportive social policies (for example, paid parental leave, free pre-primary schooling and improvements in female education)	1.3; 4.1; 4.2; 4.5; 5.1; 8.6; 8.7

Table 3
New opportunities provided by the 2030 Agenda with reference to 6 main lines of action

	Six Main Lines of Action	Opportunities Provided by the 2030 Agenda
Building better systems for health	Intersectoral action by multiple stakeholders (see section 1.6)	Placing health in all sectors of policy-making; combining the strengths of multiple stakeholders
	Health systems strengthening for UHC (see section 1.2)	Disease-control programmes embedded in a comprehensive health system that provides complete coverage through fully staffed and well-managed health services, with financial risk protection
Enabling factors	Respect for equity and human rights (see section 1.3)	Improving health for whole populations by including all individuals ("leave no one behind") and empowering women
	Sustainable financing (see section 1.4)	Attracting new sources of funding; emphasizing domestic financing, with alignment of financial flows to avoid duplication of health system functions
	Scientific research and innovation (see section 1.5)	Reinforcing research and innovation as foundations for sustainable development, including a balance of research on medical, social and environmental determinants and solutions
	Monitoring and evaluation (see section 1.1)	Exploiting new technologies to manage large volumes of data, disaggregated to ascertain the needs of all individuals; tracking progress towards SDG 3 and all other health-related targets

From World Health Statistics 2017: monitoring health for the SDGs, sustainable development goals. Geneva: World Health Organization; 2017. License: CC BY-NC-SA 3.0 IGO. Available at: http://apps. who.int/iris/bitstream/handle/10665/255336/9789241565486-eng.pdf?sequence=1. Accessed June 6, 2018.

The WHO 2030 agenda is stressing interprofessional education (IPE) and training of midlevel health workers. This could possibly be accomplished with innovations in health care training platforms, such as the Yale Online Physician Assistant Program. The Yale Online Program has a collaborative technology partner, 2U Inc. This structure has been able to provide education to students in rural Montana and South Dakota and to students on Indian reservations. With the partnership with 2U, they will create an online IPE working with six other online universities to encompass public health, physical therapy, occupational therapy, advanced practice nurses, social work, and speech and language pathology.

Models such as MOOCs and university training programs can be looked at to provide quality education in underserved areas internationally as well as outreach via social media and corporate programs.

SUMMARY

Providers must be sensitive when working with the underserved abroad. They must take into account everything from their personal safety and well-being, to licensure, to liability to their role. Donations and medications should be carefully assessed.

While working and living in Africa, I will never forget a woman who looked to me and said, "I know people in your country and the rest of the world feel sorry for us and think we do not have everything that they have, but we are happy here. Please go back to your country, travel, and tell the world that, just because we do not have anything, we are happy." Every provider should respect cultural differences and remember to make the most out of every resource.

Every small difference is still a difference.

Mary Showstark, MS, PA-C
Physician Assistant Online Program
Yale University
100 Church Street South, Suite A230
New Haven, CT 06520, USA

E-mail address:
Mary.showstark@yale.edu

REFERENCES

1. Doherty GW. Cross-cultural counseling in disaster settings. The Australasian Journal of Disaster and Trauma Studies 1999;1999(2). Available at: http://www.massey.ac.nz/~trauma/issues/1999-2/doherty.htm. Accessed June 6, 2018.
2. World Health Organization. Education and training. 2013. Available at: https://whoeducationguidelines.org/sites/default/files/uploads/WHO_EduGuidelines_20131202_web.pdf. Accessed June 6, 2018.
3. World Health Organization. Global health observatory data. 2016. Available at: http://apps.who.int/gho/data/node.main.A1444. Accessed June 6, 2018.
4. United Nations. World populations prospect 2017. Available at: https://esa.un.org/unpd/wpp/Publications/Files/WPP2017_DataBooklet.pdf. Accessed June 6, 2018.
5. Ballweg R. History of the profession and current trends. In: Physician assistant: a guide to clinical practice. 6th edition. Philadelphia: Elsevier; 2018. p. 6–24.
6. Kuhns D. International development of the physician assistant profession. In: Physician assistant: a guide to clinical practice. 6th edition. Philadelphia: Elsevier; 2018. p. 25–36.
7. Atiyeh BS, Gunn SWA. Refugee camps, fire disasters, and burn injuries. Ann Burns Fire Disasters 2017;30(3):214–7.
8. AAPA. Guidelines for ethical conduct for the PA profession. 2013. Available at: https://www.aapa.org/wp-content/uploads/2017/02/16-EthicalConduct.pdf. Accessed June 6, 2018.
9. AAPA. American Academy of Physician Assistants Policy Manual. 2016. Available at: https://www.aapa.org/wp-content/uploads/2017/02/International-Policy.pdf. Accessed June 6, 2018.
10. FEMA. National incident management system. An introduction. Available at: https://emilms.fema.gov/is700anew/index.htm. Accessed June 6, 2018.
11. National Incident Management System. Homeland Security. 2008. Available at: https://www.fema.gov/pdf/emergency/nims/NIMS_core.pdf. Accessed June 6, 2018.
12. FEMA. Department of Homeland Security. 2012. Available at: https://training.fema.gov/emiweb/is/icsresource/assets/so_pcl.pdf. Accessed June 6, 2018.
13. National Guard Regulation 500-3/Air National Guard Instruction 10-2503. Emergency employment of army and other resources. Weapons of mass destruction

civil support team management. Unclassified. 2011. Available at: http://www.ngbpdc.ngb.army.mil/pubs/10/angi10_2503.pdf. Accessed June 6, 2018.

14. Kuhns D. International health care. In: Physician assistant: a guide to clinical practice. 6th edition. Philadelphia: Elsevier; 2018. p. 581–90.

15. AAPA. The physician assistant in disaster response. 2006. Available at: http://www2.wpro.who.int/internet/files/eha/toolkit/web/Technical%20References/Human%20Resources/The%20Physician%20Assistant%20in%20Disaster%20Response%20Guidelines.pdf. Accessed June 6, 2018.

16. Pardun JT. Good Samaritan laws: a global perspective. 20 Loy. L.A. Int'l & Comp. L. Rev. 591. 1998. Available at: http://digitalcommons.lmu.edu/ilr/vol20/iss3/8. Accessed June 6, 2018.

17. Malinowski HJ, Westelinck A, Sato J, et al. Same drug, different dosing: differences in dosing for drugs approved in the United States, Europe, and Japan. J Clin Pharmacol 2008;48(8):900–8.

18. Arnold FL, Kusama M, Ono S. Exploring differences in drug doses between Japan and Western countries. Clin Pharmacol Ther 2010;87(6):714–20.

19. WHO. Guidelines for medicine donations. 2010. Available at: http://apps.who.int/iris/bitstream/handle/10665/44647/9789241501989_eng.pdf?sequence=1. Accessed June 6, 2018.

20. WHO. Guidelines for health care equipment donations. 2000. Available at: http://www.who.int/medical_devices/publications/en/Donation_Guidelines.pdf. Accessed June 6, 2018.

21. Health and Human Services. NDMS 2060. Personal gear for deployments. Unclassified. 2013. Available at: https://respondere-learn.hhs.gov/file.php/123/N_2060/NDMS-N-2060-Full-b_Rev_2013.pptx, https://respondere-learn.hhs.gov/mod/resource/view.php?id=4302. Accessed June 6, 2018.

22. Health and Human Services. NDMS 2040. Cultural awareness. Unclassified. 2018. Available at: https://respondere-learn.hhs.gov/file.php/123/NDMS-NC-2040-Full-rev1.pps, https://respondere-learn.hhs.gov/mod/resource/view.php?id=4300. Accessed June 6, 2018.

23. Manguvo A, Mafuvadze B. The impact of traditional and religious practices on the spread of Ebola in West Africa: time for a strategic shift. Pan Afr Med J 2015; 22(suppl 1):9.

24. Wanacott P. Africa's village healers complicate Ebola fight; 20. Available at: http://www.wsj.com/articles/africas-village-healers-complicate-ebola-fight-1416268426. Accessed June 17, 2018.

25. Frecska E, Bokor P, Winkelman M. The therapeutic potentials of ayahuasca: possible effects against various diseases of civilization. Front Pharmacol 2016;7:35.

26. Honma M, Endo N, Osada Y, et al. Disturbances in equilibrium function after major earthquake. Sci Rep 2012;2:749.

27. Fadiman A. The spirit catches you and you fall down. 1st edition. New York: Farrar, Straus and Giroux; 1997.

28. Ballweg R. Dealing with stress and burnout. In: Physician assistant: a guide to clinical practice. 6th edition. Philadelphia: Elsevier; 2018. p. 467–75.

29. Maslach C, Leiter MP. Understanding the burnout experience: recent research and its implications for psychiatry. World Psychiatry 2016;15(2):103–11.

30. Romney DA, Alfalasi RB, et al. A systematic review of fitness requirements for DMAT teams. West J Emerg Med 2017;18(8):58.

31. Romney DA, Alfalasi RB, Sarin RR, et al. A Systematic Review of Fitness Requirements for DMAT Teams. Western Journal of Emergency Medicine: Integrating

Emergency Care with Population Health 2017;18(6.1). Available at: https://escholarship.org/uc/item/85d9m6zk. Accessed June 16, 2018.

32. WHO. World Health Statistics 2017. Available at: http://apps.who.int/iris/bitstream/handle/10665/255336/9789241565486-eng.pdf?sequence=1. Accessed June 4, 2018.

33. United Nations. General Assembly. 2016. Available at: http://www.un.org/en/development/desa/population/migration/generalassembly/docs/A_RES_71_1_E.pdf. Accessed June 12, 2018.

34. Coca Cola. The last mile. 2018. Available at: https://www.coca-colacompany.com/project-last-mile. Accessed June 14, 2018.

35. Huicho L, Dieleman M, Campbell J, et al. Increasing access to health workers in underserved areas: a conceptual framework for measuring results. Bull World Health Organ 2010;88:357–63.

36. WHO. Guideline Development Group (GDG) convenes in Geneva for its first meeting on forthcoming WHO guidelines on policy and system support for community-based health worker programmes. 2017. Available at: http://www.who.int/hrh/news/2016/policy-system-support_gdg-group/en/. Accessed June 2, 2018.

37. WHO. Mapping educational opportunities and resources for health-care workers to learn about antimicrobial resistance a (Human Resources for Health Observer Series No. 21). Available at: http://apps.who.int/iris/bitstream/handle/10665/259362/9789241512787-eng.pdf?sequence=1. Accessed June 6, 2018.

38. Crisp N, Chen L. Global supply of health professionals. N Engl J Med 2014;370:950–7.

39. Young J. This Mongolian teenager aced a MOOC. Now he wants to widen their impact. The chronicle of higher education. 2016. Available at: https://www.chronicle.com/article/This-Mongolian-Teenager-Aced-a/236362. Accessed June 3, 2018.

APPENDIX 1: DENSITY OF NURSING AND MIDWIFERY STAFF AND PHYSICIANS

Nursing and midwifery personnel — 2012 or later, Pre-2012
Physicians — 2012 or later, Pre-2012

AFR
Mauritius
Algeria
Seychelles
South Africa
Cabo Verde
Gabon
Botswana
Nigeria
Namibia
Kenya
Benin
Swaziland
Angola
Côte d'Ivoire
Madagascar
Mauritania
Congo
Gambia
Ghana
Uganda
Democratic Republic of the Congo
Zambia
Mali
Cameroon
Guinea-Bissau
Zimbabwe
Guinea
Senegal
Rwanda
Togo
Mozambique
Burkina Faso
Central African Republic
Chad
Ethiopia
Sierra Leone
Liberia
United Republic of Tanzania
Niger
Malawi
South Sudan
Sao Tome and Principe
Lesotho
Eritrea
Equatorial Guinea
Comoros
Burundi

AMR
Cuba — 8.4, 7.5
Uruguay
Argentina
United States of America
Canada — 9.9
Bahamas
Mexico
El Salvador
Brazil — 7.4
Trinidad and Tobago
Colombia
Ecuador
Panama
Dominican Republic
Paraguay
Costa Rica
Peru
Chile
Nicaragua
Guatemala
Belize
Bolivia (Plurinational State of)
Jamaica
Guyana
Saint Lucia
Venezuela (Bolivarian Republic of)
Suriname
Saint Vincent and the Grenadines
Saint Kitts and Nevis
Honduras
Haiti
Grenada
Dominica
Barbados
Antigua and Barbuda

SEAR
Maldives — 6.2
Democratic People's Republic of Korea
Sri Lanka
India
Nepal
Myanmar
Bangladesh
Thailand
Bhutan
Indonesia
Timor-Leste

EUR
Monaco — 20.5
San Marino — 9.1
Greece
Austria — 8.3
Georgia
Portugal
Norway — 17.9
Lithuania — 6.1
Switzerland — 18.2
Germany — 13.1
Sweden — 11.9
Belarus — 11.4
Italy
Bulgaria
Russian Federation — 8.7
Malta — 9.1
Spain
Iceland — 15.2
Andorra
Czechia — 8.4
Denmark — 17.9
Israel
Netherlands — 10.5
Slovakia
Estonia
Azerbaijan
Kazakhstan — 6.5
France — 10.6
Latvia
Republic of Moldova
Finland — 12.0
Croatia
Hungary
Belgium — 11.1
Ukraine
Ireland — 12.4
Luxembourg — 12.3
The former Yugoslav Republic of Macedonia
United Kingdom — 8.4
Slovenia — 8.8
Armenia
Romania
Cyprus
Serbia
Uzbekistan — 12.1
Montenegro
Turkmenistan
Poland
Bosnia and Herzegovina
Kyrgyzstan
Turkey
Tajikistan
Albania

EMR
Jordan
Kuwait
Saudi Arabia
Lebanon
Libya
Qatar
Oman
United Arab Emirates
Syrian Arab Republic
Iran (Islamic Republic of)
Tunisia
Pakistan
Bahrain
Iraq
Egypt
Morocco
Sudan
Yemen
Afghanistan
Djibouti
Somalia

WPR
Australia — 12.6
Mongolia
New Zealand — 11.1
Japan — 11.3
Republic of Korea
Singapore
Niue — 9.4
China
Brunei Darussalam
Malaysia
Nauru
Tuvalu
Cook Islands
Palau
Fiji
Viet Nam
Tonga
Lao People's Democratic Republic
Marshall Islands
Samoa
Kiribati
Micronesia (Federated States of)
Solomon Islands
Vanuatu
Cambodia
Papua New Guinea
Philippines

From World Health Organization. 2016. Global Health Observatory Data. Available at: http://apps.who.int/gho/data/node.main.A1444.

APPENDIX 2: ABBREVIATED PACK LIST

- Water filtration devices, like SteriPENs, Waves4Water Filtration kits
- A collapsible bucket to retrieve river water for sterilization

- Fire starters
- Duct tape
- Tent and tarp
- Insect repellent
- Sleeping bag
- Hat
- Sarong
- Tweezers
- Camel back
- Stethoscope
- Toilet paper in a plastic bag
- Cipro
- Headphones
- Flashlights
- Baby wipes ("because that's how you shower")
- Shovel
- Wire saw
- Emergency radio
- Pots and pans
- Book
- Camera
- Water tablets, iodine
- Vaccines
- Passport
- Zip ties
- Currency
- Batteries
- Solar-powered hot water shower bag
- Satellite phone or global data plan
- Emergency blankets ("have saved my life in rain storms and the monsoon floods that happened after the earthquake in Nepal")
- Clothing: 3Ws
- Sturdy shoes

Editorial

Medical Care for Refugee Patients

INTRODUCTION

In recent years, immigration policy has taken center stage in the political arena. Regulations have been passed; processes have changed, and bans have been placed and lifted. It is not always clear the long-term impact this changing political landscape will have on US citizens or the hundreds of thousands of people trying to immigrate to the United States each year. In times of uncertainty, one thing remains true: people need health care. Medical providers receive training in a myriad of topics related to culturally competent care, but not much of this is traditionally focused specifically on refugee populations. Although many of the same principles apply to this group as other vulnerable populations, there are also distinct differences that need to be considered. This article seeks to highlight these additional considerations that must be made for refugee patients.

CONTENT
Defining Legal Status

How and why an individual comes to the United States helps determine their legal status and impacts their ability to receive various health benefits. Understanding the differences between these terms is key to navigating the US health care system with a patient (**Table 1**).[1] This article focuses on discussion to the refugee population (**Box 1**).[2]

Words from a provider
A patient who was a refugee once explained to me that it was difficult to assimilate to life in the US because living here was not a dream she had growing up. Moving to the US became a necessity, a choice to live, when it was no longer safe to stay in her home city.

—Stephanie L. Neary, PA-C

Refugee Numbers

Between 2001 and 2016, almost 900,000 refugees resettled in the United States. Although this number seems large, refugee numbers are very small in comparison to the close to 1 million legal immigrants who come to the United States annually.[3] The process of gaining refugee status by the US Refugee Admissions Program takes an average of 18 to 24 months and includes biographical data collection, a medical screen, an in-person interview, and a joint security screen by the Department of State, the Department of Homeland Security, the National Counterterrorism Center, and the Department of Defense.[4] The United States resettles more refugees than all other nations combined (**Box 2**).[5] The United States does not discriminate or rank individuals during this resettlement process; all individuals, regardless of age, health, or work experience, are considered equally (see **Box 2**).

Physician Assist Clin 4 (2019) xli–xlviii
https://doi.org/10.1016/j.cpha.2018.08.014

Table 1
Legal status in the United States

Term	Definition
US national	An individual who has ties to outlying possessions of the United States. As of 2018, this only includes American Samoa and the Commonwealth of the Northern Mariana Islands
US citizen	Individual born in the United States, Puerto Rico, Guam, the US Virgin Islands, or individual whose parent is a US citizen
Alien	An individual who is not a US citizen or US national
Immigrant (lawful permanent resident)	An individual granted the right to reside permanently in the United States by the USCIS
Nonimmigrant	An individual who legally resides temporarily in the United States
Undocumented alien	An alien who has entered the United States illegally, did not obtain the proper documentation or authorization, or has overstayed set time limitations
Refugee status	Status granted to an individual who left their country seeking refuge or asylum, typically for persecution or fear of persecution. Status if granted before entering the United States
Asylum status	Protection granted to people who meet the definition of refugee but are already living within the United States or seeking admission at a US port of entry

Abbreviation: USCIS, US Citizenship and Immigration Services, a component of the US Department of Homeland Security.

Data from Immigration terms and definitions involving aliens. Internal Revenue Service. Available at: https://www.irs.gov/individuals/international-taxpayers/immigration-terms-and-definitions-involving-aliens. Accessed May 30, 2018.

US Health Care for Refugee Patients

The Cash and Medical Assistance Program is a 100% federally funded program that reimburses states for services, including administrative costs, provided to refugee patients. Individuals must first be determined ineligible for Temporary Assistance for Needy Families and Medicaid before gaining eligibility for Refugee Cash Assistance

Box 1
Department of Homeland Security's 5 protected grounds

To be considered for refugee status in the US, a well-founded fear of persecution must be met for one of the Department of Homeland Security's (DHS) five protected grounds:

- Religion
- Political opinion
- Race
- Nationality
- Membership in a particular social group

Data from U.S. Refugee Admissions Program FAQs. US Department of State. Available at: https://2009-2017.state.gov/j/prm/releases/factsheets/2016/264449.htm. Accessed May 30, 2018.

Box 2
Top 5 countries sending refugees to the United States (2001-2016)

- Burma
- Iraq
- Somalia
- Bhuatan
- Iran

Data from By the numbers: the United States of refugees. Smithsonian.com. 2017. Available at: https://www.smithsonianmag.com/history/by-numbers-united-states-refugees-180962487/. Accessed May 23, 2018.

---

or Refugee Medical Assistance programs. Patients must apply to their individual state within 8 months of the date of final granting of asylee status or of arrival in the United States as a refugee.[6] After 8 months, individuals must navigate the complexities of the US health care system without the assistance of the Office of Refugee Resettlement (ORR) (**Fig. 1**). There are many volunteer organizations available to continue assisting

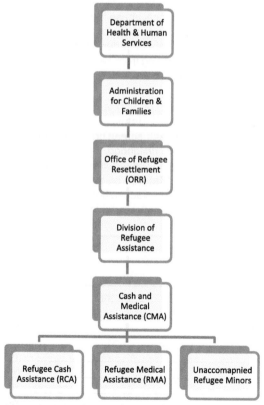

Fig. 1. Refugee support structure. (*From* About cash & medical assistance. Office of Child Care | ACF. 2018. Available at: https://www.acf.hhs.gov/orr/programs/cma/about. Accessed May 25, 2018; with permission.)

refugee patients through this resettlement process, but given the time and intricacy of most cases, there are often lapses in coverage and care.

Health Care Marketplace Eligibility

The Health Insurance Marketplace was created under the Patient Protection and Affordable Care Act (PPACA) to provide private health insurance options for individuals who make between 100% and 400% of the federal poverty level (FPL). For a family of 4 in 2018, this range is $24,600 to $98,400.[7] Individuals who qualify are eligible for federally funded tax credits to reduce the cost burden of health insurance premiums. Individuals making below 138% of the FPL in states that expanded Medicaid coverage under PPACA are eligible for Medicaid, while individuals making below 100% of the FPL in states that did not expand Medicaid may be left without coverage.[7] Eligibility also varies based on legal satus in the United States (**Table 2**).[8]

International Health Screen

As mentioned, individuals must undergo a medical examination before being accepted to resettle in the United States. Those who are found to have class A conditions are not permitted to resettle, but certain class A infectious conditions, like tuberculosis, are able to be treated and reclassified to class B, allowing a travel waiver to be granted that outlines any necessary follow-up.[5] Examples of class A conditions include tuberculosis, syphilis, gonorrhea, Hansen disease (leprosy), mental disorders with harmful behaviors, and substance abuse.[9] In general, class A conditions are communicable diseases or conditions that are of specific public health significance. Class B typical conditions are those that interfere with an person's ability to work or care for themselves.[5] Individuals traveling from certain regions must also undergo presumptive treatments for common, treatable endemic conditions.

Domestic Health Screen

Within 30 days of arriving in the United States, it is recommended that every refugee patient receive a comprehensive health screening by a primary care provider. Most refugee patients who did not receive childhood vaccinations started this process as part of their international health screen but require additional vaccinations at specific intervals after arriving in the United States to be considered fully immunized. For children, it is important to be aware of state vaccination requirements; this may delay their ability to enroll in public school. A comprehensive history and physical examination

Table 2 Health care marketplace eligibility	
	Marketplace Eligible?
US nationals	Yes
US citizens	Yes
Immigrants (lawful permanent residents)	Yes
Nonimmigrants	Yes
Undocumented aliens	No
Refugees	Yes
Asylees	Yes

Data from Healthcare.gov. Immigration status and the Marketplace. Available at: https://www.healthcare.gov/immigrants/immigration-status/. Accessed May 30, 2018.

should be performed, with special consideration given to conditions that are not common in the United States but very common in other regions (**Boxes 3** and **4**).

Words from a Provider

About 3 PM, I looked at the board and saw my next room, grabbed the superbill and walked in to find a family of 8 sitting across from me. After 6 months of working at a non-English, non-Spanish family medicine clinic serving solely refugee patients, I was used to seeing entire families together. My translator handed me the father's lab report he had brought from the county hospital and I began reviewing the details. I explained that his cholesterol and blood glucose were elevated and he would need to begin exercising and change his diet and we would continue to monitor. I explained the importance of lifestyle changes and the basis of a healthy, balanced diet. After a few minutes of discussion, the translator interrupted and stated, "He would like to let you know that he and his family came to the US 3 days ago. They are living with his sister and her family of 5, 13 in one apartment. Their family was separated for the past year and just reunited last week in Turkey. He has no job, he does not speak English and brought nothing with him when he and his family came to the US." In that moment, I realized that I had become numb to my surroundings. I worked with this vulnerable population every day and I had let their struggles become routine because this was the norm in my clinic. I failed to recognize the unique struggles of each patient, of each family, and let this impact the quality and attention given to the patient in front of me. I had been through this difficult transition many times with my patients, I knew we had services and support available, but this was the first time my patient was going through it and I lost sight of that reality. It is easy to get lost in the daily shuffle of life in a clinic, but this encounter changed my persepctive as a provider and remains in the forefront of my mind each time I meet a new patient.

—Stephanie Neary, PA-C

Unique Struggles for Refugee Patients

There are challenges to treating any patient population, and refugee patients are no exception (**Fig. 2**). From language barriers and lack of transportation to overcrowded housing and untreated chronic medical conditions, there are many factors that confound the traditional patient encounter. Being aware of these factors, discussing them openly with the patient, and knowing the resources available to aid in care are

---

Box 3
Recommended screening for all patients

- Mental health
- Prior abuse or mutilation
- CBC
- CMP
- HIV 1 and 2 antibodies
- Vaccine titers
- STD
- HbA1c
- Fasting lipid profile

Data from Annamalai A. Refugee health care: an essential medical guide. New York: Springer; 2014.

> **Box 4**
> **Specific conditions to consider**
>
> - Tuberculosis
> - Thalessemia
> - Hepatitis B
> - Strongyloidiasis
> - Schistosomiasis
> - B12 deficiency
> - Lead poisoning
>
> *Data from* Annamalai A. Refugee health care: an essential medical guide. New York: Springer; 2014.

very useful in the resettlement process. Small changes like having female translators available for sensitive gynecologic examinations can help make a patient feel more comfortable and ease anxiety to these often very foreign screenings. Nonemergency medical transportation services are available for most Medicaid beneficiaries and can help patients keep appointments without having to navigate a confusing or nonexistent public transportation system. Most large cities have volunteer refugee assistance organizations to help connect individuals with employers, with English classes, and for securing stable housing. Understanding this network of resources in your own community will help ease the transition for a refugee patient when they present to your clinic (**Box 5**).[10]

Local Resources

The ORR offers an online state resource locating service to connect individuals with local volunteer affiliates to aid in the resettlement process.[11] Nationwide, there are approximately 350 volunteer affiliate organizations working with a group of national nongovernmental agencies all contracted with the Department of State and the Department of Health and Human Services. Together, these groups adhere to a Cooperative Agreement, signed each year, to aid in the initial resettlement process by helping to provide access to basic needs and assist processes such as securing health insurance, food stamps, and social security cards.[5,11]

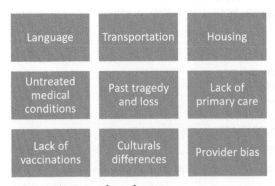

Fig. 2. Factors impacting patient care for refugees.

Box 5
Top 10 refugee native languages (fiscal years 2008-2018)
• Arabic
• Nepali
• Somali
• Sqaw Karen
• Spanish
• Kiswahili
• Chaldean
• Burmese
• Armenian
• Farsi
Data from Admissions & arrivals. Refugee Processing Center. 2018. Available at: http://www.wrapsnet.org/admissions-and-arrivals/. Accessed May 27, 2018.

SUMMARY

Having a foundational knowledge of refugee populations in your community, common cultural practices, and the local organizations available to help can provide a more smooth transition into the US health care system while still respecting the cultural values of the individual patient.

Stephanie L. Neary, MPA, MMS, PA-C
Yale Physician Assistant Online Program
PO Box 208004, 100 Church Street South
Suite A230, Room A235
New Haven, CT 06520, USA

E-mail address:
Stephanie.neary@yale.edu

REFERENCES

1. Immigration terms and definitions involving aliens. Internal Revenue Service. Available at: https://2009-2017.state.gov/j/prm/releases/factsheets/2016/264449.htm. Accessed May 30, 2018.
2. U.S. Refugee Admissions Program FAQs. US Department of State. Available at: https://www.state.gov/j/prm/releases/factsheets/2018/277838.htm. Accessed May 30, 2018.
3. Megan Alpert. By the numbers: the United States of refugees. Smithsonian.com; 2017. Available at: https://www.smithsonianmag.com/history/by-numbers-united-states-refugees-180962487/. Accessed May 23, 2018.
4. Philbrick AM, Wicks CM, Harris IM. Make refugee health care great again. Am J Public Health 2017;107(5):656–8.
5. Annamalai A. Refugee health care: an essential medical guide. New York: Springer; 2014.
6. About cash & medical assistance. Office of Child Care | ACF; 2018. Available at: https://www.acf.hhs.gov/orr/programs/cma/about. Accessed May 25, 2018.

7. Federal Poverty Level (FPL)—HealthCare.gov Glossary. HealthCare.gov. Available at: https://www.healthcare.gov/glossary/federal-poverty-level-FPL/. Accessed May 30, 2018.

8. Find out what immigration statuses qualify for coverage in the Health Insurance Marketplace. HealthCare.gov. Available at: https://www.healthcare.gov/immigrants/immigration-status/. Accessed May 30, 2018.

9. Volume 8—Admissibility, Part B—Health-related grounds of inadmissibility. USCIS; 2018. Available at: https://www.uscis.gov/policymanual/HTML/PolicyManual-Volume8-PartB-Chapter2.html. Accessed May 30, 2018.

10. Admissions & arrivals. Refugee Processing Center; 2018. Available at: http://www.wrapsnet.org/admissions-and-arrivals/. Accessed May 27, 2018.

11. ORR Network Resources. Office of Child Care | ACF. 2018. Available at: https://www.acf.hhs.gov/orr/resource/orr-network-resources. Accessed May 30, 2018.

Primary Care in Underserved Populations Definitions, Scope, Challenges and Future Considerations

Vincent Morelli, MD

KEYWORDS

- MUA • MUP • HPSA • Underserved area • Underserved population • Allostatic load
- Socioeconomic status

KEY POINTS

- Medically underserved areas (MUAs) and medically underserved populations (MUPs) are determined by the Health Resources and Services Administration (HRSA) by measuring 4 variables: (1) ratio of primary care physicians (PCPs) per 1000 population, (2) infant mortality rate, (3) percentage of the population below the poverty level, and (4) percentage of the population age 65 or over.
- In a given area or population, each of these variables is measured and then converted to a weighted value using conversion tables.
- In 2015, more than 16% of the US population lived in poverty, up from 14.3% in 2009; approximately 14% of seniors and 18% of children are impoverished.
- Low socioeconomic status (SES) has been linked to poorer metabolic profiles (eg, body mass index [BMI], fasting glucose, glycosylated hemoglobin, and lipid profiles), higher blood pressure, lower heart rate variability, higher levels of inflammatory markers, more risky behaviors (eg, smoking, drinking, and drug use), and higher overall higher allostatic load (AL).

INTRODUCTION

MUAs and MUPs are determined by the HRSA by measuring 4 variables: (1) ratio of PCPs per 1000 population, (2) infant mortality rate, (3) percentage of the population below the poverty level, and (4) percentage of the population age 65 or over.

This article is an update of an article that originally appeared in *Primary Care: Clinics in Office Practice*, Volume 44, Issue 1, March 2017.

The author of this work reports no direct financial interest in the subject matter or any material discussed in this article.

Department of Family Medicine and Community Medicine, Meharry Medical College, Nashville, TN 37208, USA

E-mail address: vmorelli@mmc.edu

In a given area or population, each of these variables is measured and then converted to a weighted value using conversion tables (see HRSA MUA/Ps: Index of Medical Underservice Data Tables at: http://www.hrsa.gov/shortage/mua/imutables.html). The 4 weighted values are then totaled to obtain an "underserved score." Areas or populations that score below 62 are designated as medically underserved, with lower scores indicating greater need. Areas and populations scoring above 62 (from 62 to 100) are designated as adequately served. Federally Qualified Health Centers, which include Community Health Centers and Rural Health Clinics, often provide care in underserved areas/populations and are eligible for federal support.

Despite concerns over the limitations of the HRSA definition of "underserved,"[1,2] for the purposes of this publication, the HRSA definition is used, as stated previously. This article focuses on areas/populations with a disproportionate number of elderly, high infant mortality rates, low access to primary care, and high poverty rates.

SCOPE OF THE PROBLEM: A CLOSER LOOK AT THE VARIABLES MEASURED IN DESIGNATING MEDICALLY UNDERSERVED AREAS AND MEDICALLY UNDERSERVED POPULATIONS

Poverty

In 2015, more than 16% of the US population lived in poverty, up from 14.3% in 2009. Approximately 14% of seniors and 18% of children are impoverished.[3] In 2013, United Nations International Children's Emergency Fund (UNICEF) found the United States to have the second highest child poverty rates of the 35 developed countries studied.[4] Currently in the United States, poverty is defined as earnings of less than $11,700 for an individual or less than $24,250 for a family of 4.

The most recent international data[5] document that, in 2012, 12.7% of the world's population lived at or below $2 a day (purchasing power parity), meaning that close to a billion people were impoverished. This is a vast improvement from the 37% impoverished in 1990, when almost 2 billion people lived in World Bank–defined poverty. This astounding improvement is largely accounted for by China's remarkable economic turnaround. Still, global poverty remains a significant issue with significant public health issues.

The Elderly

United States census data documented an elderly population of 43.1 million in 2012 and predicts that it will double to 83.7 million by 2050.[6] Internationally, population aging, resulting from decreasing mortality and declining fertility, is also taking place. The number of people over age 60 increased from 9.2% in 1990 to 11.7% in 2013 and will reach 21.1% by 2050. By that year, the number of older people will have doubled – from 841 million in 2013 to more than 2 billion.[7]

Infant Mortality

Defined as deaths of infants under 1 year of age per 1000 live births, this ratio is often used as an indicator of the level of health in a country. Worldwide, the infant mortality rate is approximately 42/1000 to 50/1000 live births.[8] The overall US infant mortality rate is 5.3/1000 live births,[9] with higher rates occurring in underserved areas. This article focuses on select underserved populations both in the Untied States and internationally, with infant mortality rates on the higher end of the spectrum.

Primary Care Physician Shortages

Currently, there are 778,000 practicing physicians in the United States. Approximately one-half of them are engaged in primary care, but approximately one-half are over the age of 50; almost one-third are projected to retire in the next 10 years.[10] Compounding the problem is that currently, just 25% of medical school graduates go into and remain in primary care.[11] The reasons for this are no secret: lower primary care salaries, busier work load, perceived lifestyle, high medical school debt, excessive administrative requirements, and relative lack of prestige.

In 2006, in response to the projected shortage of PCPs, medical schools agreed to increase enrollment by 30%. Congress, however, in its 1997 Balanced Budget Act, froze residency training funds (Congress/Medicare funds 80% of residency training slots), leaving the country with an increased number of medical school graduates and a looming shortage of residency training slots. It is projected that by 2017 there will not be enough residency slots for US medical school graduates,[10] resulting in little impact on PCP shortages — an unfathomable error in policy and an egregious disservice to expectant medical students and underserved populations.

For this article, it is important to define what is meant by a primary care shortage. For federal grant funding purposes, the HRSA designates a Health Professional Shortage Area (HPSA) as one with a PCP-to-population ratio of less than 1 PCP per 3500 residents. HRSA notes, however, that this ratio, used since the 1970s, is used for federal granting purposes only and that the primary care needs of a community vary depending on age, poverty levels, percentage of underserved, and so forth. HRSA also notes that their estimates do not take into account the availability of ancillary care providers, such as nurse practitioners (NPs) or physician assistants (PAs). Although the 1:3500 ratio has been a long-standing norm used to identify high-need areas in the United States, HRSA notes that there is no universally accepted critical shortage ratio. With this in mind, when designating underserved areas and populations for this publication, it is probably best to use the combined MUA and MUP index, as stated previously, rather than rely solely on a specific physician-to-population ratio.

Internationally the World Health Organization (WHO) differs in degree with the HRSA figures that designate HPSAs and advocates at least 1 PCP per 1000 people to sufficiently care for populations in developed countries.[12] Again, the 1/1000 ratio is likely a gross underestimation of need for disproportionately elderly populations with complicated medical conditions or in impoverished areas, where patients have more critical presentations and a greater burden of disease.

The WHO designates countries with a total physician/patient ratio of less than 1.13/1000 as having a critical physician shortage; 44% of WHO Member States report falling in this category, most in Africa, Southeast Asia, or Central America. Currently, the United States has approximately 2.5 total doctors per 1000 people but has 10 states with fewer than 1 PCP per 1000 residents.[13]

Note: in absolute numbers, the 2013 HRSA Health Workforce report[14] predicts that despite an 8% increase in the number of PCPs by 2020, there will still be a shortage of 20,000 such physicians — with the caveat that NPs and PAs will fill much of this gap. With a projected 30% increase in NPs and 60% increase in PAs, the Workforce report predicts the shortage of primary care providers nationwide will be cut down to just 6000.[14] Currently, the WHO also estimates a shortage of 4.3 million physicians, nurses and other health workers worldwide.[12]

UNINSURED THUS UNDERSERVED

Data from 2015 document approximately 37 to 43 million uninsured Americans,[15] down from 48 to 50 million uninsured prior to the implementation of the Patient Protection and Affordable Care Act.[16]

KEY CONCEPTS FOR PRIMARY CARE PHYSICIANS WORKING IN UNDERSERVED AREAS

It is important to review concepts of SES, AL, and structural violence. SES, usually defined by lower educational achievement, substandard income attainment, and/or low occupational status, is an important contributor to health. Low SES has been linked to poorer metabolic profiles (eg, BMI, fasting glucose, glycosylated hemoglobin, and lipid profiles),[17–19] higher blood pressure, lower heart rate variability,[20] higher levels of inflammatory markers,[21,22] more risky behaviors (eg, smoking, drinking, and drug use), and higher overall higher AL (discussed later).[23,24]

The concept of AL was born out of the realization that social, environmental, and economic stressors can significantly and simultaneously affect the functioning of multiple interconnected biologic systems (eg, endocrine, immune, digestive, neurologic, and cardiovascular) and that an objective measurement of SES effect would be useful.[25]

The basic idea of AL is that stress-induced changes (eg, secreted hormones and blood pressure increases) that are adaptive in the short run can cause changes leading to disease over the longer term. McEwen[26] found that one of the most potent of stressors (contributors to AL) was competitive interaction between animals of the same species and that this stress contributed to the formation of dominance hierarchies, where lower-ranking animals have been found to have impaired cognitive function and higher burdens of disease.

The quantification of AL has evolved and improved over time. Early methods, such as measured by Evans,[27] quantified 6 factors that documented the effect of stress on the body: resting systolic blood pressure, resting diastolic blood pressure, BMI, overnight urinary cortisol, overnight urinary epinephrine, and overnight urinary norepinephrine. Later and more comprehensive methods, such as those used by Zilioli and colleagues,[28,29] measured up to 24 biomarkers across 7 physiologic domains (ie, cardiovascular, lipid metabolism, glucose metabolism, inflammation, sympathetic nervous system response, parasympathetic nervous system response, and hypothalamic pituitary axis) to assess AL. As with SES, multiple studies[30–32] have documented that higher ALs are associated with negative health outcomes — many of which are discussed in the articles that follow.

It is important for PCPs to realize that both lower SES and higher AL experienced in childhood carry their untoward effects into adulthood,[29,33–35] where AL has been documented to increase negative adult health outcomes and increase all-cause mortality.[36] AL has been proved a stronger predictor of morbidity and mortality than SES or any single health parameter.[37,38] This is because AL accounts for stressors that accumulate with prolonged exposure; thus, what may be small changes in individual parameters will, over time, be accounted for in a more comprehensive fashion by measurement of the cumulative AL, all of which is to say that AL is a significant predictor of dysregulation and untoward health effects and that PCPs working in underserved environments need to be aware of the concept and its potential health effects.[30,31,39]

That being said, PCPs should be encouraged by the knowledge that interventions geared toward the reductions in AL may significantly decrease morbidity and mortality.[38] Because decreased AL has been documented in those with religious ties,[40] stronger social connections,[41] and a greater sense of meaning/purpose,[28,42] holistic interventions taking such factors into consideration are important in health promotion in underserved communities.

Closely related to AL, is the concept of "structural violence." Structural violence is any suffering caused by the structure and institutions of a society that put individuals (especially marginalized individuals) in harm's way. PCPs should be cognizant of the outcomes of structural violence — unequal access to wages, resources, political power, education, health care, or legal standing and so forth — that can contribute to poor health. Some investigators argue that not only can structural violence lead to physical violence[43] but also structural violence alone can produce suffering and death as often as direct violence, although the damage is more insidious, more widespread, and more difficult to repair.[44]

As discussed in the articles that follow, structural violence, SES, and AL play a contributory role in several maladies, including sleep disorders,[45–48] substance abuse,[49,50] psychological disorders,[51–54] appetite dysregulation and obesity,[55,56] and cardiovascular disease.[57,58]

Although much structural violence and AL may be caused or alleviated by governmental policy, it is important for PCPs to be aware of the effects of low SES and high AL if they are to ameliorate untoward individual health effects and provide optimal service when working in underserved areas or with underserved populations.

In the articles that follow, underserved areas are examined, both rural and urban, and issues are highlighted that PCPs working in these environments should be aware of. Disease entities and social and psychological issues that PCPs should be prepared for are spotlighted, to help them focus their attention and best allocate their resources.

In addition to examining underserved areas, underserved peoples are looked at. Health issues that occur disproportionately in underserved populations are discussed — again with the intent to make physicians working with these populations aware of their unique medical challenges. The populations addressed are immigrants, the elderly, underserved children, the homeless, and underserved women.

The last main section of this issue takes an in-depth look at disease categories that overly affect underserved individuals. Infectious diseases, occupational and sleep issues, cardiovascular risks, psychological conditions, substance use problems, cancer risks, diet and obesity disparities, environmental inequities, and exercise questions and sedentary lifestyle in these populations are explored. These articles highlight the "neglected diseases of the underserved" so that PCPs working in these areas will be more aware of their likelihood. For example, the infectious disease article discusses Chagas disease, an underappreciated cause of heart failure in underserved populations in the United States (see Samuel Neil Grief and John Paul Miller's article, "Infectious Disease Issues in Underserved Populations," in this issue). It discusses cysticerosis presenting as headaches or seizures; toxocariasis, the helminth infection caused by ingestion of soil infected with cat or dog feces, with its links to diminished lung and cognitive function; toxoplasmosis, with possible links not only to HIV but also to psychiatric and mood disorders; and trichomoniasis, which has a 10-times higher incidence than among Mexican-American or non-Hispanic white women. Such infectious diseases of the underserved are fully discussed and their unrecognized links to cardiovascular, respiratory, and psychiatric maladies and so forth (conditions ordinarily thought of as noncommunicable diseases) are explored.[59]

The final article discusses the changing morbidity and mortality trends in underserved communities worldwide (see Vincent Morelli and Paul Hutchinson's article, "International Comparisons in Underserved Health: Issues, Policies, Needs and Projections," in this issue). Policy change recommendations are made to address these shifting patterns of disease. In an ever-shrinking world of increasing international travel, both diseases and social ills will continue to cross geographic boundaries and disproportionately affect the most vulnerable underserved peoples. International cooperation and coordination of policy focused on primary care of the underserved is important to avert future public health crises and continue to build a socially aware and enfranchising world.

REFERENCES

1. Kviz FJ, Flaskerud JH. An evaluation of the index of medical underservice. Results from a rural consumer survey. Med Care 1984;22:877–89.
2. Goldsmith LJ, Ricketts TC. Proposed changes to designations of medically underserved populations and health professional shortage areas: effects on rural areas. J Rural Health 1999;15:44–54.
3. Short, Kathleen, "The research supplemental poverty measure: 2012" U.S. Census Bureau, P60–247, Current Population Reports, 2013. Available at: www.census.gov/prod/2013pubs/p60-247.pdf. Accessed December 1, 2015.
4. Adamson P. Child well-being in rich countries: A comparative overview. Innocenti Report Card 11. Florence (Italy): UNICEF Office of Research; 2013. p. 7. Available at: http://www.unicef-irc.org/publications/pdf/rc11_eng.pdf. Accessed December 1, 2015.
5. The World Bank: Poverty overview. Available at: http://www.worldbank.org/en/topic/poverty/overview. Accessed December 1, 2015.
6. Ortman JM, Velkoff VA, Hogan H. United States Census Bureau. An aging nation: The older population in the United States. Population estimates and projections, 2014. Available at: www.census.gov/prod/2014pubs/p25-1140.pdf. Accessed December 1, 2015.
7. United Nations, Department of Economic and Social Affairs, Population Division, 2013. World Population Ageing, page xii. Available at: http://www.un.org/en/development/desa/population/publications/pdf/ageing/WorldPopulationAgeing2013.pdf. Accessed December 1, 2015.
8. Wikipedia: the free encyclopedia. List of countries by infant mortality rate. Available at: https://en.wikipedia.org/wiki/List_of_countries_by_infant_mortality_rate. Accessed December 3, 2015.
9. United Nations, Department of Economic and Social Affairs, Population Division, page 7. World population prospects, the 2015 revision. Available at: esa.un.org/unpd/wpp/publications/files/key_findings_wpp_2015.pdf. Accessed December 1, 2015.
10. Frisch S. The primary care physician shortage. BMJ 2013;347:f6559.
11. Chen C, Petterson S, Phillips RL, et al. Toward graduate medical education (GME) accountability: Measuring the outcomes of GME institutions. Acad Med 2013;88:1267–80.
12. World Health Organization. Models and tools for health workforce planning and projections. Geneva (Switzerland): Human Resources for Health Observer; 2010. Issue No. 3. Available at: http://apps.who.int/iris/bitstream/10665/44263/1/9789241599016_eng.pdf. Accessed December 1, 2015.
13. United Health Foundation. America's Health Rankings. Primary care physicians: United States. Available at: http://www.americashealthrankings.org/all/pcp. Accessed December 1, 2015.
14. U.S. Department of Health and Human Services. HRSA Health Workforce. Projecting the supply and demand for primary care practitioners through 2020, November 2013. Available at: http://bhpr.hrsa.gov/healthworkforce/supplydemand/usworkforce/primarycare/primarycarebrief.pdf. Accessed December 1, 2015.
15. Karman KG, Eibner C. Changes in health insurance enrollment since 2013: evidence from the RAND health reform opinion study. Santa Monica (CA): The Rand Corporation; 2014. Available at: http://www.rand.org/pubs/research_reports/RR656.html. Accessed December 1, 2015.

16. Levy J, editor. U.S., Uninsured rate dips to 11.9% in first quarter. Washington, DC: Gallup; 2015. Available at: http://www.gallup.com/poll/182348/uninsured-rate-dips-first-quarter.aspx. Accessed December 1, 2015.

17. Loucks EB, Magnusson KT, Cook S, et al. Socioeconomic position and the metabolic syndrome in early, middle, and late life: Evidence from NHANES 1999–2002. Ann Epidemiol 2007;17:782–90.

18. McLaren L. Socioeconomic status and obesity. Epidemiol Rev 2007;29:29–48.

19. Senese LC, Almeida ND, Fath AK, et al. Associations between childhood socioeconomic position and adulthood obesity. Epidemiol Rev 2009;31:21–51.

20. Sloan RP, Huang MH, Sidney S, et al. Socioeconomic status and health: Is parasympathetic nervous system activity an intervening mechanism? Int J Epidemiol 2005;34:309–15.

21. Loucks EB, Pilote L, Lynch JW, et al. Life course socioeconomic position is associated with inflammatory markers: The Framingham Offspring Study. Soc Sci Med 2010;71:187–95.

22. Gruenewald TL, Cohen S, Matthews KA, et al. Association of socioeconomic status with inflammation markers in black and white men and women in the Coronary Artery Risk Development in Young Adults (CARDIA) study. Soc Sci Med 2009;69: 451–9.

23. Crimmins EM, Kim JK, Seeman TE. Poverty and biological risk: The earlier "aging" of the poor. J Gerontol A Biol Sci Med Sci 2009;64:286–92.

24. Seeman TE, Singer BH, Rowe JW, et al. Price of adaptation – allostatic load and its health consequences: MacArthur studies of successful aging. Arch Intern Med 1999;159:1176.

25. Gerdes L, Tegeler CH, Lee SW. A groundwork for allostatic neuro-education. Front Psychol 2015;6:1224.

26. McEwen BS. Protective and damaging effects of stress mediators. N Engl J Med 1998;338:171–9.

27. Evans GW. A multimethodological analysis of cumulative risk and allostatic load among rural children. Dev Psychol 2003;39:924–33.

28. Zilioli S, Slatcher RB, Ong AD, et al. Purpose in life predicts allostatic load ten years later. J Psychosom Res 2015;79:451–7.

29. Gruenewald TL, Karlamangla AS, Hu P, et al. History of socioeconomic disadvantage and allostatic load in later life. Soc Sci Med 2012;74:75–83.

30. McEwen BS. Protection and damage from acute and chronic stress: Allostasis and allostatic overload and relevance to the pathophysiology of psychiatric disorders. Ann N Y Acad Sci 2004;1032:1–7.

31. McEwen BS. Physiology and neurobiology of stress and adaptation: central role of the brain. Physiol Rev 2007;87:873–904.

32. Diez Roux AV. Conceptual approaches to the study of health disparities. Annu Rev Public Health 2012;33:41–58.

33. Tamayo T, Herder C, Rathmann W. Impact of early psychosocial factors (childhood socioeconomic factors and adversities) on future risk of type 2 diabetes, metabolic disturbances and obesity: A systematic review. BMC Public Health 2010;10:525.

34. Widom CS, Horan J, Brzustowicz L. Childhood maltreatment predicts allostatic load in adulthood. Child Abuse Negl 2015;47:59–69.

35. Tomasdottir MO, Sigurdsson JA, Petursson H, et al. Self reported childhood difficulties, adult multimorbidity and allostatic load. A cross-sectional analysis of the Norwegian HUNT Study. PLoS One 2015;10(6):e0130591.

36. Seeman TE, McEwen BS, Rowe JW, et al. Allostatic load as a marker of cumulative biological risk: MacArthur studies of successful aging. Proc Natl Acad Sci U S A 2001;98:4770–5.
37. Karlamangla AS, Singer BH, McEwen BS, et al. Allostatic load as a predictor of functional decline. MacArthur studies of successful aging. J Clin Epidemiol 2002;55(7):696–710.
38. Karlamangla AS, Singer BH, Seeman TE. Reduction in allostatic load in older adults is associated with lower all-cause mortality risk: MacArthur studies of successful aging. Psychosom Med 2006;68:500–7.
39. McEwen BS. Stress, adaptation, and disease: Allostasis and allostatic load. Ann N Y Acad Sci 1998;840:33–44.
40. Maselko J, Kubzansky L, Kawachi I, et al. Religious service attendance and allostatic load among high-functioning elderly. Psychosom Med 2007;69:464–72.
41. Seeman TE, Singer BH, Ryff CD, et al. Social relationships, gender, and allostatic load across two age cohorts. Psychosom Med 2002;64:395–406.
42. Lindfors P, Lundberg O, Lundberg U. Allostatic load and clinical risk as related to sense of coherence in middle-aged women. Psychosom Med 2006;68:801–7.
43. Copp JE, Kuhl DC, Giordano PC, et al. Intimate partner violence in neighborhood context: the roles of structural disadvantage, subjective disorder, and emotional distress. Soc Sci Res 2015;53:59–72.
44. Winter DA, Leighton DC. Structural violence. In: Christie DJ, Wagner RV, Winter DA, editors. Peace, conflict, and violence: peace psychology for the 21st century. Englewood Cliffs (NJ): Prentice-Hall; 2001. p. 99–201.
45. McEwen BS, Karatsoreos IN. Sleep deprivation and circadian disruption: Stress, allostasis, and allostatic load. Sleep Med Clin 2015;10:1–10.
46. Juster RP, McEwen BS. Sleep and chronic stress: new directions for allostatic load research. Sleep Med 2015;16:7–8.
47. Clark AJ, Dich N, Lange T, et al. Impaired sleep and allostatic load: Cross-sectional results from the Danish Copenhagen Aging and Midlife Biobank. Sleep Med 2014;15:1571–8.
48. Chen X, Redline S, Shields AE, et al. Associations of allostatic load with sleep apnea, insomnia, short sleep duration, and other sleep disturbances: Findings from the National Health and Nutrition Examination Survey 2005 to 2008. Ann Epidemiol 2014;24:612–9.
49. Chen E, Miller GE, Brody GH, et al. Neighborhood poverty, college attendance, and diverging profiles of substance use and allostatic load in rural African American youth. Clin Psychol Sci 2015;3:675–85.
50. Doan SN, Dich N, Evans GW. Childhood cumulative risk and later allostatic load: Mediating role of substance use. Health Psychol 2014;33:1402–9.
51. Juster RP, McEwen BS, Lupien SJ. Allostatic load biomarkers of chronic stress and impact on health and cognition. Neurosci Biobehav Rev 2010;35:2–16.
52. Pettorruso M, De Risio L, Di Nicola M, et al. Allostasis as a conceptual framework linking bipolar disorder and addiction. Front Psychiatry 2014;5:173.
53. Hintsa T, Elovainio M, Jokela M, et al. Is there an independent association between burnout and increased allostatic load? Testing the contribution of psychological distress and depression. J Health Psychol 2016;21(8):1576–86.
54. Misiak B, Frydecka D, Zawadzki M, et al. Refining and integrating schizophrenia pathophysiology - relevance of the allostatic load concept. Neurosci Biobehav Rev 2014;45:183–201.
55. Sinha R, Jastreboff AM. Stress as a common risk factor for obesity and addiction. Biol Psychiatry 2013;73(9):827–35.

56. Katz DA, Sprang G, Cooke C. The cost of chronic stress in childhood: Understanding and applying the concept of allostatic load. Psychodyn Psychiatry 2012;40:469–80.
57. Ippoliti F, Canitano N, Businaro R. Stress and obesity as risk factors in cardiovascular diseases: A neuroimmune perspective. J Neuroimmune Pharmacol 2013;8: 212–26.
58. Sabbah W, Watt RG, Sheiham A, et al. Effects of allostatic load on the social gradient in ischaemic heart disease and periodontal disease: Evidence from the Third National Health and Nutrition Examination Survey. J Epidemiol Community Health 2008;62:415–20.
59. Hotez PJ. Neglected parasitic infections and poverty in the United States. Plos Negl Trop Dis 2014;8:e3012.

Primary Care Issues in Rural Populations

Konstantinos E. Deligiannidis, MD, MPH, FAAFP

KEYWORDS

- Rural • Determinants of health • Prevention • Treatment • Adherence • Access
- Training • Retention

KEY POINTS

- Rural populations have different demographics and health issues compared with metropolitan populations, with higher rates of mortality.
- Rural primary care physicians (PCPs) must be familiar with treating and counseling for conditions faced more commonly in their patient population, such as occupational respiratory illness.
- Rural PCPs can address treatment, prevention, and social determinants of health.
- Multiple strategies can be used by rural PCPs to address access, such as the use of mid-level health care professionals, electronic visits, and other technology.

INTRODUCTION

The Institute of Medicine defines primary care as "the provision of integrated, accessible health care services by clinicians who are accountable for addressing a large majority of personal health care needs, developing a sustained partnership with patients, and practicing in the context of family and community."[1] Primary care physicians (PCPs) have the benefit of caring for patients from a longitudinal perspective and developing rapport and relationships with patients and their families, often across generations. Physicians receive a great benefit from assisting patients with multiple medical and psychosocial issues, both acute and chronic. However, along with these benefits that primary care gives to the physician, the specialty also presents challenges in addressing the health of patients, families, and communities. Moreover, these challenges are particularly prominent in rural communities. This article discusses some of the issues that rural PCPs face, such as health problems that are more common in rural populations, disease prevention and adherence issues, access to health care services, and educational issues.

This article originally appeared in Primary Care: Clinics in Office Practice, Volume 44, Issue 1, March 2017.
Disclosure: The author has nothing to disclose.
Northwell Health Solutions, House Calls Program, 1983 Marcus Avenue, Suite C102, New Hyde Park, NY 11042, USA
E-mail address: kdeligiann@northwell.edu

Physician Assist Clin 4 (2019) 11–19
https://doi.org/10.1016/j.cpha.2018.08.001
2405-7991/19/© 2018 Elsevier Inc. All rights reserved.

HEALTH PROBLEMS FACED IN RURAL POPULATIONS

Rural populations have a different population demographic and face a different set of medical issues, which bring about challenges for family physicians. Statistics compiled in the Rural-Urban Chartbook in 2014 revealed that there are differences between metropolitan and nonmetropolitan (including both micropolitan and rural) areas. For instance, as populations move from metropolitan areas to nonmetropolitan areas, the age distribution tends to get older, and the percentage of population in the rural counties that is 65 years old or older is higher in nonmetropolitan counties compared with metropolitan counties. This pattern is seen in all regions of the United States.[2] Furthermore, the highest levels of poverty in the South and West regions of the United States are in rural counties (whereas the highest levels in the Midwest and the Northeast were in large metropolitan counties).[2]

Substance Use

Tobacco use also affects nonmetropolitan counties more than metropolitan counties. The highest percentage of men and women who smoke are in nonmetropolitan and rural counties. Furthermore, the highest percentage of adolescents who smoke is in the rural and nonmetropolitan counties. Again, this is true for all regions of the United States, except the West, where adolescent smoking was the second highest percentage.[2]

Self-reported alcohol consumption varies across the regions of the United States, with the highest percentage of individuals who report alcohol consumption living in the nonmetropolitan/rural areas in the West, whereas in the South it is the smallest percentage (compared with metropolitan counties).[2]

Moreover, substance use treatment admission rates are higher in nonmetropolitan areas for stimulants, although treatment admission rates are lower for opiates in rural areas. The challenge with this statistic is that the rate of opiate use disorder may not correlate with the treatment admission rates. Although there is evidence that the availability of prescription opiates has increased, and more so in rural areas,[3] care must be taken in interpreting these statistics, because 94% of people who are prescribed opiates do not develop opiate use disorder.[4,5]

Obesity and Physical Inactivity

The highest percentages of the population that are obese are in the nonmetropolitan/rural counties in all regions of the United States.[2] Perhaps surprisingly, the highest percentages of the population who are physically inactive are in the nonmetropolitan/rural populations of the Midwest and the South. The large metropolitan counties in the Northeast are an exception.[2]

Mental Health

Nationally, mental illness in men and women is more prevalent in nonmetropolitan and rural counties, with a higher percentage of women with mental illness compared with men. Similar rates also occurred for serious mental illness, which is defined as mental/behavioral/emotional disorder that results in serious functional impairment.[2]

Other Medical Issues

Other health issues seen in primary care are also more prominent in rural communities. Adolescent birth rates are highest in nonmetropolitan/rural areas nationally, especially in the South and the West.[2] Limitation of activity because of chronic health conditions is highest nationally in rural counties.[2] In addition, the percentage of the population with edentulism (the condition of being toothless) is highest in nonmetropolitan/rural counties, regardless of income level.[2] This may be because the supply of dentists in rural areas decreases as urbanization increases, with approximately one-third as many dentists in rural counties as in large metropolitan counties.[2]

MORTALITY

Nationally, infant mortalities are higher in rural counties, but this varies by region. All-cause death rates are greater in children and young adults (1–24 years old) in nonmetropolitan/rural counties compared with their metropolitan counterparts nationally (with some variation among regions for male gender).[2] Nationally, all-cause mortalities for working-age adults (25–64 years old) and elderly (≥65 years old) are higher in nonmetropolitan/rural counties than metropolitan counties.[2]

Mortality Causes

The death rate from ischemic heart disease rates for men and women is highest in rural counties, as is the chronic obstructive pulmonary disease (COPD)–related death rate.[2] Similarly, death rates from unintentional injuries and motor vehicle accidents (for both genders 1–42 years old) is highest in nonmetropolitan/rural areas, with the number of male deaths approximately double the number of female deaths.[2] Furthermore, suicide rates were highest in nonmetropolitan/rural areas in each of the 4 regions of the United States.[2]

SPECIFIC RURAL ISSUES, WITH THEIR PREVENTION AND COUNTERMEASURES

PCPs have a unique position in counseling, preventing, and treating common issues that are specific to rural populations, such as motor vehicle accidents, unintentional injuries, pesticide poisoning, and occupational respiratory illnesses.

Motor Vehicle Accidents and Unintentional Injuries

Although "one-third of all motor vehicle accidents occur in rural areas, two-thirds of motor vehicle deaths occur on rural roads."[6] Furthermore, "rural residents are also nearly twice as likely as urban residents to die from unintentional injuries other than motor vehicle accidents."[6] Unintentional injuries may occur from farm equipment; working with livestock; and falls from ladders, grain binds, and other heights. PCP in rural areas should therefore help with addressing this by counseling on safe driving and on preventing occupational hazards that are specific to their location. In addition, physicians should have a fundamental knowledge of trauma care (eg, laceration repair, care of fractures) and be readily able to communicate with emergency medical services (EMS). Communication with EMS regarding medical records and medical history has been identified as a need to address, especially with electronic medical records and electronic communication.[7]

Organophosphate Poisoning

Organophosphate poisoning usually occurs as a form of intentional exposure (eg, suicide attempt), and rarely as accidental exposure. Note that adults and children are affected differently. Exposure, and subsequent poisoning, can occur via absorption through the skin, inhalation, or ingestion. Although exposures are declining because of the phasing out by the Environmental Protection Agency of the common household and agricultural organophosphate insecticides,[8] it still is important for PCPs to be aware of the signs, symptoms, and treatment of organophosphate poisoning. Symptoms in adults include muscarinic effects (eg, diaphoresis, diarrhea, urinary incontinence, miosis, bradycardia, bronchospasm, emesis, excess lacrimation, salivation), nicotinic effects (eg, fasciculations, cramping, weakness), and central nervous system effects (eg, anxiety, emotional lability, confusion, ataxia, tremors, and seizures). In children, seizure and coma are the most common presentations. Physical examination findings include decreased (or increased) respirations, bradycardia, tachycardia, hypotension or hypertension, and paralysis, as well as impaired memory, confusion, irritability, lethargy, and psychosis. Removal from exposure is paramount. PCPs or EMS personnel need to control the airways and administer oxygen, and possibly even need to intubate the patient, although atropine administration may eliminate the need for intubation. Central lines should be established, pulse oximetry and electrocardiography should be monitored, and arrhythmias should be treated accordingly.

Tick-borne Illnesses

Several tick-borne illnesses are found in rural areas, and are variable in different regions of the United States. The Northeast and upper Midwest of the United States are likely to encounter anaplasmosis, babesiosis, Powassan disease, tularemia, and Lyme disease (either from *Borrelia burgdorferi*, *Borrelia mayonii*, or *Borrelia miyamotoi*).[9] The Pacific coast can also experience anaplasmosis, Lyme, tick-borne relapsing fever (TBRF), tularemia, and 364D rickettsiosis.[9] Rocky Mountain states may see Colorado tick fever, TBRF, and tularemia. Southern tick-associated rash illness (STARI) can be seen in southeastern and eastern states; TBRF can be seen in the western half of the United States. Ehrlichiosis is seen in south-central and southeastern states.[9]

PCPs should be aware of the most common symptoms of tick-related illnesses, such as fever and chills, headache, fatigue, and muscle aches. Also, rashes may occur, such as erythema migrans (in Lyme, STARI), small pink nonpruritic macules to petechiae (in Rocky Mountain spotted fever), or skin ulcers (in tularemia). Most of these tick-borne illnesses can be treated with antibiotics, and prompt start of antibiotics when indicated may help reduce the severity of symptoms.

Occupational Respiratory Illnesses

Other issues that can occur specific to rural areas include farmer's hypersensitivity pneumonitis (FHP, or farmer's lung), organic dust toxicity syndrome (ODTS, or silo unloader's syndrome), silo filler's disease, and asthma. These conditions have different causes. For instance, FHP is related to the inhalation of mold spores. Thus, it is important for physicians to counsel patients to reduce the exposure to spores (eg, by avoiding working in confined dusty areas; by increasing ventilation to remove spores; by using mold inhibitors; and by harvesting, baling, and storing grains in a manner to reduce mold growth). Similar recommendations can be made for ODTS, which occurs from organic dust. Silo filler's disease occurs from the inhalation of nitrogen dioxide, so it is important for PCPs to counsel patients on reducing the risk of developing this, such as never entering the silo 2 to 3 days after filling, using portable gas monitors to monitor levels in the silo, and wearing an N95-rated dust mask if entering the silo after the 3-week postfilling period.[10] In addition, counseling with regard to these issues also helps with reducing the risk for asthma exacerbation. Further information is available online.[10,11]

Stress/Anxiety

Although droughts, floods, pests, natural disasters, financial instability, and isolation occur at every location, people living or working in rural environments may be especially vulnerable. Practicing rural PCPs should be aware of mental health issues and be able to offer counseling and support. Furthermore, the US Preventive Services Task force issued a grade B recommendation that "screening for depression in the general adult population should be implemented with adequate systems in place to ensure accurate diagnosis, effective treatment, and appropriate follow-up."[12] Although screening is important, PCPs should also be able to provide treatment or referral to mental health professionals. However, given the disparity between rural and urban areas with regard to access to mental health providers, PCPs may need to use other strategies to address this issue (discussed later).

Other Common Medical Conditions

In a recent National Health Report, the 10 leading causes of death in the United States were cardiovascular disease, cancer, chronic pulmonary disease, stroke, unintentional injuries, Alzheimer, diabetes, pneumonia and influenza, kidney disease, and suicide.[13] Some have been shown to have a major difference in rates of occurrence between rural and metropolitan areas (as discussed earlier). However, there are others (pneumonia and influenza), for which there are no readily available statistics that differentiate incidences between rural and urban communities, and so it is difficult to extrapolate whether there are major differences between the two areas.

PREVENTION IN RURAL AREAS

As mentioned earlier, there are many health issues that are more prominent in rural areas compared with urban areas. The top 20 Rural Healthy People 2020 national objectives that are recognized as priorities by rural stakeholders are the following: access to quality health services, nutrition and weight status, diabetes, mental health, substance abuse, heart disease and stroke, physical activity and health, older adults, maternal and child health, tobacco use, cancer, education and community-based programs, oral health, quality of life and well-being, immunizations and infectious diseases, public health infrastructure, family planning and sexual health, injury and violence prevention, social determinants of health, and health communication and health IT.[14] Although it is important to treat illnesses, it is also important to help prevent some illnesses by addressing social determinants of health.

For instance, in order to prevent heart disease, stroke, COPD, and lung cancer, smoking cessation and prevention are important. Public policy measures (eg, cigarette tax, age limits to purchase), motivational interviewing (for behavior change), nicotine replacement therapy, and other types of pharmacotherapy (bupropion, varenicline) all play a role. Furthermore, physical inactivity and obesity are important to prevent by counseling behavior change. Motivational interviewing is helpful but must also be met with resources in the area. Rural PCPs must be able to use creativity in helping patients be physically active and improve on dietary changes. For instance, walking/running clubs are used in some rural areas of the United States, as well as cooking classes coordinated by medical professionals and community members.

ADHERENCE

Adherence to lifestyle modification is challenging, no matter the behavior change. Likewise, adherence to medical advice and guidelines is also challenging. For instance, in patients who are breast cancer survivors, physical activity is associated with a decreased all-cause mortality, breast cancer mortality, and recurrence.[15,16] However, only 19% of rural breast cancer survivors meet physical activity guidelines.[17] Recommendations for clinicians that have been suggested include targeting self-efficacy and prescribing physical activity regimens that are tailored to the patient and the patient's abilities.[17]

Another study [18] showed that in a Latino population with diabetes in rural California, food insecurity was independently associated with not receiving foot examinations, dilated eye examinations, medication underuse, and not having control of a composite measure of diabetes control. The recommendation for "clinicians and health systems is to aggressively address social issues such as food insecurity in addition to improving standard diabetes medical management."[18] This recommendation includes "screening of patients at high risk for food insecurity and aggressively referring patients to nutrition services. and rethinking target A1c goals for patients with food insecurity."[18] As is evident with the previous 2 medical issues, social determinants of health are key influences of health, and rural PCPs need to be creative in addressing social issues to improve the health of the population.

ADDRESSING ACCESS IN RURAL AREAS
Improving Access to Medical Care

Just as there are differences between rural and metropolitan areas in rates of medical conditions, there are also differences in the supply of physicians. The supply of almost every subspecialty is less in nonmetropolitan areas compared with metropolitan areas. Large metropolitan counties have approximately 380.5 physicians per 100,000 population, whereas rural counties have approximately 118.3 per 100,000 population.[2] As mentioned earlier, the highest priority for Rural Healthy People 2020 is access to quality health services.[14] Improving access is addressed later.

Personnel

There are several steps that communities and policy makers have taken to address access to primary care in rural communities. First is the use of midlevel or advanced practice clinicians, such as nurse practitioners and physician assistants who can see patients, usually as part of a team. Another important aspect to the clinical team approach to patient care is the use of nurses, including visiting nurses or town nurses, to visit patients between visits with their clinicians. Other clinical team approaches involve pharmacists with a pharmacist collaborative practice agreement, by which pharmacists are authorized to provide medication management under protocol. However, the scope of authorization varies throughout the United States.

Visit types

Another approach that rural PCPs use to address access is the use of home visits and group visits. Some patients struggle with transportation, or are disabled, so that leaving their homes requires a taxing effort, making it difficult for them to get to their health care facilities. To address this access problem, rural PCPs can go to the homes of patients. The benefit to this approach is that PCPs are able to learn more about their patients and about their lives, environment, and context, further enabling them to take better care of their patients. Group visits can be held for patients who have a common condition (eg, diabetes, obesity, asthma). In this scenario, education and even clinician visits can be used to address multiple patients at the same time, thereby increasing access by seeing more patients in the time in which a clinician would typically see an individual. This approach improves access and also provides a social network for patients to teach each other how they manage their chronic conditions and help each other in their illnesses.

Technology

With the rapid development of technology, other methods have been added to the clinician's toolkit in caring for the rural population. One strategy is the use of e-visits. E-visits, whether they are part of the electronic medical record or a separate secure messaging program, involve patients entering their relevant clinical information into the message, which the PCP receives. The provider makes an assessment and communicates the clinical decision to the patient electronically. A possible scenario is one in which a female patient with no significant past medical history has dysuria, urinary frequency, and urgency, similar to her urinary tract infections in the past. She sends a message to her PCP who then may decide to call in an antibiotic for her.

Another technological advancement is the role of telemedicine, which is being used in areas where subspecialist access is limited. For example, PCPs may connect patients with dermatologists or psychiatrists via telemedicine platforms to assist them in diagnosis and treatment of conditions for which their subspecialist involvement is needed. Furthermore, the use of Project ECHO (Extension for Community Healthcare Outcomes; http://echo.unm.edu) networks may assist rural PCPs in the diagnosis and management of conditions such as hepatitis C, human immunodeficiency virus, and even chronic pain so that the issue can be treated by rural PCPs.

In addition, there has been a shift in the health care marketplace with the development of urgent care clinics. Urgent care clinics (some affiliated with drug-store chains, some independent, and some affiliated with hospital systems) have had the effect of increasing access to health care and avoidance of the emergency departments for nonemergency health care needs. However, these centers can also lead to fragmented care if used frequently.

Improving Training and Retention of Rural Primary Care Physicians

Rural areas experience physician shortages, as mentioned earlier, but this is not new, and has been a concern for decades.[19] This shortage has been the focus of many programs to increase the supply of both medical students and residents interested in practicing in rural areas, as well retaining them after graduation. This goal poses a challenge, not just because of the patient demographics in the rural communities but also because of the challenges of "lower reimbursements for services, clinician lifestyle considerations, spousal career needs, and, for those physicians with children, school quality."[20]

In order to help with recruitment and retention of physicians to rural areas, the federal government has used 3 approaches: Area Health Education Centers (AHECs), National Health Service Corps (NHSC), and Federally Qualified Health Centers (FQHCs). AHECs provide connections with academic institutions to allow training experiences in the ambulatory setting, not just for medical students but for all health professions students. The NHSC provides scholarships and loan repayment programs to physicians from allopathic and osteopathic schools practicing in underserved areas (not just rural but also urban). In addition, FQHCs are health centers that provide comprehensive primary care to patients with limited access to health care, not just in rural areas but in urban areas as well. Furthermore, some states offer loan repayment programs and scholarship programs for those interested in, and committed to, rural practice.

According to the American Academy of Family Physicians, "two of the strongest predictors that a physician will choose rural practice are specialty and background: family physicians are more likely than those with less general training to go into rural practice, and physicians with rural backgrounds are more likely to locate in rural areas than those with urban backgrounds."[21] Other factors that correlate with an increased likelihood that a physician will choose rural practice include training at a medical school with a mission to train rural physicians, osteopathic training, training that includes rural components, and participation in the NHSC. However, those who are prepared not just to practice medicine but also to live in a rural area are more likely to stay in the rural area long term.[22]

SUMMARY

Rural PCPs know their patients and their communities well, being key members of their communities. They also are positioned to be involved what the Institute of Healthcare Improvement calls the Triple Aim: optimizing health system performance with improving the patient experience of care (including quality and satisfaction), improving the health of populations, and reducing the per capita cost of health care.[23] Although rural populations have higher rates of medical conditions than their metropolitan counterparts, and have less access to quality health care, rural PCPs can use technology and health care professionals in a team-based approach to improve the health of their community. However, it is critical to note that policy makers are also key to improving rural health, because policies can produce changes to determinants of health. In this current climate of using quality metrics for pay for performance, many metrics have limited evidence and may not lead to better health outcomes. Therefore, policy makers need to transform the current system of metrics to include metrics that are patient centered, evidence based, and address social determinants of health.[24]

REFERENCES

1. Donaldson MS, Yordy KD, Lohr KN, et al, editors. Primary care: America's health in a new era. Washington, DC: Committee on the Future of Primary Care Services, Division of Health Care Services, Institute of Medicine. National Academy Press; 1996.
2. Meit M, Knudson A, Gilbert T, et al. The 2014 update of the rural-urban Chartbook. Bethesda (MD): Rural Health Reform Policy Research Center, University of North Dakota Center for Rural Health and the NORC Walsh Center for Rural Health Analysis; 2014. Available at: https://ruralhealth.und.edu/projects/health-reform-policy-research-center/pdf/2014-rural-urban-chartbook-update.pdf.
3. Keyes KM, Cerda M, Brady JE, et al. Understanding the rural-urban differences in nonmedical prescription opioid use and abuse in the United States. Am J Public Health 2014;104(2):e52–9.
4. Substance Abuse and Mental Health Services Administration, Results from the 2011 National Survey on Drug Use and Health: Summary of National Findings, NSDUH Series H-44, HHS Publication No. (SMA) 12-4713. Rockville (MD): Substance Abuse and Mental Health Services Administration; 2012. Available at: http://www.samhsa.gov/data/NSDUH/2k11Results/NSDUHresults2011.pdf.
5. Jones CM, Paulozzi LJ, Mack KA. Sources of prescription opioid pain relievers by frequency of past-year nonmedical use United States 2008-2011. JAMA Intern Med 2014;174(5):802–3.
6. Goins RT, Williams KA, Carter MW, et al. Perceived barriers to health care access among rural older adults: a qualitative study. J Rural Health 2005;21(3):206–13. Available at: http://ruralhealth.stanford.edu/health-pros/factsheets/disparities-barriers.html.
7. National Conference of State Legislatures. Emergency medical services in rural areas: how can states ensure their effectiveness? Rural Health Brief. Denver (CO): National Conference of State Legislatures; 2000.

8. Sudakin DL, Power LE. Organophosphate exposures in the United States: a longitudinal analysis of incidents reported to poison centers. J Toxicol Environ Health A 2007;70(2):141–7.
9. Centers for Disease Control and Prevention. Available at: http://www.cdc.gov/ticks/diseases/index.html. Accessed March 8, 2016.
10. Murphy DJ. Farm respiratory hazards. University Park (PA): Pennsylvania State University College of Agricultural Sciences Publication; 2013. Available at: http://extension.psu.edu/business/ag-safety/health/e26.
11. Occupational Safety and Health Administration. Safety and Health Topics. United States Department of Labor. Available at: https://www.osha.gov/dsg/topics/agriculturaloperations/hazards_controls.html. Accessed March 8, 2016.
12. Final update summary: Depression in adults: screening. U.S. Preventive Services Task Force. 2016. Available at: http://www.uspreventiveservicestaskforce.org/Page/Document/UpdateSummaryFinal/depression-in-adults-screening1. Accessed March 8, 2016.
13. Johnson NB, Hayes LD, Brown K. National Health Report: leading causes of morbidity and mortality and associated behavioral risk and protective factors – United States, 2005-2013. MMWR Suppl 2014;63(04):3–27.
14. Bolin JN, Bellamy G, Ferdinand AO, et al, editors. Rural healthy people 2020, vol. 1. College Station (TX): Texas A&M Health Science Center School of Public Health, Southwest Rural Health Research Center; 2015. p. i–xii.
15. Friendenreich CM, Gregory J, Kopciuk KA, et al. Prospective cohort study of lifetime physical activity and breast cancer survival. Int J Cancer 2009;124:1954–62.
16. Holick CN, Newcomb PA, Trentham-Dietz A, et al. Physical activity and survival after diagnosis of invasive breast cancer. Cancer Epidemiol Biomarkers Prev 2008;17:379–86.
17. Olson EA, Mullen SP, Rogers LQ, et al. Meeting physical activity guidelines in rural breast cancer survivors. Am J Health Behav 2014;38(6):890–9.
18. Moreno G, Morales LS, Isiordia M, et al. Latinos with diabetes and food insecurity in an agricultural community. Med Care 2015;53(5):423–9.
19. Mareck DG. Federal and state initiatives to recruit physicians to rural areas. Virtual Mentor 2011;13(5):304–9.
20. Rosenblatt RA, Chen FM, Lishner DM, et al. Final report 125: the future of family medicine and implications for rural primary care physician supply. Seattle (WA): WWAMI Rural Health Research Center, University of Washington; 2010.
21. Martin JC, Avant RF, Bowman MA, et al. The future of family medicine: a collaborative project of the family medicine community. Ann Fam Med 2004;2(Suppl 1): S3–32.
22. Rural practice, keeping physicians in (Position Paper). AAFP 2002, 2014 COD. Available at: http://www.aafp.org/about/policies/all/rural-practice-paper.html. Accessed March 8, 2016.
23. Berwick DM, Nolan TW, Whittington J. The triple aim: Care, health, and cost. Health Aff (Millwood) 2008;27(3):759–69.
24. Saver BG, Martin SA, Adler RN, et al. Care that matters: Quality measurement and health care. PLoS Med 2015;12(11):e1001902.

Primary Care Issues in Inner-City America and Internationally

Ramon Cancino, MD, MSc

KEYWORDS

- Inner city • Population • Disparities • Primary care • Cancer

KEY POINTS

- Inner-city patient populations are at high risk for poor outcomes, including increased risk of mortality.
- Barriers to delivering high-quality primary care to inner-city patients include lack of access, poor distribution of primary care providers, competing demands, and financial restraints.
- Health care issues prevalent in this population include obesity, diabetes, cancer screening, asthma, infectious diseases, and obstetric and prenatal care.
- Population health management and quality improvement activities must target disparities in care.
- Partnering with patients and focusing on social determinants of health and medical care are key areas in which to focus to improve overall health outcomes in this population.

The gap between rich and poor continues to widen. According to the Bureau of Labor Statistics, the minimum amount of income the top 10% of full-time wage and salary workers earned was nearly four times as much as what the lowest 10% earned in 1979; this ratio increased to five times by 2014.[1]

Inner-city populations are affected by this gap. The Urban Health Penalty is the observation that "inner city residents suffer the same chronic conditions as people everywhere, but that their situations are made worse by poverty, poor housing conditions, unemployment and other socioeconomic problems."[2] Delivering high-quality primary care to inner-city patients is important and challenging.

PRIMARY CARE IN INNER CITIES

The definition of "primary care" varies, but its principles remain consistent. The World Health Organization (WHO) defines primary care as first-contact, accessible, continued, comprehensive, and coordinated care.[3] Other descriptions build on this

This article originally appeared in *Primary Care: Clinics in Office Practice*, Volume 44, Issue 1, March 2017.
Disclosure Statement: The author has nothing to disclose.
Primary Care Center, UT Health San Antonio, 7422 Hovingham, San Antonio, TX 78257, USA
E-mail address: ramon.cancino@gmail.com

Physician Assist Clin 4 (2019) 21–32
https://doi.org/10.1016/j.cpha.2018.08.017
2405-7991/19/© 2018 Elsevier Inc. All rights reserved.

description adding emphasis on partnership,[4] disease prevention, advocacy,[5] and involvement of family and community, along with the patient.[6]

Inner-cities are usually older densely occupied, deteriorating, and populated by poor, often minority, groups. The Initiative for a Competitive Inner City defines inner-city as a geographic area that has a poverty rate of 20% or higher or a poverty rate of 1.5 times higher than the metropolitan statistical area and an unemployment rate of 1.5 the metropolitan statistical area and/or a median household income of 50% or less than the metropolitan statistical area.[7]

In the United States, about 25% of inner-city inhabitants are middle class, whereas roughly 60% are working class or working poor.[8] Poverty rates for African American and Hispanic populations living in inner-cities can be four to five times that of suburban rates. Disparities exist within cities. One study found 17.5% of inner-city residents were poor compared with 9.1% in other urban areas.[9]

Challenges to delivering primary care to the inner-city include the following:

1. Racism: 16% of whites, 35% of blacks, and 30% of Latinos believe racism in health care is a major problem.[10]
2. Low literacy: 12% to 28% of those ages 16 to 24 are out of school and chronically out of work.[8] Low health literacy contributes to misunderstanding of physician instructions, adherence, and becoming lost to follow-up.[11–13]
3. Competing demands: Personal challenges and economic factors, such as taking time off work, finding child care, and transportation, make accessing care challenging, even when available.[14]
4. Lack of physician resources: Inner-city physicians note financial barriers affect ability to provide medications, equipment, training, and patient education.[15]
5. Poor access:
   a. One in four inner-city residents did not have health insurance as of 2012.[16]
   b. Uninsured adults and those with Medicaid are less likely to get care as soon as wanted compared with adults with private insurance.[17]
   c. Pediatric patients with only Medicaid or Children's Health Insurance Program are less likely to get care as soon as wanted compared with children with any private insurance.[17]
   d. Provider-shortages compound the problem of access.[14] There are only 84 PCPs per 100,000 patients in urban areas.[18] Therefore, there exists a poor distribution of PCPs, which disproportionately affects inner-city areas.[19] In fact, inner-city communities require nearly 13,500 more physicians.[18]
   e. Distance to and long waits contribute to patients' avoidance of care.[14]

The most common health needs facing the inner-cities are explored next. A PCP should be aware of these health issues.

OBESITY

Obesity, defined as body mass index of greater than or equal to 30.0 in adults and as gender-specific weight-for-length greater than or equal to 95th percentile in children, is linked to increased risk for diabetes,[20] cardiovascular disease,[21] cancer,[22] and mortality.[23] Among adults, obesity prevalence increased from 13% to 32% between the 1960s and 2004.

There is an association between urban sprawl and obesity.[24] The inner-city prevalence of overweight and obesity is 21.7% and 22.5%, respectively.[25] Inner-city minority and low-socioeconomic-status groups are disproportionately affected at all ages.

Eleven percent to 16% of inner-city children and adolescents are overweight, and 34% are at risk of overweight.[26,27]

In the inner cities, fresh produce is unavailable or expensive. Inhabitants have less access to safe settings for exercise, increased reliance on television for entertainment of adults and children, easy access to fast-food vendors, and economic pressures limiting time for family meals at home. Children in inner-city schools rely on high fat–high carbohydrate foodstuffs in lunch programs at the same time that school budget cuts often reduce or eliminate physical education programs.[28–30]

DIABETES

The Centers for Disease Control and Prevention estimates 29.1 million people in the United States have diabetes. Of these people, 8.1 million are undiagnosed.[31] A total of 24% of patients admitted to an inner-city hospital were found to have undiagnosed diabetes, so the prevalence of diabetes and of people with diabetic complications may be higher in the inner city.[32] One study demonstrated 33.6% of inner-city patients had diabetic retinopathy.[33]

PCPs should address barriers to adherence among inner-city patients with diabetes. Inner-city inhabitants have poor access to healthy food and safe exercise areas. As many as one in six inner-city inhabitants have a drinking problem.[34] Alcohol intake is associated with poor adherence to recommendations for self-care behaviors among inner-city patients with diabetes.[35] The WHO estimates adherence to long-term therapies is as low as 50% in the developing world, and far lower in less developed countries.[36] Overall, diabetes medication adherence ranges from 25% to 40%.[37,38] Poor adherence to insulin therapy is the leading cause of recurrent diabetic ketoacidosis in inner-city patients.[39]

ASTHMA

The overall US prevalence of asthma is 7.0% in adults and 8.3% in children.[40] The prevalence is 10.9% for those adults and children living below 100% of federal poverty level.[40] The asthma prevalence rate in poor inner-city communities in the United States is twice the national prevalence rate.[41] Those living in inner-city environments experience higher asthma-related morbidity and mortality.[42,43] Furthermore, hospitalization rates for asthma are highest in inner-city neighborhoods. One cause of the increased hospitalizations is the lack of (high cost) inhaled anti-inflammatory medication.[44]

PCPs should address housing and environmental triggers in the asthma patient population. The inner-city housing environment plays a major role in the growing asthma burden in these areas. Environmental concerns include mold, rodent, cockroach, pet, and dust mite allergens.[45] Further contributing to asthma morbidity are the higher concentrations of air pollutant particulate matter and nitrogen dioxide, and secondhand smoke found in inner-city homes.[45,46]

CANCER SCREENING

Cancer screening is a complicated process, lending itself to risk of failure. Patients with low socioeconomic status have a disproportionally higher burden of gastrointestinal diseases (eg, colorectal cancer) that are commonly prevented, diagnosed, or treated with endoscopy.[47–49] Inner-city patients avoid attending appointments for invasive screening procedures. One study reported a nonattendance rate of 21% at an inner-city teaching hospital in London.[50] Another study at a large safety-net health care system found a 42% no-show rate.[51] Screening for other cancers, such as breast and cervical cancers, is also low in the inner-city.[52]

Previous studies have concluded language barriers,[53] socioeconomic status,[54] attitudes,[55] cost,[56] fear,[56] lack of knowledge,[57] and lack of insurance[58] contribute to lower screening rates. The PCP, therefore, plays an important role in communicating the importance of cancer screening and should develop systems to ensure proper patient education and follow-up of referrals and appointments.

HUMAN IMMUNODEFICIENCY VIRUS

There is an estimated 1.2 million persons aged 13 and older with human immunodeficiency virus (HIV) in the United States.[59] With a prevalence of 2.4%, low-income inner-city residents are at greater risk for HIV than those living above the poverty line.[60,61]

Drug use in the inner-city contributes to this problem. Crack cocaine users, and women who have sex in exchange for money or drugs, are at high risk for HIV infection. Drug use also promotes the indirect transmission of HIV via such sexual exchanges.[62] Advances in HIV treatment have had a positive impact on most risk groups in an HIV clinical setting,[63] and care and life expectancy have improved dramatically,[64] but these improvements have not been shared equally. Persons of low income strata have not benefitted from improvements.[65]

Infection rates are particularly high in the inner cities especially among African Americans,[66] persons below the poverty line,[67] and injection drug users.[68] Therefore, PCPs should standardize HIV screening, which can also decrease stigma. Furthermore, providers should develop therapeutic relationships with HIV-positive patients. In inner-city populations, challenges include access, retention in care, and adherence to treatment regimens.[65]

VIOLENCE

Violence is one of the leading causes of death in all parts of the world for ages 15 to 44.[69] Many large cities have a high prevalence of gang homicides and victims of gang homicides are often younger. Between 27% and 42% of victims are 15 to 19 years.[70] Between 50% and 96% of inner-city youth have been exposed to community violence, which is higher than other environments.[71,72]

Intimate partner violence (IPV), including rape and assault, affects 1.5 million women and 834,700 men in the United States annually.[73] Nearly 50% report experiencing IPV, with more than 18% reporting IPV during the previous year.[74] Inner-city single-mother households have increased risk of prolonged poverty, child abuse, and violence.[8]

PCPs to inner-city patients should speak to their patients about home and neighborhood safety, because the PCP may be the patient's only access to reliable advice.

MENTAL ILLNESS

In the United States 7.6% of persons 12 years of age and older self-reported depression in any 2-week period 2009 to 2012.[75] The same report showed that those living below the poverty level were nearly 2.5 times more likely to have depression than those at or above the level of poverty.

The inner-city environment plays a role. Community violence exposure increases risk of posttraumatic stress, aggression, and other mental health problems.[76,77] Other inner-city conditions that increase the prevalence of mental health conditions include being lower income and social class, especially among urban, predominantly ethnic minority youth.[78-80] In inner-cities, an association between depression, substance abuse, IPV, and HIV infection rates has been documented.[81]

The PCP should make screening for depression and substance abuse part of standard practice of the clinical examination. Doing so can help to decrease stigma around such diagnoses.

OTHER HEALTH ISSUES

Although overall smoking prevalence rates have declined over the past three decades,[82] prevalence rates for inner-city African Americans remain high (33%–54%). Prevalence in one inner-city is 60% in health care settings and 52% in housing developments.[83,84]

Homes painted between 1884 and 1978 can have high lead levels. There is no safe level of lead exposure and elevated levels result in lower scores in intelligence scales,[85] poor schooling outcomes,[86] and increased risk for antisocial and delinquent behavior.[87] Lead levels have been found to be higher in inner-city areas disproportionately affecting the children and minority populations.[88-90]

Obstetric outcomes are important markers of population health. Low birth weight (<2500 g) increases outcome of fetal and neonatal death, respiratory distress syndrome, blindness, deafness, and hydrocephaly. One inner-city population had a sixfold increase in the risk of low birthweight in association with financial problems.[91] Inner-city sub-Saharan Africa found a 10.2% incidence of low birth weight children.[92]

SOCIAL DETERMINANTS OF HEALTH MUST BE ADDRESSED BY PRIMARY CARE PROVIDERS

PCPs should be aware that clinical disease is not the only factor that can impact health. Issues that should be addressed include social determinants of health, which include stress, social exclusion, unemployment, social support, food, and transport.[93] Initiatives, such as that described in the report *Promoting Health Equity: A Resource to Help Communities Address Social Determinants of Health*, have given guidance to community health centers and organizations to address social determinants of health to improve outcomes.[94]

QUALITY IMPROVEMENT AND POPULATION HEALTH MANAGEMENT CAN HELP IMPROVE PATIENT OUTCOMES

The 2010 National Healthcare Disparities Report emphasizes the need for "improvements in quality and progress reducing disparities with respect to certain populations, including residents of inner-city areas." Awareness of disparities in inner-city health outcomes allows the PCP to focus care delivery. This is especially important with increasing momentum to tie financial reimbursement to quality of care delivered to patient populations.

Quality of care metrics can include diabetes control and cancer screening. Inner-city practices tie QI activities to quality metrics. Many inner-city practices form QI committees and teams to develop projects to improve quality of care. One method that is often used in QI activities is the Institute for Healthcare Improvement's Model for Improvement. Examples of projects include using measures as indicators of improvement in community health centers to show significant improvement in prevention and screening measures for chronic diseases, such as diabetes and asthma[95-97]; and focusing on communication, teamwork, process, and workflow to improve delivery of patient services.[98] Social determinants of health impact health care quality in the inner-city but is not often enough linked to QI activities.[99]

Inner-city PCPs can use quality metrics to target populations at risk for health care disparities and allocate resources to improve health. Targeted breast health navigators have been shown to improve outcomes in inner-city women.[100,101] Case management improved glycemic control, blood pressure, and cholesterol in a population of inner-city patients with diabetes.[102]

PARTNERSHIPS

An inner-city PCP should understand how partnerships with federal, state, and community-based organizations can facilitate delivery of services to patients. The National Center for Medical Legal Partnership has partnered with multiple entities to decrease housing violations, which are often tied to poor outcomes in inner-city pediatric asthma patients.[103] The South Bronx Asthma Partnership used asthma education and empowerment to work with patients and families in partnership with health care providers and community programs.[104] Navigation programs in inner-city hospitals have enhanced cancer treatment and education.[101,105] The WHO cites collaboration between primary care, community services, and specialty care as key to delivering care to these patients.[106]

As the name suggests, the PCP can be a patient's first contact with the health care system, but delivering high-quality primary care to inner-city patients is fraught with challenges. Poor access, mistrust, miscommunication, low health literacy, and competing priorities can result in poor outcomes for pediatric and adult inhabitants. These outcomes include increased risk of mortality, malignancy, and hospital utilization. Nevertheless, these sorts of outcomes highlight the important role PCPs play in using all tools available to identify, contact, and treat patients in this high-risk population. These outcomes also suggest the PCP's importance in providing comprehensive preventive care and in partnering with communities to educate patients of all ages on health-related topics. As care delivery models evolve, the PCP is entrusted to ensure that voice is given to inner-city populations such that these models decrease rather than magnify the disparities of care delivered to this population.

REFERENCES

1. A look at pay at the top, the bottom, and in between: Spotlight on statistics: U.S. Bureau of Labor Statistics. Available at: http://www.bls.gov/spotlight/2015/a-look-at-pay-at-the-top-the-bottom-and-in-between/home.htm. Accessed January 24, 2016.
2. Inner-city health care. American College of Physicians. Ann Intern Med 1997; 126(6):485–90.
3. Main terminology. 2016. Available at: http://www.euro.who.int/en/health-topics/Health-systems/primary-health-care/main-terminology. Accessed January 24, 2016.
4. Donaldson M, Yordy K, Vanselow N. Defining primary care: an interim report. Washington, DC: National Academies Press; 1994. Available at: http://www.nap.edu/catalog/9153. Accessed January 24, 2016.
5. American Academy of Family Physicians. Primary Care. AAFP's definition of primary care related terms and appropriate usage recommendations. Available at: http://www.aafp.org/about/policies/all/primary-care.html#use. Accessed February 15, 2016.
6. Starfield B, Shi L, Macinko J. Contribution of primary care to health systems and health. Milbank Q 2005;83(3):457–502.
7. In America's War on Poverty, Inner Cities Remain the Front Line | @icicorg. Available at: http://www.icic.org/connection/blog-entry/blog-in-americas-war-on-poverty-inner-cities-remain-the-front-line. Accessed March 12, 2016.

8. Patterson O. The real problem with America's inner cities. The New York Times 2015. Available at: http://www.nytimes.com/2015/05/10/opinion/sunday/the-real-problem-with-americas-inner-cities.html. Accessed March 13, 2016.

9. Weinberg D. Poverty estimates for places in the United States. Washington, DC: Center for Economic Studies, U.S. Census Bureau; 2005. Available at: https://ideas.repec.org/p/cen/wpaper/05-12.html. Accessed March 12, 2016.

10. Lillie-Blanton M, Brodie M, Rowland D, et al. Public perceptions race, ethnicity, and the health care system: public perceptions and experiences. Med Care Res Rev 2000;57(Suppl 1):218–35.

11. Beitler JJ, Chen AY, Jacobson K, et al. Health literacy and health care in an inner-city, total laryngectomy population. Am J Otolaryngol 2010;31(1):29–31.

12. Schillinger D, Piette J, Grumbach K, et al. Closing the loop: physician communication with diabetic patients who have low health literacy. Arch Intern Med 2003;163(1):83–90.

13. Paasche-Orlow MK, Riekert KA, Bilderback A, et al. Tailored education may reduce health literacy disparities in asthma self-management. Am J Respir Crit Care Med 2005;172(8):980–6.

14. Heaman MI, Sword W, Elliott L, et al. Barriers and facilitators related to use of prenatal care by inner-city women: perceptions of health care providers. BMC Pregnancy Childbirth 2015;15:2.

15. Lara M, Allen F, Lange L. Physician perceptions of barriers to care for inner-city Latino children with asthma. J Health Care Poor Underserved 1999;10(1):27–44.

16. Targeting inner cities will increase the Nation's Insured | @icicorg. Available at: http://www.icic.org/connection/blog-entry/blog-targeting-inner-cities-will-increase-the-nations-insured. Accessed March 27, 2016.

17. 2014 National Healthcare Quality & Disparities Report. 2015. Available at: http://www.ahrq.gov/research/findings/nhqrdr/nhqdr14/index.html. Accessed February 15, 2016.

18. Graham Center Policy One-Pagers: Unequal distribution of the U.S. primary care workforce - American Family Physician. Available at: http://www.aafp.org/afp/2013/0601/od1.html. Accessed March 13, 2016.

19. Reynolds PP. A legislative history of federal assistance for health professions training in primary care medicine and dentistry in the United States, 1963-2008. Acad Med 2008;83(11):1004–14.

20. Egede LE, Zheng D. Modifiable cardiovascular risk factors in adults with diabetes: prevalence and missed opportunities for physician counseling. Arch Intern Med 2002;162(4):427–33.

21. Wang G, Zheng ZJ, Heath G, et al. Economic burden of cardiovascular disease associated with excess body weight in U.S. adults. Am J Prev Med 2002;23(1):1–6.

22. Bhaskaran K, Douglas I, Forbes H, et al. Body-mass index and risk of 22 specific cancers: a population-based cohort study of 5·24 million UK adults. Lancet 2014;384(9945):755–65.

23. Calle EE, Thun MJ, Petrelli JM, et al. Body-mass index and mortality in a prospective cohort of U.S. adults. N Engl J Med 1999;341(15):1097–105.

24. Lopez R. Urban sprawl and risk for being overweight or obese. Am J Public Health 2004;94(9):1574–9. Available at: http://www.ncbi.nlm.nih.gov/pmc/articles/PMC1448496/. Accessed January 25, 2016.

25. Isasi C, Whiffen A, Campbell E, et al. High prevalence of obesity among inner-city adolescent boy in the Bronx, New York: forgetting out boys. Prev Chronic

Dis 2011;8(1):A23. Available at: http://www.cdc.gov/pcd/issues/2011/jan/10_0009.htm. Accessed January 25, 2016.

26. Wang Y, Beydoun MA. The obesity epidemic in the United States—gender, age, socioeconomic, racial/ethnic, and geographic characteristics: a systematic review and meta-regression analysis. Epidemiol Rev 2007;29(1):6–28.

27. Pan L, May AL, Wethington H, et al. Incidence of obesity among young US children living in low-income families, 2008–2011. Pediatrics 2013;132(6):1006–13.

28. Lopez RP, Hynes HP. Obesity, physical activity, and the urban environment: public health research needs. Environ Health 2006;5:25.

29. Leyden KM. Social capital and the built environment: the importance of walkable neighborhoods. Am J Public Health 2003;93(9):1546–51.

30. Candib LM. Obesity and diabetes in vulnerable populations: reflection on proximal and distal causes. Ann Fam Med 2007;5(6):547–56.

31. 2014 Statistics Report | Data & Statistics | Diabetes | CDC. Available at: http://www.cdc.gov/diabetes/data/statistics/2014statisticsreport.html. Accessed January 25, 2016.

32. Weijers RN, Bekedam DJ, Oosting H. The prevalence of type 2 diabetes and gestational diabetes mellitus in an inner city multi-ethnic population. Eur J Epidemiol 1998;14(7):693–9.

33. Broadbent DM, Scott JA, Vora JP, et al. Prevalence of diabetic eye disease in an inner city population: the Liverpool Diabetic Eye Study. Eye (Lond) 1999;13(Pt 2):160–5.

34. Simon DDG, Eley JW, Greenberg RS, et al. A survey of alcohol use in an inner-city ambulatory care setting. J Gen Intern Med 1991;6(4):295–8.

35. Johnson KH, Bazargan M, Bing EG. Alcohol consumption and compliance among inner-city minority patients with type 2 diabetes mellitus. Arch Fam Med 2000;9(10):964–70.

36. Geest SD, Sabaté E. Adherence to long-term therapies: evidence for action. Eur J Cardiovasc Nurs 2003;2(4):323.

37. Feldman BS, Cohen-Stavi CJ, Leibowitz M, et al. Defining the role of medication adherence in poor glycemic control among a general adult population with diabetes. PLoS One 2014;9(9):e108145.

38. Cramer JA. A systematic review of adherence with medications for diabetes. Diabetes Care 2004;27(5):1218–24.

39. Randall L, Begovic J, Hudson M, et al. Recurrent diabetic ketoacidosis in inner-city minority patients behavioral, socioeconomic, and psychosocial factors. Diabetes Care 2011;34(9):1891–6.

40. CDC - Asthma - Most Recent asthma data. Available at: http://www.cdc.gov/asthma/most_recent_data.htm. Accessed February 6, 2016.

41. Crain EF, Weiss KB, Bijur PE, et al. An estimate of the prevalence of asthma and wheezing among inner-city children. Pediatrics 1994;94(3):356–62.

42. Bryant-Stephens T. Asthma disparities in urban environments. J Allergy Clin Immunol 2009;123(6):1199–206 [quiz: 1207–8].

43. Gold DR, Wright R. Population disparities in asthma. Annu Rev Public Health 2005;26(1):89–113.

44. Gottlieb DJ, Beiser AS, O'Connor GT. Poverty, race, and medication use are correlates of asthma hospitalization rates. A small area analysis in Boston. Chest 1995;108(1):28–35.

45. Matsui EC, Hansel NN, McCormack MC, et al. Asthma in the inner city and the indoor environment. Immunol Allergy Clin North Am 2008;28(3):665–86.

46. Thorne PS, Kulhánková K, Yin M, et al. Endotoxin exposure is a risk factor for asthma: the national survey of endotoxin in United States housing. Am J Respir Crit Care Med 2005;172(11):1371–7.

47. Jemal A, Siegel R, Xu J, et al. Cancer statistics, 2010. CA Cancer J Clin 2010; 60(5):277–300.

48. Kinsey T, Jemal A, Liff J, et al. Secular trends in mortality from common cancers in the United States by educational attainment, 1993–2001. J Natl Cancer Inst 2008;100(14):1003–12.

49. Siegel RL, Jemal A, Thun MJ, et al. Trends in the incidence of colorectal cancer in relation to county-level poverty among blacks and whites. J Natl Med Assoc 2008;100(12):1441–4.

50. Corfield L, Schizas A, Williams A, et al. Non-attendance at the colorectal clinic: a prospective audit. Ann R Coll Surg Engl 2008;90(5):377–80.

51. Kazarian ES, Carreira FS, Toribara NW, et al. Colonoscopy completion in a large safety net health care system. Clin Gastroenterol Hepatol 2008;6(4):438–42.

52. Collins KS, Hall AG, Neuhaus C, et al. US minority health: A chartbook. 1999. Available at: http://www.commonwealthfund.org/~/media/files/publications/chartbook/1999/may/u-s-minority-health-a-chartbook/collins_usminority-pdf.pdf. Accessed March 13, 2016.

53. Green AR, Peters-Lewis A, Percac-Lima S, et al. Barriers to screening colonoscopy for low-income Latino and white patients in an urban community health center. J Gen Intern Med 2008;23(6):834–40.

54. Baquet CR, Horm JW, Gibbs T, et al. Socioeconomic factors and cancer incidence among blacks and whites. J Natl Cancer Inst 1991;83(8):551–7.

55. Chavez LR, Hubbell FA, Mishra SI, et al. The influence of fatalism on self-reported use of Papanicolaou smears. Am J Prev Med 1997;13(6):418–24.

56. Jennings K. Getting a Pap smear: focus group responses of African American and Latina women. Oncol Nurs Forum 1997;24(5):827–35. Available at: http://europepmc.org/abstract/med/9201736. Accessed February 7, 2016.

57. Meissner HI, Potosky AL, Convissor R. How sources of health information relate to knowledge and use of cancer screening exams. J Community Health 1992; 17(3):153–65.

58. Jennings-Dozier K, Lawrence D. Sociodemographic predictors of adherence to annual cervical cancer screening in minority women. Cancer Nurs 2000;23(5): 350–6 [quiz: 357–8].

59. Prevalence of diagnosed and undiagnosed HIV infection—United States, 2008–2012. Available at: http://www.cdc.gov/mmwr/preview/mmwrhtml/mm6424a2.htm?s_cid=mm6424a2_e. Accessed May 3, 2016.

60. Dinenno EA, Oster AM, Sionean C, et al. Piloting a system for behavioral surveillance among heterosexuals at increased risk of HIV in the United States. Open AIDS J 2012;6:169–76.

61. Raj A, Bowleg L. Heterosexual risk for HIV among black men in the United States: A call to action against a neglected crisis in black communities. Am J Mens Health 2012;6(3):178–81.

62. Edlin BR, Irwin KL, Faruque S, et al. Intersecting epidemics: crack cocaine use and HIV infection among inner-city young adults. N Engl J Med 1994;331(21): 1422–7.

63. Moore RD, Keruly JC, Bartlett JG. Improvement in the health of HIV-infected persons in care: reducing disparities. Clin Infect Dis 2012;55(9):1242–51.

64. van Sighem A, Gras L, Reiss P, et al. Life expectancy of recently diagnosed asymptomatic HIV-infected patients approaches that of uninfected individuals. AIDS 2010;24(10):1527–35.

65. Centers for Disease Control and Prevention (CDC). CDC health disparities and inequalities report—United States, 2011. MMWR Morb Mortal Wkly Rep Suppl 2011;60(Suppl):1–124.

66. Hall HI, Hughes D, Dean HD, et al, Centers for Disease Control and Prevention (CDC). HIV infection—United States, 2005 and 2008. MMWR Morb Mortal Wkly Rep Suppl 2011;60(Suppl):87–9.

67. Song R, Hall HI, Harrison KM, et al. Identifying the impact of social determinants of health on disease rates using correlation analysis of area-based summary information. Public Health Rep 2011;126(Suppl 3):70–80.

68. Centers for Disease Control and Prevention (CDC). HIV infection among injection-drug users—34 states, 2004-2007. MMWR Morb Mortal Wkly Rep 2009;58(46):1291–5.

69. Krug EG, Mercy JA, Dahlberg LL, et al. The world report on violence and health. Lancet 2002;360(9339):1083–8.

70. Gang homicides—five U.S. Cities, 2003–2008. Available at: http://www.cdc.gov/mmwr/preview/mmwrhtml/mm6103a2.htm. Accessed May 4, 2016.

71. Zimmerman GM, Messner SF. Individual, family background, and contextual explanations of racial and ethnic disparities in youths' exposure to violence. Am J Public Health 2013;103(3):435–42.

72. Gibson CL, Morris SZ, Beaver KM. Secondary exposure to violence during childhood and adolescence: does neighborhood context matter? Justice Q 2009;26(1):30–57.

73. Tjaden P, Thoennes N. Full report of the prevalence, incidence, and consequences of violence against women: findings from the National Violence Against Women Survey. Washington, DC: U.S. Department of Justice, Office of Justince Programs, National Institute of Justice; 2000. Available at: https://www.google.com/search?q=Tjaden+PG%2C+Thoennes+N.+Full+Report+of+the+Prevalence%2C+Incidence%2C+and+Consequences+of+Violence+Against+Women%3A+Findings+from+the+National+Violence+Against+Women+Survey.+Washington%2C+DC%3A+U.S.+Dept.+of+Justice%2C+Office+of+Justice+Programs%2C+National+Institute+of+Justice%3B+2000.&oq=Tjaden+PG%2C+Thoennes+N.+Full+Report+of+the+Prevalence%2C+Incidence%2C+and+Consequences+of+Violence+Against+Women%3A+Findings+from+the+National+Violence+Against+Women+Survey.+Washington%2C+DC%3A+U.S.+Dept.+of+Justice%2C+Office+of+Justice+Programs%2C+National+Institute+of+Justice%3B+2000.&aqs=chrome..69i57.193j0j4&sourceid=chrome&ie=UTF-8. Accessed May 4, 2016.

74. El-Bassel N, Gilbert L, Witte S, et al. Intimate partner violence and substance abuse among minority women receiving care from an inner-city emergency department. Womens Health Issues 2003;13(1):16–22.

75. Pratt LA, Brody DJ. Depression in the US household population, 2009–2012. NCHS Data Brief 2014;(172):1–8. Available at: http://198.246.124.22/nchs/data/databriefs/db172.pdf. Accessed March 12, 2016.

76. McDonald CC, Richmond TR. The relationship between community violence exposure and mental health symptoms in urban adolescents. J Psychiatr Ment Health Nurs 2008;15(10):833–49.

77. Pastore DR, Fisher M, Friedman SB. Violence and mental health problems among urban high school students. J Adolesc Health 1996;18(5):320–4.

78. Brooks-Gunn J, Duncan GJ. The effects of poverty on children. Future Child 1997;7(2):55–71.
79. McLoyd VC. Socioeconomic disadvantage and child development. Am Psychol 1998;53(2):185–204.
80. McLeod JD, Shanahan MJ. Trajectories of poverty and children's mental health. J Health Soc Behav 1996;37(3):207–20.
81. Oldenburg CE, Perez-Brumer AG, Reisner SL. Poverty matters: contextualizing the syndemic condition of psychological factors and newly diagnosed HIV infection in the United States. AIDS 2014;28(18):2763–9.
82. Giovino GA, Henningfield JE, Tomar SL, et al. Epidemiology of tobacco use and dependence. Epidemiol Rev 1995;17(1):48–65.
83. Ahluwalia JS, McNagny SE, Clark WS. Smoking cessation among inner-city African Americans using the nicotine transdermal patch. J Gen Intern Med 1998; 13(1):1–8.
84. Resnicow K, Futterman R, Weston RE, et al. Smoking prevalence in Harlem, New York. Am J Health Promot 1996;10(5):343–6.
85. Needleman HL, Gunnoe C, Leviton A, et al. Deficits in psychologic and classroom performance of children with elevated dentine lead levels. N Engl J Med 1979;300(13):689–95. Available at: http://www.nejm.org/doi/full/10.1056/NEJM197903293001301. Accessed March 13, 2016.
86. Fergusson DM, Horwood LJ, Lynskey MT. Early dentine lead levels and educational outcomes at 18 years. J Child Psychol Psychiatry 1997;38(4):471–8. Available at: http://onlinelibrary.wiley.com/doi/10.1111/j.1469-7610.1997.tb01532.x/abstract. Accessed March 13, 2016.
87. Needleman HL, Riess JA, Tobin MJ, et al. Bone lead levels and delinquent behavior. JAMA 1996;275(5):363–9. Available at: http://jama.jamanetwork.com/ARTICLE.ASPX?ARTICLEID=395592. Accessed March 13, 2016.
88. Mielke HW, Gonzales CR, Powell ET, et al. Environmental and health disparities in residential communities of New Orleans: the need for soil lead intervention to advance primary prevention. Environ Int 2013;51:73–81.
89. Mielke HW, Blake B, Burroughs S, et al. Urban lead levels in Minneapolis: the case of the Hmong children. Environ Res 1984;34(1):64–76. Available at: http://www.sciencedirect.com/science/article/pii/0013935184900768. Accessed March 13, 2016.
90. Mielke HW, Anderson JC, Berry KJ, et al. Lead concentrations in inner-city soils as a factor in the child lead problem. Am J Public Health 1983;73(12):1366–9.
91. Binsacca DB, Ellis J, Martin DG, et al. Factors associated with low birthweight in an inner-city population: the role of financial problems. Am J Public Health 1987; 77(4):505–6. Available at: http://ajph.aphapublications.org/doi/abs/10.2105/AJPH.77.4.505. Accessed March 13, 2016.
92. Olusanya BO, Ofovwe GE. Predictors of preterm births and low birthweight in an inner-city hospital in sub-Saharan Africa. Matern Child Health J 2010;14(6): 978–86.
93. Marmot M. Social determinants of health inequalities. Lancet 2005;365(9464): 1099–104.
94. Brennan Ramirez L, Baker E, Metzler M. Promoting health equity: a resource to help communities address social determinants of health. Atlanta (GA): U.S.: Department of Health and Human Services; Centers for Disease Control and Prevention; 2008. Available at: http://www.cabdirect.org/abstracts/20103345471.html. Accessed March 13, 2016.

95. Landon BE, Hicks LS, O'Malley AJ, et al. Improving the management of chronic disease at community health centers. N Engl J Med 2007;356(9):921–34.

96. Woods ER, Bhaumik U, Sommer SJ, et al. Community Asthma Initiative: evaluation of a quality improvement program for comprehensive asthma care. Pediatrics 2012;129(3):465–72.

97. Sequist TD, Adams A, Zhang F, et al. Effect of quality improvement on racial disparities in diabetes care. Arch Intern Med 2006;166(6):675–81.

98. Taylor CR, Hepworth JT, Buerhaus PI, et al. Effect of crew resource management on diabetes care and patient outcomes in an inner-city primary care clinic. Qual Saf Health Care 2007;16(4):244–7.

99. Fiscella K, Franks P, Gold MR, et al. Inequality in quality: addressing socioeconomic, racial, and ethnic disparities in health care. JAMA 2000;283(19):2579–84. Available at: http://jama.jamanetwork.com/article.aspx?articleid=192714. Accessed March 12, 2016.

100. Battaglia TA, Roloff K, Posner MA, et al. Improving follow-up to abnormal breast cancer screening in an urban population. Cancer 2007;109(S2):359–67.

101. Phillips C, Rothstein J, Beaver K, et al. Patient navigation to increase mammography screening among inner city women. J Gen Intern Med 2011;26(2):123–9.

102. Shea S, Weinstock RS, Starren J, et al. A randomized trial comparing telemedicine case management with usual care in older, ethnically diverse, medically underserved patients with diabetes mellitus. J Am Med Inform Assoc 2006; 13(1):40–51.

103. Public/private partnership to address housing and health care for children with asthma. Health Affairs. Available at: http://healthaffairs.org/blog/2015/07/22/publicprivate-partnership-to-address-housing-and-health-care-for-children-with-asthma/. Accessed March 13, 2016.

104. NACI: South Bronx Asthma Partnership works to empower health care providers and parents of asthma patients. Available at: http://www.nhlbi.nih.gov/health-pro/resources/lung/naci/naci-in-action/south-bronx.htm. Accessed March 13, 2016.

105. Robinson-White S, Conroy B, Slavish KH, et al. Patient navigation in breast cancer: a systematic review. Cancer Nurs 2010;33(2):127–40.

106. World Health Organization, World Organisation of National Colleges, Academies and Academic Associations of General Practitioners/Family Physicians, editors. Integrating mental health into primary care: a global perspective. Geneva (Switzerland): World Health Organization, Wonca; 2008.

Medical Care for Undocumented Immigrants

National and International Issues

Teresa L. Beck, MD[a,*], Thien-Kim Le, MD[a],
Queen Henry-Okafor, PhD, FNP-BC[b], Megha K. Shah, MD, MSc[a]

KEYWORDS

- Undocumented immigrants • Medical care • Health care • Access to care

KEY POINTS

- There are an estimated 30 to 40 million undocumented immigrants (UIs) worldwide, with more than 12 million in the United States.
- Barriers such as language, cost, and fear of deportation prevent many from seeking health care.
- Although some provisions exist in the United States and abroad to address the health needs of this population, most remain uninsured and with limited access to care.
- Medical conditions and issues specific to this population include infectious diseases, mental health, and inadequate prenatal care.

INTRODUCTION

Both nationally and internationally, medical care of undocumented immigrants (UIs) is a growing issue. Although definitions of who is undocumented vary internationally, in the United States UIs include individuals born outside the United States who are not legal residents. This definition includes those who have entered the country without documents or authorization, those who were legally authorized to enter but remain after their visa has expired, and those whose application for immigrant status has not been resolved.[1]

Although it is challenging to determine exact figures, recent estimates show that UIs make up roughly 4% of the US population, amounting to approximately 12 million individuals. Most of this group is of Hispanic origin (64%) (See Figure 4 at Henry Kaiser

This article originally appeared in Primary Care: Clinics in Office Practice, Volume 44, Issue 1, March 2017.

Disclosure: The authors have no financial disclosures.

[a] Emory Family Medicine Residency Program, Department of Family and Preventive Medicine, Emory University School of Medicine, 4500 N. Shallowford Rd, Suite B, Dunwoody, GA 30338, USA; [b] Family Nurse Practitioner Program, Vanderbilt University School of Nursing, Nashville, TN, USA

* Corresponding author.

E-mail address: tbeck@emory.edu

Family Foundation, Health Coverage of Immirgants: https://www.kff.org/disparities-policy/fact-sheet/health-coverage-of-immigrants/) and 90% are adults between the ages of 18 and 40 years. More than 4 million people in the United States are the US-born children of UIs. About half of UIs are of Mexican origin; however, these numbers have declined over the last 5 years, from more than 6 million to 5.6 million as of 2014. California, Texas, and Florida have the largest numbers of UIs, and Nevada has the largest share, making up 8% of the state's population.[2–5]

The issue of UIs is not unique to the United States. Internationally, the United Nations Population Division estimates that there are 30 million to 40 million unauthorized immigrants worldwide, and although most are in the United States, proportionally continental Europe has a larger share.[6] Although UIs have a variety of reasons to migrate, from safety concerns to economic incentives, addressing the health needs of these populations come with unique challenges and solutions. This article provides an overview of challenges in addressing their health needs, existing methods for accessing care, health conditions specific to this population, and potential solutions to consider in both the national and international contexts, specifically in Europe.

CHALLENGES IN HEALTH CARE

Despite the better health status of the younger UI population, this advantage deteriorates over increasing time spent in the United States.[7] Various factors from socioeconomic status to fear of deportation affect the UI population's health both domestically and internationally and deter UIs from seeking care. The UI population is often of lower socioeconomic status, which adds to the difficulties accessing health care. Given that most of the federal insurance plans are unavailable to the UI population, UIs are susceptible to higher out-of-pocket costs for care. In addition, because of undocumented status, they may not have sick leave days and may have difficulty negotiating time off from work to seek care.[8]

Decreased proficiency in the language of the host country and fear of deportation may also present barriers to health care for UIs. Studies have shown that patients with limited English language proficiency (LEP) are at higher risk of poor health and have decreased access to health care. Patients who have LEP had increased difficulty in understanding their health status as well as accessing preventive services.[9] Fear of deportation may lead to the avoidance of seeking care and risk of severe health complications,[8] and this also affects health care for US-born children of UIs. In addition, shame and discrimination are common feelings experienced by the UI population and contribute to poor access to health care globally.[8]

Many of these issues in health care are not unique to the United States. In a study by Chauvin and colleagues,[10] 22% of the UI population in Europe had access to health coverage, and, of those, only about 36% had true access because of barriers such as administrative difficulties, limited language proficiency, and lack of awareness of available services. Of the main reasons for lack of access, administrative difficulties in obtaining health care and finances were cited as the most common. France and Belgium were found to have the most complicated systems for obtaining health care and, for those who had access, the fear of deportation or imprisonment was prevalent.

ACCESS TO HEALTH CARE

The Patient Protection and Affordable Care Act (ACA), passed in 2010, required most US citizens and legal residents to have health insurance, and resulted in the expansion of Medicaid in 32 states. UIs are not eligible for Medicaid or state-based exchanges under this law.[11] Thus, although the number of overall uninsured in the United States has decreased, it is mostly US citizens and legal residents who have gained access to health insurance.[12]

In 1986, Congress approved the Emergency Medical Treatment and Labor Act (EMTALA), requiring hospitals to provide services for active labor and emergency care regardless of insurance and immigration status. In addition to EMTALA, there is emergency care under Medicaid, which is currently the only federal insurance that is available to UIs. Emergency Medicaid covers patients in active labor and those with acute medical emergencies.[13] It may only be used to stabilize patients and may not cover patients for services after the patient has been stabilized.

Federal provisions available to UIs include prenatal care and care for children funded by Maternal and Child Health Block grants and the Supplemental Food Program for Women, Infants and Children. In 2009, the Children's Health Insurance Program (CHIP) was expanded under the CHIP Reauthorization Act (CHIPRA). In 2015, federal funding for CHIP was expanded to states, which included the standard Medicaid benefit package such as the Early and Periodic Screening, Diagnostic, and Treatment services for medically necessary mental health and dental services, vaccinations and prescription drugs, and access to medical specialists and hospital care and services. Although these resources are available for a vulnerable subset of UIs, there are few resources that exist for sick, nonpregnant adults.[12]

Federally Qualified Health Centers (FQHCs) are community health centers that receive federal grant funding to support care to the uninsured without regard for immigration status. There are approximately 1200 health centers operating around the country, providing primary health care, dental, mental health, and pharmacy services on a sliding-scale basis. In addition, there are many low-cost and free community clinics that rely on private donations and volunteers to provide services to those who cannot afford to pay.[14]

ACCESS TO HEALTH CARE IN EUROPE

Europe faces similar challenges regarding access to health care for its UI population. The Platform for International Cooperation on Undocumented Migrants (PICUM) reported that Italy and Spain provided the widest coverage for UI with universal access to health care.[10] Germany, Greece, Sweden, and Switzerland only cover emergency care for UIs.[10] **Table 1** provides an overview of access to care for UIs in Europe.[15]

THE NATIONAL DEBATE ON MEDICAL CARE FOR UNDOCUMENTED IMMIGRANTS

There is ongoing political debate in the United States regarding health care services for UIs. Those in opposition maintain that using taxpayer-funded services to support individuals who enter and remain in the United States illegally undermines the legal system. However, some scholars and legislators have argued that it is both unethical and impractical to deny access to health care services for illegal immigrants living in the United States.[16] They view health care as a basic human right and an obligation of a just society to provide health care for everyone. Leading medical professional societies such as the American Medical Association (AMA), American College of Physicians (ACP), the American Academy of Family Physicians (AAFP), and the American Nurses Association (ANA) reaffirm the position that all individuals living in the United States, regardless of their immigration status, should have access to quality health care, including the opportunity to purchase insurance. These leaders maintain that providing this population with access to health insurance is an evidence-based way to reduce health care costs.[17–19]

Table 1
Health care access to undocumented migrants in 7 European countries

Country	Undocumented Migrants as Percentage of Population	Main Vehicle for Covering Undocumented Migrants	Benefits	Additional Notes
United Kingdom	1.2	NHS	Emergency care and certain infectious diseases with public health hazard. NHS requires hospitals to confirm the ability to pay of patients not covered by the NHS	Cost must either be covered by the patient or taken out of the hospital's budget, which creates a barrier
France	0.6	AME	Full range as provided in the public system	Undocumented migrants without AME eligibility are entitled to emergency care, pediatric care, and maternity care
Germany	0.6–1.8	Separate tax-funded scheme in which providers can receive reimbursement for the costs of emergency treatment	All emergency care Several categories of planned care, only accessible with a medical card	Undocumented migrants face a high barrier when applying for a medical card in the welfare office because the office must report the individual to the authorities, which could lead to deportation
Italy	0.3–1.6	Undocumented migrants can apply to a local national health service office for a temporary (ie, 6-mo) health card	Health card entitles bearer to urgent care, essential care, preventive care (including maternity care), and diagnosis/treatment of infectious diseases	There are local differences in interpretation of the law and willingness to provide services. There are reports of many people without access
Netherlands	0.4–1.4	Separate tax-funded scheme in which the government pays providers for undocumented migrant care at 80% of normal fees for costs that cannot be recovered from the patient	Full range as provided in the public system	The requirement that patients be billed and the limited number of contracted providers for services provided on referrals may create barriers to care

Spain	0.8	Undocumented migrants are covered by the national health service if they have registered as residents of the municipality	Full range as provided in the public system	The requirements for registration with a municipality (valid passport, a proven residency) and police having access to registers constitute the greatest barriers
Switzerland	1.0–1.3	Undocumented migrants are required to purchase insurance in the statutory health insurance system provided by private insurers. There are income-related subsidies	Full range as provided in the public system	High premiums, cost-sharing requirements, and administrative procedures may seriously hamper undocumented migrants' ability to purchase insurance. Undocumented migrants mostly rely on basic health care provided by the cantons

Abbreviations: AME, State Medical Assistance; NHS, UK National Health Service.

Data from Country-specific reports from the Nowhereland Project and the Platform for International Cooperation on Undocumented Migrants (PICUM). PICUM submission to the UN Committee on the Protection of the Rights of All Migrant Workers and Members of Their Families: day of general discussion on the role of migration statistics for treaty reporting and migration policies. 2013. Available at: http://www.ohchr.org/Documents/HRBodies/CMW/Discussions/2013/DGDMigrationData_PICUM_2013.pdf. Accessed February 14, 2016.

Another argument, from a cost perspective, is that many UIs will benefit from preventive care and early treatment of chronic diseases before they advance to life-threatening and costly complications.[20,21] Proponents of this strategy advocate for improving health literacy and vaccination rates, and offering health screenings to the UI population to try to prevent long-term adverse health outcomes and control cost. Moreover, UIs may harbor infections such as tuberculosis (TB), which, when undetected, can easily be transmitted to the general public, thus posing a public health risk.[22]

In contrast, some have argued that treating UIs creates more expenditures for the United States while saving their countries of origin the costs of providing health care.[23] Furthermore, they argue that sharing inadequate health care resources with UIs will reduce the availability of those scarce resources for US citizens. In the last 2 decades, several states have attempted to advance legislation designed to deny UIs access to publicly funded health services. One such initiative was California's Proposition 187. This law, later deemed unconstitutional, required health care professionals to verify immigration status and report UIs to authorities.[24]

In addition, some believe that continued unabated treatment of UIs is an incentive for persistent violation of the immigration laws and threatens national security in the post-9/11 era.[25] Proponents of this argument suggest that denying health care to UIs will discourage others from attempting to immigrate without proper documentation.[24]

COMMON MEDICAL CONDITIONS IN UNDOCUMENTED IMMIGRANTS

There are significant gaps in the literature on the health status of the UI population. Immigrants in general, and the undocumented in particular, report lower levels of cancer, heart disease, arthritis, depression, hypertension, and asthma than do the native born.[26] Factors thought to contribute to lower rates of reported chronic diseases include the young immigrant population and the process of migration, which, especially in cases of undocumented individuals, positively selects for those healthy enough to make the often arduous journey (ie, the so-called healthy immigrant effect).[7,26] In addition, little is known about the long-term health of the children of UIs, particularly related to the adverse effects of inadequate prenatal care and the stressors related to undocumented status, which has been shown to negatively affect children regardless of their own legal status.[12]

Most of the emergency health care services used by UIs are for childbirth. A study of emergency Medicaid expenditures for undocumented and recent immigrants in North Carolina between 2001 and 2004 found that more than 82% of health care spending was related to childbirth and complications of pregnancy. Of the remaining health care expenditures, one-third was spent on the treatment of acute injuries and poisoning, possibly related to exposure to pesticides or other toxins in the workplace.[27] These uses of health care services reflect not only the young age of most UIs but also the type of work that they perform.[28] Beyond pregnancy and acute injury, chronic renal failure, cerebrovascular disease, and heart disease were major contributors to emergency Medicaid use.[27]

Various factors associated with undocumented status are thought to erode the health advantage of the undocumented at a faster rate than their documented counterparts. Specifically, limited access to quality health care; increased vulnerability caused by low income and occupational status; and the stressors associated with undocumented status, such as fear of deportation, have been implicated.[29] In addition,

UIs with chronic and infectious medical conditions are negatively affected because of poor access to care.[30–32]

Perinatal health of undocumented women and their US-born children is a specific area of concern. Consistent with much of the health literature, several studies have found that undocumented women engage in few health risk behaviors while pregnant and seem to have low rates of low-birth-weight or preterm babies.[33–36] However, the beneficial effects of better health behaviors during pregnancy are counteracted by the effects of lower rates of prenatal care among UIs. Poor (and late) prenatal care has been associated with higher risk for adverse perinatal outcomes.[36,37]

In addition, stressors related to undocumented status, such as fear of deportation or experiences of discrimination and stigma, may adversely affect the physical and emotional health of UIs, with potential consequences for their US-born children.[38,39] Findings from a qualitative study of 85 immigrant families experiencing the arrest of at least 1 parent by immigration authorities, showed an increase in the children's behavioral problems, speech and developmental concerns, and declines in school performance.[40]

There is a public health concern over UIs bringing infectious diseases into the United States. Legal immigrants and refugees are required to have a medical examination for migration to the United States, while they are still overseas. This examination is the responsibility of the Centers for Disease Control and Prevention (CDC), which provide instructions to the panel physicians who conduct the medical examinations. The procedure consists of a physical examination, an evaluation (skin test/chest radiograph examination) for TB, and a serologic evaluation for syphilis. Requirements for vaccination are based on recommendations from the Advisory Committee on Immunization Practices.[41]

Individuals who fail the examination because of certain health-related conditions are not admitted to the United States. Such conditions include drug addiction or communicable diseases of public health significance, such as TB, syphilis, gonorrhea, leprosy, and a changing list of current threats such as polio, cholera, diphtheria, smallpox, or severe acute respiratory syndromes.[42] There is a growing concern that UIs crossing into the United States illegally could bring any of these threats. The most prevalent infectious diseases are hepatitis B, latent and active TB, filariasis, intestinal helminth infections, malaria, intestinal protozoa infections, hepatitis C, other nonparasitic infections, sexually transmitted diseases, and human immunodeficiency virus.[43]

Little is known about the mental health issues of UIs. However, the literature suggests that UIs have a unique risk profile that may contribute to different mental health outcomes compared with their documented counterparts. Themes specific to UIs include failure in the country of origin, dangerous border crossings, limited resources, restricted mobility, marginalization/isolation, stigma/blame and guilt/shame, vulnerability/exploitability, fear and fear-based behaviors, and stress and depression.[44]

One study compared the diagnoses and mental health care use of undocumented Latin American immigrants (15%) with those of documented (73%) and US-born Latin Americans (12%) treated in this clinical setting. The undocumented Latin Americans were more likely to have a diagnosis of anxiety, adjustment, and alcohol abuse disorders. The UIs also had a significantly greater mean number of concurrent psychosocial stressors compared with documented immigrants and US-born groups, and they were more likely to have psychosocial problems related to occupation, access to health care, and the legal system.[45] Other studies have shown increasing rates of substance abuse, binge-eating, and conduct disorders among UIs residing longer in the United States.[7]

THE EUROPEAN EXPERIENCE

The European immigrant population comes from many different countries, with a heavy concentration from countries in Africa, the Middle East, and the former Soviet Union. The most commonly reported health care problems in this undocumented migrant population include mental health, infectious and sexually transmitted diseases, and reproductive health. Concerns about human trafficking, particularly of women and children, for commercial sexual exploitation or forced labor or slavery are more prominent in Europe.[15]

POTENTIAL SOLUTIONS

Despite the contentious debate over the ACA, a consensus has emerged that strengthening primary care will improve health outcomes and restrain the growth of health care spending. Supporting evidence comes from studies of primary care as an orientation of health systems and as a set of functions delivered by a usual source of care.[46] Although methodological concerns exist, many observational studies in the United States have found that regions with higher primary care physician-to-specialist ratios have better health outcomes, including lower mortality; fewer emergency department visits, hospitalizations, and procedures per capita; and lower costs.[46]

International comparisons between industrialized countries also suggest that countries with higher ratings of primary care orientation experience better health care outcomes and incur lower health care costs than countries with lower degrees of primary care orientation.[46] These finding suggest that reducing barriers to primary care for UIs may ultimately improve the quality and cost of delivering health care for all countries struggling to manage their growing immigrant populations.

MODELS FOR OFFERING COMPREHENSIVE CARE

Several US cities and states with large immigrant populations have attempted to address their health care needs by providing access to primary care. New York City has the nation's largest public health system, composed of the Health and Hospitals Corporation (HHC) and Community Health Care Association of New York State, whose members include FQHCs and migrant health programs. These organizations provide much of the health care for uninsured and undocumented patients. Both systems rely on Medicaid (and, to a lesser extent, Medicare) reimbursements. They also depend on federal Disproportionate Share Hospital funding and other sources of state Indigent Care Pool funding. In addition to primary and preventive health care, HHC ambulatory centers offer uninsured patients access to on-site pharmacies and referrals to medical specialists and diagnostic and other services located in HHC medical centers.[47]

California offers a Medi-Cal health insurance plan that provides a full range of low-cost health care options for uninsured Californians, with some benefits provided regardless of immigration status. In addition, Kaiser Permanente offers a Child Health Program for uninsured California children younger than 19 years who do not have access to Medi-Cal or other coverage, regardless of immigration status. My Health LA (MHLA) is a no-cost health care program that offers comprehensive health care for low-income, uninsured Los Angeles county residents, regardless of immigration status or medical condition. It offers care through 164 community clinic medical home sites, where patients receive primary and preventive health care services and some diagnostic services. Los Angeles County Department of Health Services facilities also provide county clinic medical home sites, plus emergency, diagnostic, specialty, inpatient services, and pharmacy services. Healthy San Francisco (HSF) is a low-income program for San Francisco County residents regardless of employment status, immigration status, or medical condition. Unlike MHLA, HSF charges a participation fee and point-of-service fee to all patients except for those at less than 100% of the federal poverty level and those who are homeless.[47]

The Harris County Health System, which includes the city of Houston, Texas, offers Access Care, a financial assistance program open to uninsured and undocumented Harris County residents, and provides access to discounted health care at more than 20 community clinics, a dental clinic, and surgical and other subspecialty clinics. The Harris Health System has a dialysis clinic as well as a long-term care facility.[47]

In Massachusetts, all immigrants are eligible for some form of health coverage. There is 1 application for all available programs, including the insurance marketplace. Mass Health Limited is the state version of emergency Medicaid. It is available to UIs and some immigrants who are PRUCOL (Permanent Residence Under Color of Law), defined as aliens who are living in the United States with the knowledge and permission of the federal government, and whose departure the agency does not contemplate enforcing.[47]

In Nevada, the nonprofit Access to Healthcare Network (AHN) offers medical discount programs, specialty care coordination, a health insurance program, nonemergency medical transportation services, a pediatric hematology/oncology practice, and a toll-free statewide call center. AHN has 35,000 members, more than half of whom are presumed to be undocumented.[47]

ADDRESSING BARRIERS TO CARE FOR UNDOCUMENTED IMMIGRANTS

A study by Hacker and colleagues[8] identified 5 areas to address barriers to care for UIs: advocacy for policy, insurance options, expansion of the safety net, training of providers, and education of UIs on navigating the system (**Table 2**).

Table 2
Recommendations for improving barriers

Category	Description
Advocacy/legal change	• Expand health care access to all, regardless of status • Make UIs documented and give full rights to health care
Insurance	• Allow all residents to have access to state-funded limited network health plan and paid or subsidized insurance options, or provide insurance to all workers regardless of status
Expansion of the safety net	• Expand the capacity of public, nonprofit, and free clinics to render care to the population • Provide health and education in nonprofit social service or faith-based organizations • Enhance support for safety-net providers through state-funded vehicle
Training providers	• Train providers to better understand the needs of their immigrant patients • Train providers and update them on legal mandates within the country
Education and outreach to UIs	• Outreach to specific immigrant communities to educate on the current laws and the system, especially education regarding rights to health care • Provide culturally appropriate navigators in health care environments

POTENTIAL SOLUTIONS IN EUROPE/INTERNATIONAL CONTEXT

Nearly all industrialized countries provide some form of government-supported health care to all of its residents, including those who are undocumented (see **Table 1**). Although countries in the European Union have significantly fewer UIs, their models may offer insights on the options and challenges of addressing this health care dilemma facing the United States.

SUMMARY

Medical care for UIs is a complex area involving challenges for accessing care, barriers in financing care, and unique medical conditions. Fear, stigma, cost, and cultural barriers often prevent UIs from seeking medical care. UIs make up a small but substantial portion of the population in the United States and internationally, and there is an emerging interest in finding solutions to address their health care needs. In the United States, cities with large numbers of immigrants have models that provide health care to their uninsured regardless of immigration status, and could potentially be expanded to other areas of the country experiencing increasing growth of their immigrant populations. International approaches may also inform on policies to address the health care needs of UIs.

REFERENCES

1. Internal Revenue Service. Immigration terms and definitions involving aliens. Available at: https://www.irs.gov/Individuals/International-Taxpayers/Immigration-Terms-and-Definitions-Involving-Aliens. Accessed February 14, 2016.
2. Passel JS. Unauthorized migrants: numbers and characteristics. Background briefing prepared for Task Force on Immigration and America's Future. 2005. Available at: http://www.pewhispanic.org/files/reports/46.pdf. Accessed April 29, 2016.
3. Artiga S, Damico A, Young K, et al. Health coverage and care for immigrants. 2016. Available at: http://kff.org/disparities-policy/issue-brief/health-coverage-and-care-for-immigrants/. Accessed February 14, 2016.
4. Hoefer M, Rytina N, Baker B. Estimates of the unauthorized immigration population residing in the United States: January 2011. 2012. Available at: https://www.dhs.gov/xlibrary/assets/statistics/publications/ois_ill_pe_2011.pdf. Accessed April 28, 2016.
5. Krogstad JM, Passel JS. 5 facts about illegal immigration in the U.S. 2015. Available at: http://www.pewresearch.org/fact-tank/2015/11/19/5-facts-about-illegal-immigration-in-the-u-s/. Accessed April 29, 2016.
6. Platform for International Cooperation on Undocumented Migrants (PICUM). PICUM submission to the UN Committee on the Protection of the Rights of All Migrant Workers and Members of Their Families: day of general discussion on the role of migration statistics for treaty reporting and migration policies. 2013. Available at: http://www.ohchr.org/Documents/HRBodies/CMW/Discussions/2013/DGDMigrationData_PICUM_2013.pdf. Accessed February 14, 2016.
7. Teruya SA, Bazargan-Hejazi S. The immigrant and Hispanic paradoxes: a systematic review of their predictions and effects. Hispanic J Behav Sci 2013; 35(4):486–509.
8. Hacker K, Anies M, Folb BL, et al. Barriers to health care for undocumented immigrants: a literature review. Risk Manag Healthc Policy 2015;8:175.

9. Sentell T, Braun KL. Low health literacy, limited English proficiency, and health status in Asians, Latinos, and other racial/ethnic groups in California. J Health Commun 2012;17(Suppl 3):82–99.

10. Chauvin P, Parizot I, Simonnot N. Access to healthcare for undocumented migrants in 11 European countries, vol. 70. Paris: CLUMIC; 2009. p. 93–102. Available at: http://www.epim.info/wp-content/uploads/2011/02/Access-to-healthcare-for-Undocumented-Migrants-in-11-EU-countries-2009.pdf. Accessed February 11, 2016.

11. Medicare.gov. Affordable Care Act. 2012. Available at: https://www.medicaid.gov/affordablecareact/affordable-care-act.html. Accessed February 11, 2016.

12. Wallace SP, Torres J, Sadegh-Nobari T, et al. Undocumented immigrants and health care reform. Final report to The Commonwealth Fund 2012.

13. Congressional Budget Office. The impact of unauthorized immigrants on the budgets of state and local governments. 2007. Available at: https://www.cbo.gov/sites/default/files/110th-congress-2007-2008/reports/12-6-immigration.pdf. Accessed February 11, 2016.

14. Centers for Medicare/Medicaid Services. CMS issues proposed changes in conditions of participation requirements and payment provisions for rural health clinics and federally qualified health centers. 2008. Available at: https://www.cms.gov/Newsroom/MediaReleaseDatabase/Fact-Sheets/2008-Fact-sheets-items/2008-06-26.html. Accessed April 29, 2016.

15. Gray BH, van Ginneken E. Health care for undocumented migrants: European approaches. Issue Brief (Commonwealth Fund) 2012;33:1–12.

16. Fowler N. Providing primary health care to immigrants and refugees: the North Hamilton experience. CMAJ 1998;159(4):388–91.

17. Kline M. National immigration policy and access to health care: American College of Physicians - a position paper 2011. 2011. Available at: https://www.acponline.org/acp_policy/policies/natl_immigration_policy_access_healthcare_2011.pdf. Accessed April 22, 2016.

18. Stream GR, American Academy of Family Physicians: STRONG MEDICINE for America. 2013. Available at: http://www.aafp.org/dam/AAFP/documents/advocacy/coverage/aca/LT-ReidMcConnellImmigrationReform-062113.pdf. Accessed April 22, 2016.

19. Godfrey T. Nursing beyond borders: access to health care for documented and undocumented immigrants living in the US. 2010. Available at: http://www.nursingworld.org/MainMenuCategories/Policy-Advocacy/Positions-and-Resolutions/Issue-Briefs/Access-to-care-for-immigrants.pdf. Accessed April 22, 2016.

20. Kuruvilla R, Raghavan R. Health care for undocumented immigrants in Texas: past, present, and future. Tex Med 2014;110(7):e1.

21. Chernin G, Gal-Oz A, Schwartz IF, et al. Care of undocumented-uninsured immigrants in a large urban dialysis unit. BMC Nephrol 2012;13:112.

22. Seybolt LM, Christiansen D, Barnett ED. Diagnostic evaluation of newly arrived asymptomatic refugees with eosinophilia. Clin Infect Dis 2006;42(3):363–7.

23. Phillips CB, Benson J. Better primary health care for refugees - catch up immunisation. Aust Fam Physician 2007;36(6):440–2, 444.

24. Schuck PH. The message of 187: facing up to illegal immigration. Am Prospect 1995;(21):85–92.

25. Flechner SM, Leeser D, Pelletier R, et al. Do the right thing. it will gratify some people and astonish the rest. Am J Transpl 2015;16(3):1039–40.

26. Footracer KG. Immigrant health care in the United States: what ails our system? JAAPA 2009;22(4):33–6.
27. DuBard CA, Massing MW. Trends in emergency Medicaid expenditures for recent and undocumented immigrants. JAMA 2007;297(10):1085–92.
28. Gusmano M. Undocumented immigrants in the United States: use of health care. Garrison (NY): The Hastings Center. Available at: http://undocumentedpatients. org/issuebrief/health-care-use/.
29. Heyman JM, Nunez GG, Talavera V. Healthcare access and barriers for unauthorized immigrants in El Paso County, Texas. Fam Community Health 2009;32(1): 4–21.
30. Coritsidis GN, Khamash H, Ahmed SI, et al. The initiation of dialysis in undocumented aliens: the impact on a public hospital system. Am J Kidney Dis 2004; 43(3):424–32.
31. Achkar JM, Sherpa T, Cohen HW, et al. Differences in clinical presentation among persons with pulmonary tuberculosis: a comparison of documented and undocumented foreign-born versus US-born persons. Clin Infect Dis 2008;47(10): 1277–83.
32. Dang BN, Giordano TP, Kim JH. Sociocultural and structural barriers to care among undocumented Latino immigrants with HIV infection. J Immigr Minor Health 2012;14(1):124–31.
33. Dang BN, Van Dessel L, Hanke J, et al. Birth outcomes among low-income women—documented and undocumented. Permanente J 2011;15(2):39.
34. Kelaher M, Jessop DJ. Differences in low-birthweight among documented and undocumented foreign-born and US-born Latinas. Soc Sci Med 2002;55(12): 2171–5.
35. Korinek K, Smith KR. Prenatal care among immigrant and racial-ethnic minority women in a new immigrant destination: exploring the impact of immigrant legal status. Soc Sci Med 2011;72(10):1695–703.
36. Reed MM, Westfall JM, Bublitz C, et al. Birth outcomes in Colorado's undocumented immigrant population. BMC Public Health 2005;5(1):100.
37. Lu MC, Lin YG, Prietto NM, et al. Elimination of public funding of prenatal care for undocumented immigrants in California: a cost/benefit analysis. Am J Obstet Gynecol 2000;182(1):233–9.
38. Potochnick SR, Perreira KM. Depression and anxiety among first-generation immigrant Latino youth: key correlates and implications for future research. J Nerv Ment Dis 2010;198(7):470.
39. Suárez-Orozco C, Yoshikawa H, Teranishi RT, et al. Growing up in the shadows: the developmental implications of unauthorized status. Harv Educ Rev 2011; 81(3):438–72.
40. Chaudry A, Capps R, Pedroza J, et al. Facing our future: children in the aftermath of immigration enforcement. Washington, DC: The Urban Institute; 2010. Available at: http://www.urban.org/sites/default/files/alfresco/publication-pdfs/412020-Facing-Our-Future.PDF. Accessed May 18, 2011.
41. Centers for Disease Control and Prevention. Immigrant and refugee health: technical instructions for medical examination of aliens. 2012. Available at: http:// www.cdc.gov/immigrantrefugeehealth/exams/ti/panel/technical-instructions/panel-physicians/medical-history-physical-exam.html. Accessed May 2, 2016.
42. Centers for Disease Control and Prevention. Immigrant and refugee health: frequently asked questions about the final rule for the medical examination of aliens - revisions to medical screening process. 2016. Available at: http://www.cdc.

gov/immigrantrefugeehealth/laws-regs/revisions-medical-screening/faq.html. Accessed May 2, 2016.

43. López-Vélez R, Huerga H, Turrientes M. Infectious diseases in immigrants from the perspective of a tropical medicine referral unit. Am J Trop Med Hyg 2003; 69(1):115–21.

44. Sullivan MM, Rehm R. Mental health of undocumented Mexican immigrants: a review of the literature. ANS Adv Nurs Sci 2005;28(3):240–51.

45. Pérez MC, Fortuna L. Psychosocial stressors, psychiatric diagnoses, and utilization of mental health services among undocumented immigrant Latinos. J Immigrant Refugee Serv 2005;3:107–23.

46. Friedberg MW, Hussey PS, Schneider EC. Primary care: a critical review of the evidence on quality and costs of health care. Health Aff 2010;29(5):766–72.

47. Berlinger N, Calhoon C, Gusmano MK, et al. Undocumented immigrants and access to health care in New York City: identifying fair, effective, and sustainable local policy solutions: report and recommendations to the Office of the Mayor of New York City, The Hastings Center and the New York Immigration Coalition. 2015. Available at: www.undocumentedpatients.org and www.thenyic.org/healthcare. Accessed February 29, 2016.

Pediatric and Adolescent Issues in Underserved Populations

Neerav Desai, MD*, Mary Elizabeth Romano, MD, MPH

KEYWORDS

- LGBT youth • Foster/kinship care • Juvenile justice system • Refugee health
- Native American health

KEY POINTS

- Children and adolescents in underserved populations have unique health care needs.
- Resources are available for pediatric/adolescent providers to facilitate delivery of care to high-risk children/adolescents.
- Being aware of the health care issues in this underserved pediatric/adolescent population can ensure that preventive health care needs are met as well as screening for physical and mental health needs that require additional intervention.

INTRODUCTION

Children and adolescents in underserved populations experience health care disparities that are unique. These disparities include access to care, continuity of care, and confidentiality issues. This article reviews which groups are underserved, why they are underserved, and how podiatric providers can best care for them. The following pediatric populations are discussed:

- Inner city
- Rural
- American Indians and Alaskan Natives (AIAN)
- International refugees
- Lesbian/gay/bisexual/transgender/questioning/intersex (LGBT)
- Foster care/kinship care
- Juvenile detention
- Homeless

This article is an update of an article that originally appeared in *Primary Care: Clinics in Office Practice*, Volume 44, Issue 1, March 2017.
Disclosure: The authors have nothing to disclose.
Division of Adolescent Medicine & Young Adult Health, Monroe Carell Jr. Children's Hospital at Vanderbilt, Vanderbilt University Medical Center, One Hundred Oaks, 719 Thompson Lane, Suite 36300, Nashville, TN 37204, USA
* Corresponding author.
E-mail address: neerav.desai@vanderbilt.edu

Physician Assist Clin 4 (2019) 47–59
https://doi.org/10.1016/j.cpha.2018.08.018
2405-7991/19/© 2018 Elsevier Inc. All rights reserved.

Inner City Youth

Inner city areas are defined as the central section of an urbanized area in which poorer residents live, older housing structures exist, and there is the highest population density. In the United States, most inner city populations are nonwhite. Children in these areas are at higher risk for moderate to severe asthma, trauma and violence, lead poisoning, malnutrition (including obesity), psychiatric, and substance use disorders.[1] Higher rates of sexually transmitted infections (STIs) and pregnancies are also well documented in urban and inner city areas.[2]

Pediatric providers can use strategies to engage inner city youth to improve health care outcomes. They should promote the pediatric medical home model of care. This model ensures that acute visits, ongoing chronic care, sports physicals, and possibly behavioral health are managed in 1 location by the same providers who are closely familiar with each child's history. It engenders trust and cuts down on unnecessary tests and procedures usually done in retail-based or urgent care settings. Providers in retail based and urgent care settings should communicate with patient's medical home in order to achieve seamless care.[3] Another strategy is the development of school-based health centers. They augment access to care and with proper communication can fit into the medical home model of care.[4] School-based health centers have repeatedly been shown to reduce unnecessary pediatric emergency department visits and have improved quality of asthma care.[5]

Rural Pediatric Populations

Rural areas are defined as those not within a designated urban area.[6] Health care, schools, groceries, and other necessities are harder to access in these areas, presenting challenges to long-term health outcomes. Poverty rates and children and adolescents living in poverty are higher in rural areas and parental education levels are lower.[7]

Two vulnerable pediatric populations in rural areas are those that have special health care needs and those who need subspecialty care. Children with special health care needs are defined as having 1 or more of the following: limitations in performance ability, use of multiple prescription drugs, and requirement of specialized therapies or services.[7] In rural areas, they are less likely to be seen by a trained pediatric provider compared with their urban peers.[7] The data also show significant delays in access to therapists and dentists compared with their urban counterparts. Children in rural areas who need subspecialty care have the most difficulty accessing pediatrics-trained cardiologists, neurologists, gastroenterologists, and psychiatrists. Many of these families have the added burden of cost and time because they are forced to drive long distances to access specialists.

Health care systems must adapt to the disparity faced by rural children by incorporating new technology and promoting the medical home model. The increasing use of telemedicine in rural pediatrics has shown promise, especially in accessing subspecialty care.[8] The most pressing question related to implementation of telemedicine centers is the lack of standardized insurance reimbursements for these services. Moreover, according to the summary of the Pediatrician Workforce Policy Statement developed by the American Academy of Pediatrics (AAP): "More primary care pediatricians will be needed to care for the increasing number of children who have significant chronic health problems and who will require more medical and surgical care from pediatric physicians throughout their childhood. In addition, there will be an increased demand for general pediatricians" because, according to AAP, there is a "decrease in the number of family physicians providing care for children and the limited number of non-physician clinicians interested in pediatric careers."[9,10]

Native American Youth

AIAN youth are a well-studied underserved segment of the population, representing about 1% of all US children.[11] The key demographic contributors to health care disparity are emphasized in **Table 1**.[12]

The largest contributions to morbidity and mortality in AIAN youth are accidents and injuries. Data show that AIAN youth are involved in much higher rates of violent crimes, injuries, and accidents compared with the general population.[13] AIAN adolescents engage in more risk-taking behavior, including not wearing seatbelts, drinking and driving, and riding with someone who is impaired.[14]

The data focusing on physical health reveals much higher rates of obesity and dental caries, which could be affected by diet, education, and health care access.[15,16] The disparity in infant mortality and Sudden Infant Death Syndrome, and the lack of prenatal care compared with the general population, are also alarming. The AIAN community has 5 times the rate of fetal alcohol syndrome (FAS) compared with geographically similar nonnatives.[17] The burden of FAS is distributed across the entire childhood spectrum and affects adult caregivers as well.

Several mental health disparities exist between AIAN youth and their nonnative geographic peers. In one study in Appalachia, substance use was prevalent in 9% of Indian children compared with 3.8% of white children.[18] Perhaps the greatest disparity is seen in the suicide rates among AIAN youth, which are from 3 to 6 times greater than in their nonnative peers.[19,20]

Pediatric providers face a combination of these disparities and some barriers in working with AIAN children. One large barrier to engagement is the inherent distrust the Native American community has for government-backed initiatives, as mentioned in the Broken Promises Letter of Transmittal.[21] Another is a lack of funding for Indian Health Services, which in 2004 was allocated $1914 per patient per year (compared with $3803 per year spent on federal prisoners).[22] The best providers can integrate into the environment and understand which health care priorities and goals are most important to the community. In addition, culturally appropriate community and school-based education has been shown to be best adapted, as shown in health curriculums that prioritize Native American values.[23] In addition, and perhaps most importantly for pediatric providers, the role of the extended family and joint health care decision making is a key part of many Native American cultures.[24]

International Refugee Health in Pediatrics

The United States pediatric refugee population is a diverse group that varies greatly by region and city. Although the numbers vary, roughly 18,000 to 20,000 pediatric refugees are resettled to the United States every year.[25] Refugees and asylum seekers are distinct from immigrants because they have been forced to leave their countries of origin because of persecution or fear of persecution.[26] It may take up to 18 months

Table 1		
Adult demographics for American Indians and Alaskan Natives that affect child health		
	AIAN Adults (%)	**General Population Adults (%)**
Individuals below poverty	27	15.6
High school diploma	71	80
Bachelor's degree	11.5	24.4
Unemployment	14–35 (regional variation)	7

for refugee applications to be considered and approved, which results in a lag time of vulnerability.[27]

Refugee children are particularly vulnerable to inequalities in health care caused by several factors, including language and communication barriers, underinsured parents, and a complex maze of support services.[28] Pediatric providers should be aware that the most vulnerable time is between 8 and 24 months after resettlement, because of the lapse in family benefits, including stipends, vocational training, and health insurance, that occurs around 8 months after migration. Refugee families are generally undertrained in accessing school resources, health care facilities, insurance providers, and vocational prospects by the time their benefits expire.[28]

Some pediatric health care issues that have a higher prevalence in refugee patients are shown in **Box 1**.[29] Refugee children are at particularly high risk for violence in their places of origin and in refugee camps before resettlement, which predisposes them to physical and mental health issues. Providers should screen for these issues over multiple visits using culturally appropriate methods and suitable communication methods. **Box 2** provides resources for clinicians. Pediatric providers usually complete an initial domestic health assessment that is specific to each state and in conjunction with the refugee resettlement agency. Frontloading services and interventions for refugee children are recommended because of problems of access and availability.

Health Care for Lesbian, Gay, Bisexual, and Transgender Adolescents

According to Youth Risk Behavior Surveillance System (YRBS) 2015, 8% of 9th to 12th graders identify as LGB and 3.2% report questioning their sexual identity.[1] Health care disparities in the LGBT population are well documented.[30]

Box 1
Initial and ongoing screening for pediatric refugee health

Initial and ongoing health care issues in refugee children

Malnutrition

Micronutrient deficiencies

Immunization schedules

Parasitic diseases

Tuberculosis

STIs

Female genital cutting and mutilation

Dental problems

Lead screening

Emerging infectious diseases (Ebola, Zika)

Depression

Anxiety

Posttraumatic stress disorder

Rheumatic heart disease

Adapted from Seery T, Boswell H, Lara A. Caring for refugee children. Pediatr Rev 2015;36:323–38.

Box 2
Valuable resources for clinicians caring for refugee families

Ethnomed (Integrating cultural medicine into practice)
   http://ethnomed.org

Cultural Orientation Resource Center
   http://www.culturalorientation.net

BRYCS (Building Refugee Youth and Children's Services)
   http://www.brycs.org/publications/index.cfm

US Centers for Disease Control and Prevention (CDC) Refugee Health Profiles
   www.cdc.gov/immigrantrefugeehealth

Adapted from Seery T, Boswell H, Lara A. Caring for refugee children. Pediatr Rev 2015;36:323–38.

Healthy People 2010 included a companion document that outlined the need for more information about the health status of the LGBT population in order to document and address the factors that contribute to health disparities.[31] Healthy People 2020 used these data to create health goals specific to the disparities of the LGBT population.[32] These disparities include:

- LGBT youth are 2 to 3 times more likely to attempt suicide
- LGBT youth are more likely to be homeless
- Men having sex with men are at higher risk of human immunodeficiency virus (HIV) and other STIs
- Transgender individuals have a high prevalence of HIV/STIs, victimization, mental health issues, and suicide and are less likely to have health insurance than heterosexual or LGBT individuals
- LGBT populations have the highest rates of tobacco, alcohol, and other substance use[31]

Providers should identify LGBT adolescents and young adults and screen for risk and protective factors. LGBT youth must also contend with discrimination, limited social support, and limited contact with other LGBT adults. Providers should train all staff about LGBT health to create a safe clinical environment and should ensure confidentiality and proactively share these policies with patients and families, including when a breach of confidentiality is indicated. Laws vary by state and can be accessed at http://www.guttmacher.org/sections/adolescents.php.

LGBTI youth may be reluctant to use insurance for fear of disclosure to parents through explanation of benefits information. As a result, public clinics may be a preferred option and see a larger proportion of LGBT youth and young adults.

The HEADSSS (home, education/employment/eating, activities, drugs, sexuality, suicide/depression, safety) mnemonic is a useful interview tool to ensure that a thorough risk assessment is done, and this is outlined in **Table 2**.[33]

Pregnancy risk is an issue for all sexually active female patients. Teen pregnancy rates are higher in lesbian and bisexual youth than in heterosexual teens.[30] All sexually active adolescent girls should be counseled on contraceptive options and all sexually active adolescents should be educated on the use of emergency contraception.

STI screening should be done based on behaviors, not sexual orientation and gender identity. Specific STI screening and treatment guidelines are delineated by the US Centers for Disease Control and Prevention (CDC).[34] Providers should be aware and proactive about transgender youths' comfort and preferences for

Table 2	
HEADSSS psychosocial assessment tool	
H	Home: where do you live; with whom do you live; relationships at home; violence at home
E	Education: what grade are you in; school performance; changes in school performance; favorite subjects; future plans/goals; problems at school with bullying, suspension Employment: hours; effect on school performance Eating: history of dieting; concerns about weight/body; exercise habits
A	Activities: activities with friends; activities with families; extracurricular activities/sports; hobbies; television/media use
D	Drugs: tobacco, alcohol, or substance use; frequency of use; social use vs using alone; CRAFFT questionnaire if concerns for abuse
S	Sexuality: romantic relationships; interested in boys/girls/both; sexual activity (ask about types of sexual activity; have you ever used birth control; have you ever been pregnant; have you have had an STI or STI testing; is family aware of sexual activity or sexual/gender identity; safe sex practices)
S	Suicide/depression: are you more sad, irritable, or anxious than usual; do you have a lack of interest in activities or difficulty with sleep or energy; are you more isolated; any thoughts of killing yourself, hurting yourself or other; have you ever tried to kill yourself or hurt yourself?
S	Safety: seatbelt use; helmet/protective equipment use; texting and driving; ridden with someone who was impaired; exposure to violence at home, at school; history of physical or sexual abuse; bullying at school; cyber bullying; access to guns

Abbreviation: CRAFFT, car, relax, alone, forget, friends, trouble.
Adapted from Goldenring J RD. Getting into adolescent heads: An essential update. Contemp Pediatr 2004;21:64.

genitourinary examinations. Many clinics provide accessible, reliable, and accurate information through Web sites and pamphlets about sexual education for all youth, including LGBT youth.

According to the Substance Abuse and Mental Health Services Administration, substance abuse disorders among LGBT youth are almost double those of their heterosexual peers.[35] Substance use is linked to high-risk sexual behaviors, motor vehicle accidents, and suicide attempts, further putting LGBT youth at risk for morbidity and mortality. Referrals for treatment should be pursued aggressively.[34]

LGBT youth are also at risk for physical violence and bullying as documented in YRBS 2015 which showed that:

- Among LGBT youth, 17.5% reported being victims of physical dating violence versus 8.3% of heterosexual youth
- Among LGBT youth, 17.8% reported non-consensual sexual activity versus 5.4% of heterosexual youth
- Rates of non-consensual sex and physical dating violence are much higher among youth who are questioning their sexual identity, 24.5%
- Transgender and female youth report the highest rates of victimization[1]

LGBT youth have higher rates of suicide attempts compared with their heterosexual peers.[31] The risk is further increased in LGBT youth who are homeless, in foster care, or in juvenile detention centers. Providers should screen LGBT youth for depression and suicidality, assessing social support and bullying issues and asking directly about suicidal ideation. They should also ask about acceptance by family. LGBT youth who experience parental rejection are more likely to experience negative health outcomes and have issues with depression, suicidality, and substance use.[31] Providers can work with patients and families to promote acceptance strategies and increase positive support.

Health Care in the Juvenile Justice System

Adolescents in the juvenile justice system are at risk, as shown in the 2010 Survey of Youth in Residential Placement:

- Among youth offenders in custody, 69% have some type of health care need
- Dental, vision, or hearing needs were reported by 37%
- More than one-quarter of those interviewed needed care for illness, injury, or some other health care need that was not listed[36]
- Adolescents with fetal alcohol spectrum disorder (FASD) are over-represented in the juvenile justice populations: 35% of adolescents 12 years of age or older with FASD have been incarcerated at some point[37]

Health issues in this population range from common problems that have been neglected, to consequences of exposure, to violence or poor living conditions and high-risk behaviors.

Health care services received while in detention may be affected by length of stay. On admission, all juveniles should be screened for medical or mental health problems requiring immediate attention. For those that are in custody for 7 days or longer, more comprehensive adolescent health services should be provided. Adolescents in juvenile detention typically receive fragmented medical care because of inconsistent living situations, being in custody or a detention facility, and frequent running away from their home environments.[38]

Immediate health issues that should be assessed and addressed appropriately include:

- Infectious diseases, such as tuberculosis, scabies, lice
- Substance use disorders that may result in withdrawal with abrupt cessation
- Psychiatric emergencies, such as suicidal or homicidal ideation
- Chronic medical problems that require continuation of daily medications

Comprehensive evaluation should include a medical assessment that addresses vision, hearing, and dental needs. These needs are more frequently reported as unmet compared with other health care issues.[36] Adolescents in juvenile detention should be assessed for a history of traumatic injuries. These youth report higher rates of interpersonal violence and have been found to have higher rates of traumatic brain injury.[39]

They also have higher rates of risky sexual activity and pregnancy than the general adolescent population.[36] A pelvic examination may be indicated in adolescent girls with genitourinary symptoms. Pregnancy testing should be done in all postmenarchal girls. When possible, contraception should be offered to all adolescent girls. Routine vaccines, including hepatitis A and B, meningitis, and human papilloma virus should also be completed. Adolescent vaccine recommendations as per the CDC are available at http://www.cdc.gov/vaccines/hcp/acip-recs.

All adolescents should have comprehensive mental health screening by a trained mental health professional because substance use and suicide attempts are reported at higher rates in juvenile detention.[38] This screening should be done on admission and as part of ongoing care, and includes:

- Initial assessment within 24 hours of admission
- Comprehensive assessment as soon as possible

- Accessing previous records from families, schools, mental health providers
- Rescreening as part of transition/release from custody
- Regular screenings during periods of confinement[38]

An evidence-based screening tool should be used. One such tool specifically developed for adolescents and young adults in juvenile detention is the Massachusetts Youth Screening Instrument Second Version (MAYSI-2).[40] MAYSI-2 is a 52-item self-reported questionnaire. It requires 10 minutes to complete and is not biased to age, ethnicity, or gender.

Health Care for Adolescents and Children in Foster Care

The number of children and adolescents (aged 0–21 years) living in foster and kinship care has decreased from its peak in 2002.[41] Almost 614,000 children, up to age 21 years, spent some time in foster care in 2013. In 2002 that number was approximately 814,000.[41] Kinship care is a term used to designate those who, by court order, are living with extended family and not their biological parents. More than 70% of children and adolescents in foster care have a documented history of abuse and greater than 80% have had significant exposure to violence. Health care issues in this group are often the result of inconsistent access to health care, previously chaotic home environments, and a history of trauma, which includes the placement into foster care. Health care providers also encounter barriers when providing care to this population, which includes limited access to medical history, poorly identified consent protocols, and limited resources. The AAP has detailed guidelines for the provision of medical care to children and adolescents in the foster care system.[41] Whenever possible, every effort should be made to establish a medical home for children and adolescents in foster care, including:

- Obtaining a copy of signed consents from the foster care agency
- Keeping consent paperwork as part of each child's permanent health record
- Maintaining contact information for each child's caseworker in the health record
- Providing a summary of the visit to the caseworker after each health care visit

The AAP recommends evaluation by a pediatric or adolescent provider within 72 hours of placement into foster care. This evaluation should be done sooner if there are concerns for acute needs or abuse. Three visits within the first 3 months of placement are recommended with more comprehensive evaluations occurring at 30 and 60 days. **Box 3** provides a comprehensive outline of these visits.[41]

Health Care for Homeless Youth and Adolescents

According to a 2013 report, 1 in 30 children in the United States are homeless, equating to approximately 2.5 million children.[42] Homelessness includes anyone who lacks a permanent residence, lives in a place that is not designed for human living (ie, car, park), lives in temporary living arrangements, or is in imminent risk of losing housing. Populations at risk for homelessness include parents who have a history of substance use, job loss, mental illness, previous military service, or a history of domestic violence and physical or sexual abuse.[43] Among adolescents, previous placement in foster care, school expulsion, and identifying as LGBT are all risk factors for homelessness.[43]

Box 3
Health care visits for youth and adolescents in foster/kindship care

Initial health visit (within 72 hours):

- Identify health conditions requiring immediate attention
  - Review health information
  - Review trauma history
  - Review of systems
  - Symptom-targeted examination
- Identify health/behavioral conditions relevant to placement decisions
  - Child abuse screen
    - Growth parameters, vital signs
    - Skin examination
    - External genitourinary examination
  - Developmental surveillance/screen
  - Mental health screen
    - Suicidality, homicidality
    - Exposure to violence
    - Substance use/abuse
    - History of violent behaviors
  - Sexual health screen
    - Pregnancy test
    - STI screening

Comprehensive health visit (within 30 days):

- Review available health information
  - Records from previous providers, caregivers if available
  - Immunization review
  - Complete physical examination
- Identify acute and chronic health conditions
  - Child abuse screen
  - Trauma screen
  - Mental health screen for mood/conduct disorders, suicidality, behavioral issues
- Health maintenance
  - School performance
  - Adolescent risk review (sexual history, substance use history)
- Develop an individualized treatment plan
  - Dental referral
  - Hearing and vision screening/referral
  - STI screening, contraceptive counseling
  - Mental health referral
  - Psychoeducational testing
  - Laboratory screening: complete blood count, lipid panel, lead level
  - Communicate with caseworker, schedule follow-up appointments

Comprehensive health visit (within 90 days):

- Identify acute and chronic health conditions
  - Growth parameters
  - Physical examination
- Assess ongoing stressors
  - Mental health screening
  - Interaction/relationship between child and foster parents
  - Assess for abuse/neglect
- Health maintenance
  - Update immunizations
  - Reassess school performance
  - Adolescent risk review

- Update treatment plan
  - Follow up on referrals and recommendations
  - Reviewed individualized education plan
  - Communicate with caseworker, schedule follow-up appointments

Adapted from Szilagyi MA, Rosen DS, Rubin D, et al. Health care issues for children and adolescents in foster care and kinship care. Pediatrics 2015;136:e1142–66.

Children who are homeless face significant health challenges, including complicated access to care, interrupted education, and trauma. Children and adolescents who are homeless may have chosen to leave home, but many are escaping abusive or neglectful homes or rejection because of sexual orientation or gender identity. Minors have the added barrier of lacking an adult caregiver, issues with consent, and lack of access to health insurance. An exact number of uninsured homeless youth is not available. Many homeless youth are eligible for state-funded insurance programs and eligibility has increased with the Affordable Care Act. A difficult application process and disconnectedness from family can make it difficult for youth to access these services.[44] Health care providers should work with community resources to facilitate access to and enrollment in health insurance programs.

A list of common health conditions with higher prevalence in homeless youth is provided in **Box 4**.[43] Providers should screen for housing insecurity and inquire about options for storing and securing medications. Providers should offer information about insurance enrollment and, if possible, provide an avenue for access. They can use the medical home model to alleviate the fragmentation of care. Practitioners should also be mindful of communication, transportation, and cost when developing a treatment plan. Providers can obtain state-specific statistics about the homeless population in their area in the State Report Card on Homelessness at www.homelesschildrenamerica.org. Pediatric providers can advocate for homeless youth by partnering with schools, community outreaches, and caseworkers to ensure continuity and coordination of care. State-specific laws are available from the National Association for the Education of Homeless Children and Youth at http://naehcy.org/sites/default/files/pdf/State%20by%20state%20overview.pdf.

Box 4
Common conditions in homeless youth

Infectious diseases (recurrent respiratory infections, infectious diarrhea)

Malnutrition (obesity and failure to thrive)

Dermatologic disease

Asthma

Poor dentition, dental caries

Mental health disorders

Substance use/abuse

Poor academic performance

SUMMARY

A variety of children and adolescents are underserved in the United States. What stands out are the common challenges each population faces, including access to care, poverty, marginalization, vulnerability, and issues of confidentiality. This article emphasizes the essential role that pediatric and adolescent providers play in the health care of these individuals by being informed and creating a welcoming and culturally appropriate environment. It is also important to remember that underserved youth will have limited access to healthcare and every opportunity should be made to address both urgent and chronic medical needs at every health care interaction.

REFERENCES

1. CDC Youth Risk Behavior Survey. 2015. Available at: www.cdc.gov/features/yrbs. Accessed May 8, 2018.
2. Kann L, Olsen EO, McManus T, et al. Sexual identity, sex of sexual contacts, and health-risk behaviors among students in grades 9-12–youth risk behavior surveillance, selected sites, United States, 2001-2009. MMWR Surveill Summ 2011; 60(7):1–133.
3. Committee on Practice and Ambulatory Medicine. AAP principles concerning retail-based clinics. Pediatrics 2014;133(3):e794–7.
4. Council on School Health. School-based health centers and pediatric practice. Pediatrics 2012;129(2):387–93.
5. Brindis CD, Klein J, Schlitt J, et al. School-based health centers: accessibility and accountability. J Adolesc Health 2003;32(6 Suppl):98–107.
6. What is rural? Available at: https://ric.nal.usda.gov/what-rural. Accessed February 26, 2016.
7. Skinner AC, Slifkin RT. Rural/urban differences in barriers to and burden of care for children with special health care needs. J Rural Health 2007;23(2):150–7.
8. Ray KN, Demirci JR, Bogen DL, et al. Optimizing telehealth strategies for subspecialty care: recommendations from rural pediatricians. Telemed J E Health 2015; 21(8):622–9.
9. Basco WT, Rimsza ME, Committee on Pediatric Workforce, et al. Pediatrician workforce policy statement. Pediatrics 2013;132(2):390–7.
10. Committee on Pediatric Workforce. Enhancing pediatric workforce diversity and providing culturally effective pediatric care: implications for practice, education, and policy making. Pediatrics 2013;132(4):e1105–16.
11. Flores G, Res CP. Technical report: racial and ethnic disparities in the health and health care of children. Pediatrics 2010;125(4):E979–1020.
12. US Census Bureau. We the people: American Indians and Alaska Natives in the United States.
13. Manson SM, Beals J, Klein SA, et al. Social epidemiology of trauma among two American Indian reservation populations. Am J Public Health 2005;95(5):851–9.
14. Blum RW, Harmon B, Harris L, et al. American Indian–Alaska Native youth health. JAMA 1992;267(12):1637–44.
15. Jackson MY. Height, weight, and body mass index of American Indian schoolchildren, 1990-1991. J Am Diet Assoc 1993;93(10):1136–40.
16. Jones C. Indian Health Service oral health survey of American Natives. Preface. J Public Health Dent 2000;60(Suppl 1):236–7.
17. May PA, Gossage JP. Estimating the prevalence of fetal alcohol syndrome. A summary. Alcohol Res Health 2001;25(3):159–67.

18. Costello EJ, Farmer EMZ, Angold A, et al. Psychiatric disorders among American Indian and white youth in Appalachia: The Great Smoky Mountains study. Am J Public Health 1997;87(5):827–32.

19. Harrop AR, Brant RF, Ghali WA, et al. Injury mortality rates in native and non-native children: a population-based study. Public Health Rep 2007;122(3):339–46.

20. Wallace LJD, Patel R, Dellinger A. Injury mortality among American Indian and Alaska native children and youth - United States, 1989-1998. JAMA 2003; 290(12):1570–1.

21. US Commission on civil rights. Broken promises evaluating the Native American health care system. 2004. Available at: http://www.usccr.gov/pubs/nahealth/nabroken.pdf. Accessed February 26, 2016.

22. US Commission on Civil Rights. A quiet crisis: federal funding and unmet needs in Indian country. 2004. Available at: http://www.usccr.gov/pubs/na0703/na0204.pdf. Accessed February 26, 2016.

23. Stokes SM. Curriculum for Native American students: using Native American values. Read Teach 1997;50(7):576–84.

24. LaFromboise TD, Trimble JE, Mohatt GV. Counseling intervention and American Indian tradition: an integrative approach. In: Atkinson DR, Morian G, Sue DW, editors. Counseling American minorities. Madison (WI): Brown & Benchmark Publishers; 1993. p. 119–91.

25. Office of the United Nations High Commissioner for Refugees. Figures at a glance. Available at: http://www.unchr.org/pages/49c3646c11.html. Accessed February 26, 2016.

26. US Department of Homeland Security. Definition of terms. Available at: http://www.dhs.gov/definition-terms#17. Accessed February 26, 2016.

27. US Refugee Admissions Program FAQs. 2013. http://www.state.gov/j/prm/releases/factsheets/2013/210135.htm. Accessed February 26, 2016.

28. Mirza M, Luna R, Mathews B, et al. Barriers to healthcare access among refugees with disabilities and chronic health conditions resettled in the US Midwest. J Immigr Minor Health 2014;16(4):733–42.

29. Seery T, Boswell H, Lara A. Caring for refugee children. Pediatr Rev 2015;36(8): 323–38 [quiz: 339–40].

30. CDC Report. Available at: https://www.cdc.gov/lgbthealth/. Accessed February 26, 2016.

31. Gay and Lesbian Medical Association and LGBT health experts. Healthy People 2010 companion document for lesbian, gay, bisexual, and transgender (LGBT) health. Available at: http://www.glma.org/_data/n_0001/resources/live/Healthy CompanionDoc3.pdf. Accessed February 25, 2016.

32. Healthy People 2020. Available at: http://www.healthypeople.gov/2020/topics-objectives/topic/lesbian-gay-bisexual-and-transgender-health. Accessed February 25, 2016.

33. Goldenring J, Rosen D. Getting into adolescent heads: an essential update. Contemp Pediatr 2004;21(64):76–95.

34. CDC STD Treatment guidelines. 2015. Available at: http://www.cdc.gov/std/tg2015/screening-recommendations.htm. Accessed February 26, 2016.

35. Poirier JM, Francis KB, Fisher SK, et al. Practice brief 1: providing services and supports for youth who are lesbian, gay, bisexual, transgender, questioning, intersex, or two-spirit. 2008.

36. Office of Juvenile Justice and Delinquency Prevention. Youth's needs and services: findings from the survey of youth in residential placement. 2010. Available

at: https://syrp.org/images/Youth_Needs_and_Services.pdf. Accessed February 26, 2016.

37. Office of Juvenile Justice and Delinquency Prevention. 2012. Available at: http://www.ojjdp.gov/newsletter/238981/sf_2.html. Accessed February 26, 2016.

38. Golzari M, Hunt SJ, Anoshiravani A. The health status of youth in juvenile detention facilities. J Adolesc Health 2006;38(6):776–82.

39. Committee on Adolescence. Health care for youth in the juvenile justice system. Pediatrics 2011;128(6):1219–35.

40. Penn JV, Thomas C. Practice parameter for the assessment and treatment of youth in juvenile detention and correctional facilities. J Am Acad Child Adolesc Psychiatry 2005;44(10):1085–98.

41. Council on Foster Care, Adoption, Kinship Care, Committee on Adolescence, Council on Early Childhood. Health care issues for children and adolescents in foster care and kinship care. Pediatrics 2015;136(4):e1131–40.

42. The National Center on Family Homelessness. America's youngest outcasts 2014: state report card on child homelessness. Available at: www.FamilyHomelessness.org. Accessed February 26, 2016.

43. Council on Community Pediatrics. Providing care for children and adolescents facing homelessness and housing insecurity. Pediatrics 2013;131(6):1206–10.

44. English A, Scott J, Park M. Implementing the Affordable Care Act: how much will it help vulnerable adolescents and young adults? Available at: http://nahic.ucsf.edu/wp-content/uploads/2014/01/VulnerablePopulations_IB_Final.pdf. Accessed February 26, 2016.

Women's Select Health Issues in Underserved Populations

Luz M. Fernandez, MD, Jonathan A. Becker, MD*

KEYWORDS

- Breast cancer • Cervical cancer • Contraception • Health care disparities
- Underserved women

KEY POINTS

- Health care disparities exist among populations with a lack of health care resources or poorer socioeconomic status.
- Barriers to health care include transportation, distrust of the health care system, lack of access to health care, and intimate partner issues.
- There is a lack of availability of cancer screening in poorer nations.
- Creating a needs assessment and using community resources are methods used to combat health care disparities in underserved women.
- Continuity of care and use of allied health professionals improve maternal-fetal outcomes.

INTRODUCTION

Care of the medically underserved presents unique challenges to health care providers. Underserved women lack or have limited access to health care. Combatting health care disparities requires a partnership between the community, its providers, and health care advocates for developing a needs assessment so that resources are used in an effective, efficient, and economically viable manner. Women are especially vulnerable to health care disparities in both industrialized and developing nations. The basis of this is multifactorial with poor socioeconomic status, lack of appropriate cancer screening, lack of reasonable transportation, and unequal gender roles all playing a part. The focus of this article is to outline the health care disparities in underserved women and present solutions to help bridge the health care gap.

This article originally appeared in Primary Care: Clinics in Office Practice, Volume 44, Issue 1, March 2017.
The authors have nothing to disclose.
Department of Family and Geriatric Medicine, University of Louisville, Louisville, KY, USA
* Corresponding author. 201 Abraham Flexner Way, Suite 690, Louisville, KY 40202.
E-mail address: jon.becker@louisville.edu

Physician Assist Clin 4 (2019) 61–69
https://doi.org/10.1016/j.cpha.2018.08.003
2405-7991/19/© 2018 Elsevier Inc. All rights reserved.

CANCER SCREENING IN UNDERSERVED WOMEN

Cancer-related health disparities are defined by the National Cancer Institute as "adverse differences in cancer incidence cancer prevalence, cancer mortality, cancer survivorship, and burden of cancer or related health conditions that exist among specific population groups in the United States."[1] The disparity may exist due to age, disability, education, ethnicity, gender, geographic location, income, or race/ethnicity. Women who are uninsured or underinsured have higher incidence of cervical and breast cancers and a more advanced disease than the general population. In the United States, the most vulnerable groups include African Americans/blacks, Asian Americans, Hispanic/Latinos, Native Americans, Alaska Natives, and underserved whites.

CERVICAL CANCER SCREENING
Barriers to Access to Care: Transportation

Women in underserved populations are more vulnerable to cervical cancer than their counterparts due to barriers to access to care.[1,2] Few primary care clinics are situated to serve patients of lower socioeconomic status. Many of these women may not have personal vehicles for transportation, relying instead on friends and/or family or city/local buses for transportation to their clinics.[1] They may arrive late to their office visits due to late buses. Some patients may rely on transportation provided by their insurance companies, which requires calling a specific company with whom the insurance company has a contract at least 3 days in advance of an appointment to arrange transportation.[3] Arriving late to an appointment may result in a lost appointment or the necessity of rescheduling. Repeated missed appointments may result in a patient being dismissed and discharged from the practice.[1–4]

In countries of lower socioeconomic status, reliable and timely transportation may not be available. Many villages in Africa are far from industrialized areas, without dependable transportation. Women may have to travel far distances on foot through treacherous terrain to seek medical care for themselves and their children.[5]

Distrust of the Medical Providers and System

Another barrier to care includes distrust of the medical providers and the medical system in general.[6] Underserved women may have had bad experiences with the health care system and with medical providers who may not be sensitive to their individual needs. They may have experienced refusal to be seen by a medical provider due to either lack of insurance.[6,7] Some may believe that they receive treatment that was less than optimal based on their race, gender, religion, or other factors.[1,2] African American patients may recall the history of experimentation on patients of color. Modern surgical gynecology, founded by J. Marion Sims, has a gruesome foundation in its use of female slaves as his experimental subjects.[8] Still others may recall the Tuskegee Experiment[9] (US Public Health Service 1932–1972). Hispanic/Latino women residing in the United States may not seek health care services so as to not be vulnerable to inquiry about immigration status and face possible deportation.[6]

Fear of Cancer

The data show that precancerous or cancerous lesions of the cervix (and those of the breast as well) are found at more advanced stages in underserved women than in their counterparts.[2,3] The fear of diagnosis of higher-grade lesions perpetuates the avoidance of preventive health care. Many women in this population delay preventive health maintenance and seek care only when they experience symptoms. Because most cervical cancer is asymptomatic until later stages, and the symptoms may be nonspecific, there may be a remarkable delay in care. Underserved women may not understand the importance of routine health maintenance, prevention, and promotion.[2,3]

Confusion over Newer Cervical Cancer Screening Guidelines

Newer guidelines for cervical cancer screening are confusing to patients and providers (**Table 1**).[10] The most recent guidelines issued by the US Preventive Services Task Force (USPSTF) in 2012 move away from yearly Papanicolaou (Pap) smears for women who have never had an abnormal Pap smear in favor of screening with liquid-based cytology and testing for human papillomavirus (HPV), the virus implicated in most cases of cervical dysplasia and cervical cancer (especially strains HPV 16 and HPV 18). Cytology and HPV status (positive for high-risk strains vs negative) guide the screening interval. Women with an abnormal Pap smear should be screened at more frequent intervals. Some underserved women have routine Pap smears only during pregnancy or postpartum period and may not understand the need for cervical cancer screening at other intervals.[10] **Table 1** lists cervical cancer screening guidelines based on age group. These guidelines assume an average-risk woman and do not apply to those with a history of higher-grade precancerous cervical lesions or cervical cancer or who are immunocompromised.

Test Discomfort

Some women delay having a Pap smear because the test is uncomfortable. The discomfort and potential embarrassment of the examination outweigh any perceived benefit of the test.[6,7]

Lack of Availability of Papanicolaou Tests

Many developing countries do not have access to Pap smears for routine cervical cancer screening.[5] Some of these developing nations use an acetic acid solution applied to the cervix of patients to try to indirectly detect the presence of HPV; areas that turn

Table 1
Summary of US Preventive Services Task Force cervical cancer screening guidelines

Age	Screening Guideline	Screening Interval	Strength of Recommendation
<21	Not indicated	Not indicated	D
21–29	Cytology	Every 3 y	A
30–65	Cytology alone	Every 3 y	A
30–65	Cytology + HPV DNA testing	Every 5 y if HPV negative	A
>65	Not indicated	Not indicated	D
Women post-hysterectomy with removal of cervix for benign reasons	Not indicated	Not indicated	D

Adapted from Moyer V. Screening for Cervical Cancer: US Preventive Services task force recommendation statement. Ann Intern Med 2012;156:882.

acetowhite are treated as HPV lesions without cytology, HPV DNA testing, or colposcopy with biopsy of suspicious lesions.[7,11,12] Many areas in developing countries do not have physicians to perform these tests. They rely on nurses, allied health care professionals, and/or lay individuals trained in cervical cancer screening and detection and perform the acetic acid crude testing both independently and, when available, under the guidance of a remote physician or other medical provider using telemedicine.[5,11–13]

Special Considerations

Certain cultural practices can make routine female health screenings more challenging. For example, female circumcision, which results in genital mutilation. may make pelvic examinations more difficult because there may be more difficulty inserting a speculum (or it may be impossible to insert a standard speculum) and the experience may be traumatic to the patient.[14,15] The introduction of DNA testing for the detection of higher-risk strains of HPV may help increase cervical cancer screening programs in underserved areas by making DNA swabs more widely available and at a more reasonable cost. DNA swabs could be self-administered by the patients under direction of a trained health care advocate.[16]

Sexual Assault

Sexual violence against women occurs in all countries and spans all socioeconomic statuses. In many countries, sexual assault is used as a form of torture and warfare. Some women are also sold into sexual slavery.[16–18] Women who are at very high risk for cervical dysplasia may not tolerate a pelvic examination. The use of a speculum may trigger flashbacks of sexual assault. Multiple visits with use of desensitization techniques may help patients tolerate the examination over time.[18,19]

SCREENING FOR BREAST CANCER

Breast cancer remains a leading cause of cancer-related death among women worldwide.[20] The highest rates of breast cancer deaths are in areas of lower socioeconomic status with more limited resources.[20–23] These countries may not have universal breast cancer screening programs. To combat this issue, the Breast Health Global Initiative has compiled evidence-based guidelines, which take into account the economic burden of breast cancer screening and treatment.[20–22]

Screening for breast cancer has similar barriers to access for care as cervical cancer screening. Developing countries may not have access to mammography; therefore, breast cancer is generally found at later stages than in countries with a robust breast cancer screening program.[20–22] Poorer countries may use guidelines that lean more heavily on a provider's clinical breast examination and defer mammogram or diagnostic ultrasound for those with abnormal clinical breast examinations. Diagnostic ultrasound may be more available in these countries and may be the test of choice when abnormalities are detected on clinical breast examination.[20–22] DNA testing for mutations that may place women into higher-risk categories for developing breast cancer (such as BRCA mutations) may not be readily available.[21,22] As a result, early breast cancer screening as well as procedures, such as prophylactic mastectomy, prophylactic oophorectomy, and colon cancer screening, may not be available to decrease their risk of developing breast cancer, ovarian cancer, or colon cancer.[20–22]

Some developing countries have not made breast cancer screening a public health priority. This is in part because these countries have a higher incidence of infectious diseases, which take priority in terms of resource allocation. According to the World Health Organization, guidelines for breast cancer screening and treatment are not readily feasible in poor or developing countries.[20,21] **Table 2** describes methods of breast cancer screening based on resource allocation.

Recent guidelines by the USPSTF rate teaching self-breast examinations as a category D (recommend against) recommendation and clinical breast examinations as a category I recommendation (insufficient to assess the additional benefits and harms of clinical breast examination beyond screening mammography in women 40 years or older).

These guidelines are aimed at trying to detect breast cancer at earlier stages because later stages require more intensive treatments and resource allocation. Based on needs assessments, resources for breast cancer screening are allocated to areas in which overall rates are higher.[20–22]

CONTRACEPTIVE CARE IN UNDERSERVED WOMEN

Women of lower socioeconomic status may not have access to contraceptives for many reasons beyond the transportation issues and distrust of the medical system (discussed previously).

Cost

Prior to the passing of the Affordable Care Act in the United States, long-term contraception was cost-prohibitive to many underserved women of lower socioeconomic status.[24,25] Long-acting reversible contraceptive methods, such as intrauterine devices and implantable hormonal contraceptives, are expensive methods that were not affordable to those without contraceptive coverage on their insurance plans.[26] In the United States, undocumented women immigrants do not have access to insurance, including state-sponsored plans, such as Medicaid.[24,25] Clinics not requiring insurance coverage or payment may not offer long-acting reversible contraceptives or lack the necessary supply.[24,25] Methods, such as oral contraceptive pills, hormone-containing vaginal ring, hormone-containing patch, and hormone injections, may also not be readily accessible to these women.[24,25]

Differences in Contraceptive Preferences and Contraceptive Acceptance

Certain contraceptive methods are more popular in some areas than in others. For example, in Latin America and Europe, the intrauterine device is widely accepted and used.[26–28] Select contraceptive methods that provide for a monthly period (such as oral contraceptive pills, hormone pills, and hormone vaginal rings) may

Table 2 Methods for breast cancer screening based on resource allocation		
Method	**Resource Poor**	**Resource Plentiful**
Patient education	+	+
Self-breast examinations	+	+
Clinical breast examination (performed by a provider)	+/−	+
Mammography	+/−	+
Diagnostic ultrasound	+	+

Adapted from Anderson BO, Shyyan R, Eniu A, et al. Breast cancer in limited-resource countries: an overview of the Breast Health Global Initiative 2005 Guidelines. Breast J 2006;12:S9.

be preferable to some women who believe having regular menses provides reassurance that they are not pregnant.[27] Women may also prefer contraceptive methods they can use without the knowledge of their sexual partners due to social, cultural, and/or religious reasons. In some regions, women may have fear that a contraceptive device would be placed by a health care provider without their explicit informed consent. Moreover, in developing countries, there may be a precedent of experimentation on members of their population.[29–31] For example, the first clinical trials of oral contraceptive pills were performed in Puerto Rico without the explicit informed consent of women participating in the study. Likewise, several developing countries have been sites of forced sterilization. Certain groups in the United States, such as women with mental health disorders or cognitive and other impairments who were institutionalized in the past, were victims of forced sterilization.[29–31]

Perceived side effects of the various contraceptive methods are also a barrier to its use. For example, those who use the contraceptive hormone injections may experience a delay of up to 18 months after their last injection in regaining fertility and becoming pregnant.[26,27] **Table 3** describes potential side effects of contraceptives that may contribute to women's refusal of certain contraceptive methods.

INTIMATE PARTNER VIOLENCE

In the United States, intimate partner violence is prevalent in all socioeconomic groups.[17] Women experiencing physical, verbal, and/or sexual violence may experience fear and shame, which keep them from reporting the abuse to their medical providers.[17,18] Women in the United States who are of limited English proficiency may be unable to report abuses to their medical providers because interpretation of their office visits may be performed through their significant other and not a third party.[17–19] In many situations, even if a third party is present to provide medical interpretation,

Table 3 Potential side effects of contraceptive methods	
Intrauterine device, hormonal	Irregular bleeding/spotting Amenorrhea Weight gain Mood changes
Intrauterine device, copper	Increased menstrual cramping Increased menstrual flow
Hormone implant	Irregular bleeding/spotting Amenorrhea Weight gain Arm pain Mood changes
Hormone injection	Irregular bleeding/spotting Amenorrhea Weight gain Increased risk of osteopenia Delayed fertility on discontinuation Mood changes
Oral contraceptive pills	Weight gain Bloating Mood changes

the significant other may still be present for the entire medical encounter, and the patient may not feel able to recount a history of abuse. In some countries, it is socially acceptable for the male partner to use physical methods of discipline on his female partner.[17–19]

SPECIAL CONSIDERATIONS FOR MATERNAL-FETAL HEALTH

Many developing countries experience a higher rate of death during childbirth than industrialized nations, with the highest incidences in areas of Africa and Asia[32]; 90% of all maternal deaths and 80% of stillbirths are in countries that lack trained health care workers. Contributing factors to these deaths include poverty, poor overall health status, poor health literacy, lack of autonomy for medical decision making, lack of an adequately trained birth attendant, lack of an adequate referral system, inadequate transportation, and poor communication between health centers and communities.[32–34]

The programs that seem most successful in decreasing morbidity and mortality associated with pregnancy, childbirth, and the postpartum period are those that are community based.[32–34] Allied health care workers, such as midwives and volunteers, can educate women on proper care, nutrition, and vaccination (where available) during or after childbirth. Use of local, trained professionals helps increase adherence by eliminating patients' need to travel away from home for health care services.[34–36] It also helps lessen distrust in the medical providers and health care system to receive health information and care from one of their perceived peers. These workers are trained in a variety of skills that range from keeping the baby warm postdelivery and neonatal resuscitation to care of the umbilical cord stump and breastfeeding.[34–36] Studies have shown that the use of local health care advocates (described previously) helps increase breastfeeding rates for the mother and increase immunization rates in both mother and the infant.[32–34] Home visitation has also been shown to decrease antenatal hospital admissions and the rates of cesarean section births.[35–38]

In the United States, methods that have been studied to help in teenage pregnancy have included support via telephone calls, home visits, social support from friends and family, and continuity of care, such as same obstetric provider throughout the whole pregnancy, family doctor to handle prenatal care, postpartum care, and care of the infant; however, these methods have not been shown to have a statistically significant effect on infant mortality in that population.[39] Methods, such as mass media campaigns, community education, and outreach services, still lack data showing effectiveness.[39]

In industrialized, higher-income countries, the leading causes of deaths in infants are congenital anomalies, conditions related to premature birth, and sudden infant death syndrome/sudden or unexpected death in infancy.[37,38] Group antenatal visits are one intervention that may help decrease infant mortality. This is true of in both industrialized and developing countries.[38]

SUMMARY

Underserved women experience health care disparities in the United States and abroad, especially in the areas of cervical or breast cancer screening, and contraception. Additional factors relate to intimate partner violence and prenatal and postpartum care. Understanding these disparities and working with local resources within these communities are among the most promising interventions that will help health care providers and patients partner to reduce these gaps.

REFERENCES

1. Freeman HP, Wingrove BK. Excess cervical cancer mortality: a marker for low access to healthcare in poor communities. Rockville (MD): National Cancer Institute; Center to Reduce Cancer Health Disparities; 2005. NIH Pub. No. 05-5282.
2. Wharam JF, Zhang F, Xu X, et al. National trends and disparities in cervical cancer screening among commercially insured women, 2001–2010. Cancer Epidemiol Biomarkers Prev 2014;23:2366–73.
3. Health care financing administration. National Association of Medicaid Directors' Non-Emergency Transportation Technical Advisory Group. (1998, August). Designing and operating cost effective medicaid non-emergency transportation programs: a guidebook for state medicaid agencies. Available at: http://ntl.bts. gov/lib/12000/12200/12290/medicaid.pdf. Accesed July 17, 2015.
4. Hicks ML, Yap OW, Matthews R, et al. Disparities in cervical cancer screening, treatment and outcomes. Ethn Dis 2006;16:S3.
5. Haar EK, Vonder KK, Schust DJ. Adapting cervical dysplasia screening, treatment and prevention approaches to low resource settings. Int STD Res Rev 2013;1:38–48.
6. Johnson CE, Mues KE, Mayne SL, et al. Cervical cancer screening among immigrants and ethnic minorities:a systematic review using the health belief model. J Low Genit Tract Dis 2008;12:232–41.
7. Goldie SJ, Gaffikin L, Goldhaber-Fiebert J, et al. Cost-effectiveness of cervical-cancer screening in five developing countries. N Engl J Med 2005;353:2158–68.
8. Axelsen DE. Women as victims of medical experimentation: J. Marion Sims' surgery on slave women, 1845-1850. Sage 1985;2:10–3.
9. Green BL, Maisiak R, Wang MQ, et al. Participation in health education, health promotion, and health research by African Americans: effects of the Tuskegee Syphilis Experiment. J Health Educ 1997;28:196–201.
10. Moyer V. Screening for cervical cancer: US preventive services task force recommendation statement. Ann Intern Med 2012;156:880–91.
11. Murillo R, Almonte M, Pereira A, et al. Cervical cancer screening programs in Latin America and the Caribbean. Vaccine 2008;26(Suppl 11):L37–48.
12. Ditzian LR, David-West G, Maza M, et al. Cervical cancer screening in low-and middle-income countries. Mt Sinai J Med 2011;78:319–26.
13. Roger E, Nwosu O. Diagnosing cervical dysplasia using visual inspection of the cervix with acetic acid in a woman in rural Haiti. Int J Environ Res Public Health 2014;11:12304–11.
14. De Silva S. Obstetric sequelae of female circumcision. Eur J Obstet Gynecol Reprod Biol 1989;32:233–40.
15. Toubia N. Female circumcision as a public health issue. N Engl J Med 1994;331: 712–6.
16. Dzuba IG, Díaz EY, Allen B, et al. The acceptability of self-collected samples for HPV testing vs. the pap test as alternatives in cervical cancer screening. J Womens Health Gend Based Med 2002;11:265–75.
17. Gandhi S, Rovi S, Vega M, et al. Intimate partner violence and cancer screening among urban minority women. J Am Board Fam Pract 2010;23:343–53.
18. Elliott L, Nerney M, Jones T, et al. Barriers to screening for domestic violence. J Gen Intern Med 2002;17:112–6.
19. McFarlane J, Malecha A, Watson K, et al. Intimate partner sexual assault against women: Frequency, health consequences, and treatment outcomes. Obstet Gynecol 2005;105:99–108.

20. Anderson BO, Shyyan R, Eniu A, et al. Breast cancer in limited-resource countries: an overview of the Breast Health Global Initiative 2005 Guidelines. Breast J 2006;12(Suppl 1):S3–15.
21. Anderson BO, Jakesz R. Breast cancer issues in developing countries: an overview of the Breast Health Global Initiative. World J Surg 2008;32:2578–85.
22. Coughlin SS, Ekwueme DU. Breast cancer as a global health concern. Cancer Epidemiol 2009;33:315–8.
23. Bray F, McCarron P, Parkin DM. The changing global patterns of female breast cancer incidence and mortality. Breast Cancer Res 2004;6:229–39.
24. Peipert JF, Madden T, Allsworth JE, et al. Preventing unintended pregnancies by providing no-cost contraception. Obstet Gynecol 2012;120:1291–7.
25. Burlone S, Edelman AB, Caughey AB, et al. Extending contraceptive coverage under the Affordable Care Act saves public funds. Contraception 2013;87:143–8.
26. Feyisetan B, Casterline JB. Fertility preferences and contraceptive change in developing countries. Int Fam Plan Perspect 2000;26:100–9.
27. Garcia SG, Snow R, Aitken I. Preferences for contraceptive attributes: voices of women in Ciudad Juárez, México. Int Fam Plan Perspect 1997;23:52–8.
28. Narzary PK, Sharma SM. Daughter preference and contraceptive-use in matrilineal tribal societies in Meghalaya, India. J Health Popul Nutr 2013;31:278–89.
29. Bruinius H. Better for all the world: the secret history of forced sterilization and America's quest for racial purity. New York: Vintage Books; 2007.
30. Briggs L. Discourses of forced sterilization in Puerto Rico: the problem with the speaking subaltern. Differences 1998;10:30–3.
31. Hyatt S. A shared history of shame: Sweden's four-decade policy of forced sterilization and the eugenics movement in the United States. Indiana Int Comp Law Rev 1998;8:475–503.
32. Hollowell J, Oakley L, Kurinczuk JJ, et al. The effectiveness of antenatal care programmes to reduce infant mortality and preterm birth in socially disadvantaged and vulnerable women in high-income countries: a systematic review. BMC Pregnancy Childbirth 2011;11:13.
33. Lassi ZS, Das JK, Salam RA, et al. Evidence from community level inputs to improve quality of care for maternal and newborn health: interventions and findings. Reprod Health 2014;11:S2.
34. Osrin D, Prost A. Perinatal interventions and survival in resource-poor settings: which work, which don't, which have the jury out? Arch Dis Child 2010;95:1039–46.
35. Kurinczuk JJ, Hollowell J, Brocklehurst P, et al. Inequalities in infant mortality project briefing paper 1. Infant Mortality: overview and context. Oxford (United Kingdom): National Perinatal Epidemiology Unit; 2009.
36. Callaghan WM, MacDorman MF, Rasmussen SA, et al. The contribution of preterm birth to infant mortality rates in the United States. Pediatrics 2006;118:1566–73.
37. Rosano A, Botto LD, Botting B, et al. Infant mortality and congenital anomalies from 1950 to 1994: an international perspective. J Epidemiol Community Health 2000;54:660–6.
38. Ickovics JR, Kershaw TS, Westdahl C, et al. Group prenatal care and preterm birth weight: results from a matched cohort study at public clinics. Obstet Gynecol 2003;102:1051–7.
39. Little M, Gorman A, Dzendoletas D, et al. Caring for the most vulnerable: a collaborative approach to supporting pregnant homeless youth. Nurs Womens Health 2007;11:458–66.

Medical Care of the Homeless
An American and International Issue

Sheryl B. Fleisch, MD[a], Robertson Nash, PhD, ACNP, BC[b],*

KEYWORDS

- Homelessness • Environment • Smoking • Diabetes mellitus • HIV • Dental
- Sexually transmitted infections • Cardiac disease

KEY POINTS

- Homeless persons die significantly younger than their housed counterparts.
- In many cases, relatively straightforward primary care issues (obesity, hypertension, diabetes mellitus, sexually transmitted infections, urinary tract infections, upper and lower respiratory infections, chronic obstructive pulmonary disease, depression, and poor dental hygiene) escalate into life-threatening, expensive emergencies.
- Poor health outcomes driven by negative interactions between comorbid symptoms meet the definition of a health syndemic in this population.
- Successful primary care of patients struggling with homelessness may result in long-term lifesaving measures along with decreased expenditure to hospital systems.
- This primary prevention requires patience, creativity, and acknowledgment that the source of many confounders may lay outside the control of these patients.

INTRODUCTION

Homeless persons die significantly younger than their housed counterparts.[1] In many cases, relatively straightforward primary care issues (obesity, hypertension, diabetes mellitus, sexually transmitted infections, urinary tract infections, upper and lower respiratory infections, chronic obstructive pulmonary disease [COPD], depression, and poor dental hygiene) escalate into life-threatening, expensive emergencies. The goal of this article is to provide the interested reader with insights gained from serving

This article originally appeared in Primary Care: Clinics in Office Practice, Volume 44, Issue 1, March 2017.

Disclosure: The authors of this work report no direct financial interest in the subject matter or any material discussed in this article.

[a] Vanderbilt University School of Medicine, 2215 Garland Avenue, Light Hall, Nashville, TN 37232, USA; [b] Vanderbilt Comprehensive Care Clinic, Vanderbilt Health at One Hundred Oaks, 719 Thompson Lane, Suite 37189, Nashville, TN 37204, USA

* Corresponding author.

E-mail address: Robertson.nash@vanderbilt.edu

https://doi.org/10.1016/j.cpha.2018.08.004
2405-7991/19/© 2018 Elsevier Inc. All rights reserved.

physicianassistant.theclinics.com

homeless patients, on the street and in shelters. The focus is to highlight factors that exacerbate diseases and complicate care. The authors also hope to provide readers with clinically proven methods to improve the lives of homeless patients.

ENVIRONMENT AS A HEALTH CHALLENGE
Pearl

The outside environment, where homeless people spend most of their time, is a risk factor and driver of poor health outcomes.

For individuals struggling with homelessness, the outside environment is where they will spend most of their time. The outdoors is where they work, sleep, socialize, and live out the functions of daily life. No matter whether hot, cold, raining, or snowing, they must learn how to survive in the environment that surrounds them. It is often this environment that becomes a risk factor and driver of poor outcomes because of exposure-related injuries.

Approximately 700 individuals experiencing homelessness or at risk of homelessness will die from hypothermia yearly in the United States.[2] Signs and symptoms of hypothermia include exhaustion, numbness, cold sensation, shivering, pale, or flushed skin, decreased hand coordination, slurred speech, and confusion.[3] Hypothermia can occur before extreme cold, especially when clothes are wet.

Frostbite, like hypothermia, is a medical emergency. Superficial frostbite often presents with tingling and numbness, whereas deep frostbite that has been present for a long time can present dark and gangrenous. Affected areas could require amputation and need to be checked for infection. It is critical that cities prepare for cold weather, including provision of emergency shelter beds. This includes admission of all homeless persons to shelters no matter their sobriety status or whether they have previously been banned.[4]

Just as cold weather poses significant risks, hot weather does as well. High humidity makes thermoregulation difficult because it is more challenging for sweat to evaporate. Heat cramps, heat exhaustion, and heat stroke are all potential risks, with heat stroke being the most serious. The person will often present with inability to sweat and become hot and dry. He or she may experience chest pain, shortness of breath, headache, abdominal pain, and confusion. This person will require cooling via any means necessary.[5]

Given that homeless persons frequently stay outdoors or within shelters, exposure to insect bites or parasitic infestations is 3 times higher than in the general population.[6] Homeless persons staying in shelters are at particular risk for exposure to scabies, lice, and bedbugs. Lice and scabies are highly contagious and can spread in the confines of close quarters. Spiders, mosquitoes, ticks, fleas, and ants may affect persons staying outdoors, so provision of repellant and proper tenting is important. It is critical to do a thorough history on exposure to insects, particularly those that are communicable, to provide the best medical care to homeless persons.[5]

In addition to weather-related hazards, there are challenges by virtue of simply living on the streets, including being the victim of physical and sexual crimes. From 1999 to 2013, the National Coalition for the Homeless documented 1437 acts of violence against homeless persons, including 375 acts that resulted in death. These acts of violence occurred in 47 states, Puerto Rico, and Washington, DC. Perpetrators were generally male, under 30 years old, and commonly teenagers. It is thought that these numbers are an underrepresentation of hate crimes against homeless persons. Additionally, in a racially diverse sample of homeless mothers, 92% reported experiencing severe physical and/or sexual violence at some point in their lives, with 43% reporting sexual abuse in childhood and 63% reporting intimate partner violence in adulthood.[7]

OCULAR CARE
Pearl

Decreased visual acuity, combined with lack of access to eyeglasses, increases the risk of trauma and sexual assaults in this population based on affected individual's impaired ability to safely avoid or navigate potentially dangerous situations.

Poor visual acuity is known to be correlated with reduced earning potential and reduced well-being.[8] In a study of 960 homeless adults, 41% reported an unmet need for eyeglasses,[9] with need for eyeglasses in homeless children ranging from 13% to 26%.[10] Studies done in both the United States[11] and Canada[12] show increased risk of ocular morbidity in homeless samples. Despite having access to universal health care, only 14% of homeless Canadian study participants reported visiting an ocular specialist in the last year versus 41% of the general population. Eighty-nine percent of participants stated that if ocular services were brought to them, they would use such services.[13]

The most common eye conditions in persons who are homeless are the same as those in the general population, including macular degeneration, cataracts, diabetic eye disease, glaucoma, dry eyes, and low vision. However, persons who are homeless and struggle with low visual acuity are at increased risk of traumatic injuries due to inability to see an intruder at a campsite or an oncoming vehicle. Poor eyesight can lead to inability to negotiate food and shelter, safe sexual practices, and employment. All of these can lead to further homelessness, criminalization, and victimization.

PULMONARY DISEASES
Pearl

Although smoking is recognized as a significant health threat, focusing on smoking cessation in marginalized populations may erode the therapeutic relationship that providers seek to build with their homeless patients.

According to data published by the Centers for Disease Control and Prevention (CDC), an estimated 900,000 Americans die prematurely every year from 5 causes of death: heart disease, cancer, stroke, lung disease, and unintentional injury. Smoking is implicated as a modifiable risk factor in 4 of these 5 preventable causes of death.[14] Although the overall prevalence of smoking in the United States is estimated at around 20%, the prevalence of smoking among those living below the federal poverty level in 2009 was around 31%.[15] Studies investigating the prevalence of smoking among homeless populations have documented prevalence rates as high as 80%.[16] In 1 study, investigators found rates of obstructive lung disease as high as 15% (95% CI 8%–26%) in a population of urban homeless.[17] A cluster analysis of 2733 homeless veterans found that 1 of 4 unique disease clusters was marked by elevated rates of cardiopulmonary disease, including COPD.[18]

These data beg the question of why smoking, an admittedly expensive habit, is so prevalent among the poorest members of the society. In 1 qualitative study regarding attitudes toward smoking in California family homeless shelters, participants reported that smokers associated relief from stress and boredom and higher levels of social inclusion with cigarette smoking.[19] Given the highly unpredictable and stressful environment of homelessness, it may not be unreasonable to view smoking as having more short-term benefit than long-term cost. Although smoking cessation education is considered a bedrock principle of primary care, in this population, advocacy of smoking cessation without appreciation for the larger content of homeless people's lives may actually erode versus enhance the therapeutic relationships on which all care rests.

Asthma is another pulmonary disease frequently encountered among homeless persons. In 1 small study (N = 67), 24% indicated a previous diagnosis of asthma, with 40% reporting wheezing and 20% affirming dyspnea on exertion.[17] In comparison, the American Lung Association reports asthma prevalence rates in US community-dwelling adults between 6.4 and 12%.[20] Extended exposure to both cold and heat, walking for hours at a time, and elevated levels of stress may all lead to asthma exacerbation.[21] In the authors' experience, the prohibitive cost of multidose albuterol inhalers increases the likelihood of adverse outcomes in this population, and drives the costs of unreimbursed care for asthma and COPD exacerbations. The bulk of portable nebulizers and lack of ready access to electricity make that modality of care impractical in this population. One easily implemented technique that might minimize aerosolized transmission would be arranging beds so that shelter residents slept head to toe versus head to head.[4]

CARDIAC DISEASE
Pearl

Obesity is the leading cause of death in both homeless and nonhomeless persons. Awareness of cardiac risk factors and barriers to obtaining treatment is critical in providing successful preventive management of obesity and hypertension in this vulnerable population.

Every year, approximately 600,000 people will die of heart disease in the United States. It is the leading cause of death for both men and women.[22] Middle-aged homeless men are more likely to die of heart disease than age-matched nonhomeless men, and heart disease is the leading cause of death in older homeless men.[23] Homeless persons have similar cardiac risk factors to the general population, such as smoking, hypertension, and obesity, but they have less ability to combat risk factors. For instance, diet often consists of high fat and cholesterol foods due to affordability and availability. In a study based in Toronto, Canada, 202 homeless adults were assessed for cardiac risk factors. In this study, 78% smoked, 35% had hypertension (with only 33% aware they had hypertension), and 46% were obese (body mass index >25). Approximately 30% of persons used both alcohol and cocaine.[24] This highlights the incredible need for preventive cardiology services for individuals who are homeless.

However, persons who are homeless will often delay seeking care, undergo fewer procedures, decline medications, and obtain less follow-up care. Reasons include lack of transportation, poor understanding of the seriousness of the condition, lack of finances, and often distrust of the medical system.[25] There seems to be an inverse relationship between socioeconomic status and 1-year mortality rate in individuals with cardiac disease.[26] In the authors' opinions, barriers to treating cardiac disease in homeless persons can only be overcome through some of the following mechanisms: mobile vans and clinics (addressing transportation and trust issues), meticulous patient education (addressing the poor understanding of health issues), education to hospital systems about the rates of cardiac disease in homeless persons and the systemic effect it has on hospital admissions (addressing 1 side of the financial barriers), and creative discharge planning that includes a combination of patience, appropriate follow-up care, and medications at bedside (addressing financial and trust issues).

DENTAL CARE
Pearl

Poor dentition can have a negative impact on nutrition, physical health, and on self-efficacy and mental health. There are far too few dental care resources available for homeless people.

Malnutrition, poor dental hygiene, tobacco use, and facial trauma are frequent causes of disfigured, decayed, and missing teeth. Access to dental care is generally difficult due transportation challenges and affordability of procedures. In the General Accounting Office Report to Congress, it was reported that more than half of homeless persons reported not seeking dental care in the preceding 2 years and one-third did not seek dental care in their lifetime.[27] In a Boston shelter, 90% of homeless persons had untreated dental caries.[28] Poor oral hygiene is 10 times higher in homeless children than an age-matched population.[29]

In persons who are homeless, lack of oral hygiene can result in multiple dental caries and periodontal disease that can lead to infection and loss of teeth. Medical conditions that are more common in homeless persons, such as diabetes, human immunodeficiency virus (HIV), or acquired immunodeficiency syndrome (AIDS), can exacerbate oral disease and make healing more difficult. Persons with poor dentition struggle with poor self-esteem and self-worth, which can lead to substance use, depression, and further homelessness.[5]

Even when persons who are homeless would like to receive dental treatment, barriers to receipt of care can be mindboggling. Generally, initial appointments are cost prohibitive. Often, even free clinics will charge for more expensive procedures and, given the level of dental care required by most homeless persons, it is rare that procedures are free of charge. The most successful strategies in treating oral hygiene in homeless persons include mobile dental clinics, community organization affiliation with a dental school, and volunteer dental nights.[30] Most persons who are homeless will not seek out dental care[23] and providers must inquire, encourage, and assist in provision with these important services.

DIABETES MELLITUS
Pearl

Many shelters rely on food donations to serve their participants. Be aware that the nutritional value of donated food is often low, and that careful planning and procurement of food is needed to address the needs of diabetic homeless people.

The CDC estimates that, in 2011, an estimated 25.8 million people, 8.3% of the US population, had a diagnosis of diabetes. An additional 35% of adults older than 20 years of age were diagnosable with prediabetes, defined as a fasting hemoglobin A1C level between 5.7 and 6.4.[31] Data regarding the prevalence of diabetes in homeless populations is sparse; 1 study of homeless citizens of New York City (N = 177) found that 35% of that sample were diabetic.[32]

Challenges to the successful management of diabetes abound in homeless populations. For example, homeless people are often unable to safely store insulin and insulin syringes. Optimal management of insulin in shelters requires access to refrigeration as well as accurate labeling of insulin type and patient name, both of which may wear off of manufacturer labels. A closely related issue is access to glucometers and glucometer strips. Given the array of glucometer manufacturers and models, it would not be possible for any health care system to stock test strips to fit any glucometer. Maintaining a calibrated and regularly tested glucometer and supply of test strips at a shelter may be beyond the scope of services offered by a shelter.

Remember that asking a person to fulfill what may seem to be a simple, straightforward task such as checking and tracking their blood sugar may not be possible in the chaos of homelessness.

Poor management of diabetes among homeless populations can have unexpected, life-threatening, consequences. For example, impaired cognitive and motor function secondary to hypoglycemia may prove fatal for urban homeless people because they spend significant amounts of time navigating traffic-filled roadways. Additionally, the physical manifestations of hypoglycemia may mimic intoxication. People exhibiting dizziness, altered mental status, and nausea may be assumed to be inebriated and left to their own devices. Shelters serving intoxicated homeless people should have ready access to a glucometer to ensure that episodes of hypoglycemia are not overlooked.

Obesity and diabetes are of particular concern in homeless populations because of the extended amount of time homeless people spend walking and their lack of access to properly fitting footwear. Diabetic neuropathy increases the likelihood of tissue damage caused by ill-fitting footwear and this is exacerbated by obesity. Resulting problems, from nonhealing ulcers to Charcot disease, present sometimes unmanageable obstacles for the homeless.

DERMATOLOGIC CONCERNS

Unmanaged chronic diseases cause many of the dermatologic challenges faced by homeless people. Lack of access to bathing facilities and to clean socks leads to higher rates of tinea pedis compared with the general population. One study done in a homeless shelter in Boston, MA, found that 38% of participants had tinea pedis.[33] Maceration of tissue may lead to intradigital fissuring, which may, in turn, lead to bacterial superinfection of open wounds.

Access to clean socks is essential for homeless people. One of the authors of this article started a foot washing clinic at a homeless shelter. Once a week, people signed up for foot washing, nail and callous trimming, and clinical evaluation of comorbidities noted during foot washing. Participants with tinea pedis were given an antifungal cream donated by a local pharmaceutical nonprofit, and all participants received 3 pairs of new socks. This intervention required a minimum level of clinical staffing (1 nurse practitioner); trained volunteers did all of the foot washing and trimming or filing services.

Clothing challenges are not confined to footwear. Ill-fitting, restricting, unwashed clothing anywhere on the body increases the likelihood of cellulitis secondary to abrasion. Cellulitis and tinea in intra-abdominal skin folds are not uncommon in obese homeless people,[33] for whom access to daily bathing facilities is unavailable.

In many cases, interventions to minimize dermatologic disease are within the scope of shelters. The key is recognizing that common shelter practices may need to be adapted to meet new demands. For example, shelters that do not allow daytime occupancy are foregoing an opportunity to provide respite from the damaging effects of chronic sun exposure. Provision for foot washing in shelter settings may be possible, even when showering facilities are not available. Access to washers and dryers in shelters might also be useful interventions.

GENITOURINARY INFECTIONS
Pearl

Homeless people may not always be in a position to advocate that their sexual partners use condoms. The presence of STDs may be a marker for abuse and/or depression.

The prevalence of nonsexually transmitted genital-urinary diseases (eg, candida, vaginitis) in homeless people is unknown. It would not be unreasonable for these rates to be elevated relative to the general population, based solely on a relative lack of access to bathing and clothes washing facilities. In addition to programs that stock socks for homeless people, the authors' experiences have led to advocating for making cotton underwear available at all shelters. Cotton fabrics breathe much better than synthetics, thus minimizing the buildup of excess moisture in the genital region, thereby discouraging the growth of candida.

A thorough review of the diagnosis and treatment of sexually transmitted diseases (STDs) is well beyond the scope of this article. Interested readers are referred to the CDC's *2015 Sexually Transmitted Diseases Treatment Guidelines*, available at no cost online. That being said, there are several unique features of homelessness that exacerbate the risk of the transmission and acquisition of STDs. Awareness of these issues can help shelter administrators and staff design and deliver more effective support for safe sex.

In the authors' experiences working with homeless populations in the Southeastern United States, a basic issue for homeless people is lack of access to condoms. This leads to a higher prevalence of unprotected sex among homeless people.[34] Human beings are sexual creatures and the lack of access to condoms does not imply celibacy in homeless shelters. Rather, this lack of access implies higher rates of unprotected sex, leading to higher rates of STDs.

In the authors' opinions, another issued affecting the elevated rate of STDs in homeless populations is that of transactional sex. Anyone who has spent time with homeless persons, both men and women, is aware that sex is used as a commodity in this population to barter for food, shelter, and to achieve companionship.[35] The issue is not that people are sexually active. The issue is that transactional sex is, by definition, based on a marked asymmetry of power between 2 individuals. One of the many problematic aspects of this asymmetrical relationship is that the more powerful person may be able to ignore the less powerful person's request that a condom be used with intercourse. In addition to the obvious increase in the likelihood of transmission of STDs, this behavior only serves to amplify the powerless person's sense of shame, helplessness, and social marginalization.[36]

Shelters are not designed to provide environments for sexual activity but they can serve a powerful role by clearly advocating for an atmosphere of mutual respect among all shelter users. Shelters should strongly consider embracing a culture of inclusion and respect among all shelter users and staff. Bright, visible posters should be used to communicate intolerance for race, gender, or any other discrimination.

SUMMARY

Homelessness is a national and international problem, and the medical problems that persons who are homeless face are serious and unrelenting. Homelessness leads to poor health and poor health leads to homelessness. Common conditions, such as high blood pressure, diabetes, asthma and even a small laceration, can become life-threatening because of inability to obtain medications, unhealthy diet, or lack of access to a clean environment. Successful providers must always be cognizant of the role of structural violence in the lives of their homeless patients. This means that patients experiencing homelessness may find themselves unable to transition into housing and health, despite working 1 or more minimum wage jobs. This, in turn, serves to erode faith in the very institutions from which practitioners strive to offer care. Serving these patients requires time, patience, and a willingness to engage around nontraditional issues in clinical care, including asking about living conditions, medication access and affordability, and transportation. Other keys to care, in the authors' experiences, include a willingness to work with patients on goals that they prioritize as important. It is also helpful to set goals with homeless patients and to empower them toward greater self-efficacy at every encounter. Provision of medical care for homeless persons may require coordination with medical outreach teams, shelters, and free clinics.

REFERENCES

1. Henwood BF, Byrne T, Scriber B. Examining mortality among formerly homeless adults enrolled in Housing First: an observational study. BMC Public Health 2015;15:1209.
2. Sturgis R, Sirgany A, Stoops M, et al. Bringing our neighbors in from the cold. A report from the National Coalition for the Homeless. 2010. Available at: http://www.nationalhomeless.org/publications/winter_weather/report.html. Accessed Feburary 27, 2016.
3. CDC. Hypothermia-related deaths - United States, 1999-2002 and 2005. MMWR Morb Mortal Wkly Rep 2006;55(10):282-4.
4. O'Connell J. The health care of homeless persons: a manual of communicable diseases & common problems in shelters & on the streets. Boston: Boston Health Care for the Homeless Program; 2004.
5. Coalition NHftH. Exposure-related conditions: symptoms and prevention strategies. Nashville (TN): HCH Clinicians' Network; 2007. Available at: https://www.nhchc.org/wp-content/uploads/2012/01/Dec2007HealingHands.pdf.
6. Wright J. Health care for homeless people: evidence from the National Health Care for the Homeless Program. New York: WW Norton & Co; 1990.
7. Bassuk EL, Melnick S, Browne A. Responding to the needs of low-income and homeless women who are survivors of family violence. J Am Med Womens Assoc 1998;53(2):57-64.
8. Tielsch JM, Sommer A, Katz J, et al. Socioeconomic status and visual impairment among urban Americans. Arch Ophthalmol 1991;109(5):637-41.
9. Baggett TP, O'Connell JJ, Singer DE, et al. The unmet health care needs of homeless adults: a national study. Am J Public Health 2010;100(7):1326-33.
10. Berti LC, Zylbert S, Cable G. Comparison of health status of children utilizing a school-based health center for comprehensive care. Pediatr Res 2000;47(4):175A.
11. Ho J, Chang R, Wheeler N, et al. Ophthalmic disorders among the homeless and nonhomeless in Los Angeles. J Am Optom Assoc 1997;68(9):567-73.
12. Nia J, Wong D, Motamedinia D. The visual acuity and social issues of the homeless population in Toronto. Univ Toronto Med J 2003;80(2):84-6.
13. Noel CW, Fung H, Srivastava R, et al. Visual impairment and unmet eye care needs among homeless adults in a Canadian city. JAMA Ophthalmol 2015;133(4):455-60.
14. CDC. Leading causes of death. 2015. Available at: http://www.cdc.gov/nchs/fastats/leading-causes-of-death.htm.
15. CDC. Vital Signs: current cigarette smoking among adults aged greater than or equal to 18 years, United States 2009. MMWR Morb Mortal Wkly Rep 2010;60(35):1207-12. Available at: http://www.cdc.gov/MMWR/preview/mmwrhtml/mm6035a5.htm. Accessed February 3, 2016.

16. Tsai J, Rosenheck RA. Smoking among chronically homeless adults: prevalence and correlates. Psychiatr Serv 2012;63(6):569–76.
17. Snyder LD, Eisner MD. Obstructive lung disease among the urban homeless. Chest 2004;125(5):1719–25.
18. Goldstein G, Luther JF, Jacoby AM, et al. A taxonomy of medical comorbidity for veterans who are homeless. J Health Care Poor Underserved 2008;19(3): 991–1005.
19. Stewart HC, Stevenson TN, Bruce JS, et al. Attitudes toward smoking cessation among sheltered homeless parents. J Community Health 2015;40(6):1140–8.
20. Association AL. Asthma in adults fact sheet. 2016. Available at: http://www.lung. org/lung-health-and-diseases/lung-disease-lookup/asthma/learn-about-asthma/ asthma-adults-facts-sheet.html?referrer=https://www.google.com/.
21. Badiaga S, Richet H, Azas P, et al. Contribution of a shelter-based survey for screening respiratory diseases in the homeless. Eur J Public Health 2009; 19(2):157–60.
22. CDC. Heart disease fact sheet. 2015. Available at: http://www.cdc.gov/dhdsp/ data_statistics/fact_sheets/fs_heart_disease.htm.
23. Hwang SW, Orav EJ, Oconnell JJ, et al. Causes of death in homeless adults in Boston. Ann Intern Med 1997;126(8):625–8.
24. Lee TC, Hanlon JG, Ben-David J, et al. Risk factors for cardiovascular disease in homeless adults. Circulation 2005;111(20):2629–35.
25. Flaskerud JH, Strehlow AJ. A culture of homelessness? Issues Ment Health Nurs 2008;29(10):1151–4.
26. Alter DA, Naylor CD, Austin P, et al. Effects of socioeconomic status on access to invasive cardiac procedures and on mortality after acute myocardial infarction. N Engl J Med 1999;341(18):1359–67.
27. GAO. Oral health: dental disease is a chronic problem among low-income populations. April, 2000. (HEHS-00–72). Available at: http://www.gao.gov/new. items/he00072.pdf.
28. Kaste LM, Bolden AJ. Dental-caries in homeless adults in Boston. J Public Health Dent 1995;55(1):34–6.
29. Wright J. Children in and out of the streets. Am J Dis Child 1991;145:516–9.
30. Hale A, Allen J, Caughlan J, et al. Healing Hands: filling the gaps in dental care, vol. 3. Nashville (TN): NHC Clinicians' Network; 2003.
31. CDC. National Diabetes Fact Sheet, 2011. 2011. Available at: http://www.cdc. gov/diabetes/pubs/pdf/ndfs_2011.pdf.
32. Asgary R, Sckell B, Alcabes A, et al. Rates and predictors of uncontrolled hypertension among hypertensive homeless adults using New York City shelter-based clinics. Ann Fam Med 2016;14(1):41–6.
33. Stratigos AJ, Stern R, Gonzalez E, et al. Prevalence of skin disease in a cohort of shelter-based homeless men. J Am Acad Dermatol 1999;41(2):197–202.
34. Tucker JS, Wenzel SL, Golinelli D, et al. Understanding heterosexual condom use among homeless men. Aids Behav 2013;17(5):1637–44.
35. Towe VL, Sifakis F, Gindi RM, et al. Prevalence of HIV infection and sexual risk behaviors among individuals having heterosexual sex in low income neighborhoods in Baltimore, MD: The BESURE Study. J Acquire Immune Defic Syndr 2010;53(4):522–8.
36. Dunkle KL, Wingood GM, Camp CM, et al. Economically motivated relationships and transactional sex among unmarried African American and white women: results from a US national telephone survey. Public Health Rep 2010;125:90–100.

Occupational Health and Sleep Issues in Underserved Populations

Medhat Kalliny, MD, PhD[a],*, Judith Green McKenzie, MD, MPH[b]

KEYWORDS

- Sleep disorders • Sleep health disparities • Burden of occupational injury and illness
- Occupational hazards, injuries and illnesses in underserved worker populations
- Workers' compensation

KEY POINTS

- In the United States, substantial racial, ethnic, and socioeconomic disparities exist in sleep health.
- Poor sleep is associated with a wide range of health effects, and therefore, it is important that primary care physicians working in underserved communities are aware of this disparity and target this higher-risk group for focused evaluation and intervention.
- The workplace, home, and social environment, as well as diet and genetics among other factors, work together to affect an individual's health status.
- Workplace hazards impact one's overall health status, which in turn impact one's ability to obtain, perform, and tolerate work, as well as gain satisfaction from work.
- Primary care physicians should be familiar not only with the type of work an individual does but also with workplace hazards and their effects on individual's health and how to address them.

SLEEP DISORDERS: AN IMPORTANT PUBLIC HEALTH PROBLEM
Historical Background

Sleep and dreams have been a mystery and topics of writings by philosophers, writers, religious leaders, and scientists since the inception of the recorded history.[1] The Greeks and Romans personified sleep through their deities: Hypnos and Somus, respectively.[2] Hippocrates was likely the first writer in the ancient world to mention the

This article originally appeared in Primary Care: Clinics in Office Practice, Volume 44, Issue 1, March 2017.

The authors have no conflicts of interest to disclose.

[a] Department of Family and Community Medicine, Meharry Medical College, 1005 Dr D. B. Todd Boulevard, Nashville, TN 37208, USA; [b] Division of Occupational Medicine, Department of Emergency Medicine, Hospital of the University of Pennsylvania, First Floor, Silverstein Pavilion, Philadelphia, PA 19104-4283, USA

* Corresponding author.

E-mail address: mkalliny@mmc.edu

importance of sleep in general health.[3] In 350 BC, the Greek philosopher, Aristotle, wrote about sleep and waking, whether they are a function of the body or the soul, and the significance of dreams.[4] Interestingly, in 360 BC, historical documents described obstructive sleep apnea (OSA), for the first time: Dionysius, the tyrant of Heraclea, died "chocking on his own fat."[5] Similar writings about sleep and health are found in Egyptian, Indian, and Chinese ancient civilizations and early modern era.[6,7]

In 1836, Dickens wrote about OSA in his work the *Posthumous Papers of the Pickwick Club*, wherein he described "Joe the Fat Boy" as obese and sleepy and a snorer.[8] Thereafter, in 1956, Burwell and colleagues[9] described OSA as Pickwickian syndrome. Electroencephalography changes during sleep and rapid eye movement (REM) were described for the first time by Loomis and colleagues[10] and Aserinsky and Kleitman,[11] respectively. In 1957, Dement and Kleitman[12] identified the stages of sleep. In 1971, Konopa and Benzer[13] discovered the first circadian clock gene in Drosophila. Later in 1972, the suprachiasmatic nucleus (SCN) was discovered as the site of the body's internal circadian pacemaker.[14] Clinicians, scientists, and researchers continue to work toward a greater understanding of the cause and pathophysiology of sleep disorders. Sleep Medicine is developing into an interdisciplinary field in which integration and coordination across the traditional medical specialties, other health care providers such as dentists, and between basic and clinical science are vital.[15]

Scope of the Problem

About 50 to 70 million Americans chronically suffer from a sleep disorder. Sleep-disordered breathing (SDB), including OSA, affects more than 15% of the population and causes excessive daytime sleepiness, injuries, hypertension, cognitive impairment, metabolic syndrome, and an increased risk of heart attack, stroke, and mortality. In children, SDB is associated with cardiovascular and metabolic risk factors, attention-related behavioral problems, and poor academic performance.[16]

Nationwide, 70% of adults report insufficient sleep at least once each month and 11% report such difficulties daily.[17] Nearly 70% of high school adolescents sleep less than the recommended 8 to 9 hours of sleep on school nights.[18] Short and long sleep duration are associated with up to a 2-fold increased risk of obesity, diabetes, hypertension, cardiovascular disease, stroke, depression, substance abuse, and all-cause mortality.[19]

Chronic insomnia is the most common sleep disorder and affects more than 20% of adults. It is a risk factor for depression, substance abuse, and impaired function.[20]

Chronic circadian disorders, including shift work syndrome, affect 20% of the US workforce and is associated with significant safety hazard, increased risk of cardiovascular disease, cerebrovascular disease, breast cancer, colorectal cancer, prostate cancer, obesity, diabetes, gastrointestinal disease, motor vehicle crashes, and difficulty adhering to work schedules.[21,22]

Restless legs syndrome affects 5% of adults and causes sleep onset and maintenance insomnia and subsequent daytime sleepiness.

Another less common disorder is narcolepsy with and without cataplexy affecting 0.05% and 3.9% of population, respectively.

In addition to its deleterious health consequences, the cumulative long-term effects of sleep disorders have a significant economic impact. Billions of dollars a year are spent on direct medical costs associated with doctor visits, hospital services, prescriptions, and over-the-counter medications.[17]

Sleep Health in Underserved Population

In the United States, substantial racial, ethnic, and socioeconomic disparities exist in sleep health. Many studies found that those with longer work hours and lower socioeconomic status report less sleep duration and/or lower sleep quality.[23–25] In a survey of 15,227 Hispanics of low socioeconomic status, Cespedes and his colleagues[26] reported that 28% had insomnia, 19% were short sleepers, and 9% were long sleepers. Grandner and colleagues[27] assessed sleep complaints with a telephone survey of 159,856 participants from across the United States and found that unemployment, being unmarried, lower income, and lower educational attainment were associated with more sleep complaints. Similar findings were reported by other researchers.[28,29]

Because poor sleep is associated with all of the untoward health effects noted above, it is important that primary care physicians (PCPs) working in underserved communities are aware of this disparity and target this higher-risk group for focused evaluation and intervention.

SLEEP PHYSIOLOGY. A *BRIEF* PRIMER FOR THE PRIMARY CARE PHYSICIAN
Sleep-Wake Cycle and Circadian Rhythm

Sleep-wake cycle, which consists of roughly 8 hours of nocturnal sleep and 16 hours of daytime wakefulness, is controlled by 2 internal influences: sleep homeostasis and circadian rhythm. The period of circadian rhythms is about 24 hours in a normal light-dark cycle and is synchronized to the external physical environment and social/work schedules. In humans, light is the strongest synchronizing agent. Sleep-wake cycle is controlled by the suprachiasmatic nucleus (SCN) of the hypothalamus. In addition to providing synchronization in time between various rhythms, the SCN also helps promote wakefulness.[30–35]

It is generally agreed that sleep quality and restfulness are best when the sleep schedule is regularly synchronized to the internal circadian rhythms and the external light-dark cycle and that individuals should go to bed and wake up at around the same time each day.[36–38] Sleep loss results in the accumulation of a sleep debt that must eventually be repaid—by napping or sleeping longer in later cycles. Even the loss of 1 hour of sleep time that accumulates for several days can have a powerful negative effect on daytime performance, concentration, and mood.[39,40] One study recently quoted in the *Economist* states that sleeping 4 hours per night "has the same impact on the performance of various cognitive tasks as a blood-alcohol level of 0.1%, well over the limit for driving a car."[41]

Sleep Architecture

Sleep architecture refers to the basic structural organization of normal sleep. Cycles of non–rapid eye movement (NREM) sleep and rapid eye movement (REM) sleep are recognized by using electroencephalographic recordings. NREM sleep is divided into stages N1, N2, and N3 representing a continuum of relative depth. Each has unique characteristics, including variations in brain wave patterns, eye movements, and muscle tone.[42] The function of alternations between these 2 types of sleep is not yet understood, but irregular cycling and absent sleep stages are associated with sleep disorders. For example, instead of entering sleep through NREM, as is typical, individuals with narcolepsy enter sleep directly into REM sleep.[43]

The individual usually enters sleep through N1 within 10 to 20 minutes after lights out, progressing through stage N2, followed by stage N3, and finally, to REM. However, individuals do not remain in REM sleep the remainder of the night but, rather, cycle between stages of NREM and REM throughout the night every 90 minutes. NREM sleep constitutes about 75% to 80% of total sleep time, and REM sleep constitutes the remaining 20% to 25%.[44]

Stage N1 sleep serves a transitional role in sleep-stage cycling and constitutes 2% to 5% of total sleep. Stage N2 sleep lasts approximately 10 to 25 minutes in the initial cycle and lengthens with each successive cycle, eventually constituting between 45% and 55% of the total sleep time. Stage N3 is referred to as a slow-wave sleep (SWS), most of which occurs during the first third of the night and constitutes about 15% to 20% of sleep. N3 sleep is important for feeling well rested. It is important in restorative functions, lowering inflammatory cytokines, maintaining hormone balance, and, together with REM, in restorative memory processing.

REM sleep is defined by the presence of desynchronized (low-voltage, mixed-frequency) brain wave activity, muscle atonia, and bursts of REMs. During the initial cycle, the REM period may last only 1 to 5 minutes; however, it becomes progressively prolonged as the sleep episode progresses. The last REM period may last from 30 to 60 minutes. About 4 to 5 REM-NREM cycles occur during night sleep. As the night progresses, stage N3 sleep gets progressively less and the final sleep period is composed mainly of stage N2 and REM sleep. Dreaming is associated with REM sleep with approximately 80% of vivid dream recall resulting after arousal from this stage of sleep. REM sleep may also be important for memory consolidation.[43–48]

Sleep Variants with Age

Neither full-term nor premature neonates show clear circadian rhythm. Newborns usually sleep about 16 to 18 hours per day. Circadian rhythm begins to arise around 2 to 3 months of age, leading to sleep consolidation that manifests in greater durations of wakefulness during the day and longer periods of sleep at night. In young children, sleep amounts decrease as a child gets older. Most children discontinue napping between 3 and 5 years old. Older children are significantly more likely to experience challenges in initiating and maintaining sleep and having nightmares than younger children.[49–56]

Adolescents require 9 to 10 hours of sleep each night. More than a quarter of high school and college students were found to be sleep deprived. Slow-wave sleep (N3) progressively declines with advancing pubertal development; however, time spent in stage N2 increases. These changes are likely in part due to pubertal and hormonal changes that accompany the onset of puberty. With increasing age, the total sleep time and REM sleep decrease, leading to the emergence of normal sleep pattern in adults.[57–59]

Sleep architecture continues to change with age across adulthood. As they age, individuals tend to have earlier wake time. Older adults greater than the age of 65 typically awaken 1.33 hours earlier, and go to bed 1.07 hours earlier, than younger adults, which might be due to an advanced circadian pacemaker that accompanies age. Younger adults may experience brief awakenings, but they are usually minor and occur close to REM sleep transition; thus, sleep remains relatively consolidated. As an individual ages, slow-wave sleep (SWS) declines at a rate of about 2% per decade. Because arousal thresholds are typically highest during SWS, and because SWS declines with age, older adults experience more frequent awakenings during a sleep episode.[60–62]

Elderly show an increase in disturbed sleep that can create a negative impact on their quality of life, mood, and alertness. Although the ability to sleep becomes more difficult, the need to sleep does not decrease with age. Elderly usually suffer both sleep onset and maintenance insomnia, both of which are associated with depression, respiratory symptoms, and physical disability. The progressive decrease in SWS is one of the most prominent changes with aging; however, it appears to preferentially affect men. The reason for the gender difference is unclear.[63–66] Other prominent factors affecting sleep in the elderly (that are beyond the scope of this text) are a decrease in melatonin levels, changes in sleep latency, nighttime awakenings, inconsistency of external cues such as light exposure, irregular mealtimes, nocturia, and decreased mobility leading to a reduction in exercise.[60–66]

THE IMPACT OF SELECTED SLEEP DISORDERS—WITH SPECIFIC FOCUS ON THE UNDERSERVED
Sleep Deprivation

Sleep deprivation is defined as sleeping less than the recommended 7 to 9 hours of sleep per night. The causes of sleep deprivation are multifactorial. All 4 common sleep disorders mentioned above as well as occupational and lifestyle changes can lead to sleep deprivation.[67] The National Health and Nutrition Examination Survey showed that about 37.1% of US adults report regularly sleeping less than 7 hours per night. Short sleep duration was more common among young adults (aged 20–39 years) and non-Hispanic blacks.[68] Patients with sleep deprivation experience difficulty in concentration, impaired ability to perform daily tasks, lower mental and physical well-being, worsening of chronic diseases, and increased morbidity and mortality.[69,70] Similar findings were reported by other studies.[71,72]

In a cross-sectional survey of 9714 randomly selected subjects, effect of socioeconomic factors on sleep quality was assessed. Sleep quality was strongly associated with poverty level, employment status, and education level.[73] It is postulated that perceived discrimination is a potential cause of sleep disturbance and its resulting heath consequences. In their analysis of data of 7148 adults from Michigan and Wisconsin, Grandner and colleagues[74] found that perceived racial discrimination was associated with increased risks of sleep disturbance (odds ratio [OR] = 2.62, $P<.0001$) and daytime fatigue (OR = 2.07, $P<.0001$). Similarly, in a study of 168 Hispanic-American immigrants, perceived racism was related to increased sleep disturbance and higher levels of depressive symptoms.[75]

Sleep deprivation is associated with wide-ranging effects on the cardiovascular, endocrine, immune, and nervous systems, including obesity, diabetes, impaired glucose tolerance, cardiovascular disease, hypertension, depression, anxiety, fatigue, lack of concentration, increased inflammatory markers, and impairment of functional capacity.[76–82]

Sleep deprivation is also common among adolescents.[83] In a study of 242 healthy adolescents, Troxel and associates[84] found that adolescents from single-parent households had poorer sleep efficiency across the week and shorter sleep duration on weekends. Black adolescents from single-parent households were found to have the lowest weekend sleep efficiency. Inadequate sleep among adolescents has negative consequences for self-regulation and emotional well-being as well as poor school performance, behavioral problems, obesity, insulin resistance, and hypertension.[85,86]

Sleep-Disordered Breathing

OSA is the most common type of sleep-disordered breathing (SDB). It is characterized by loud snoring, breathing interruptions, awakenings, gasping, and choking and usually results in excessive daytime sleepiness.[87–90] OSA is common in adults, with men, older individuals, and the obese being at higher risk. The prevalence of OSA ranges between 2% and 7% with higher prevalence among non-Hispanic blacks.[91–93] In the Sleep Heart Health Study, black men and women had significantly higher Epworth Sleepiness Scores reflecting greater daytime sleepiness.[94] Snoring is the most common reported symptom of OSA; however, awareness of the predominant symptom of

OSA and knowledge of its clinical significance appear to be the lowest among minorities and those with low socioeconomic status and education.[28,95–100]

Epidemiologic and clinical studies suggest that between 35% and 91% of patients with hypertension have OSA.[101,102] A strong racial disparity exists in the prevalence and treatment of hypertension and its relationship to OSA.[103] Jean-Louis and colleagues[101] reported that hypertensive blacks have a 91% prevalence of SDB. A causal association between OSA and hypertension is supported by evidence of a dose-response relationship; the higher the apnea-hypopnea index, the greater the increase in blood pressure. Treatment of OSA by continuous positive airway pressure (CPAP) therapy can reduce blood pressure levels.[104–108] Similarly, OSA is associated with increased risk of other cardiovascular diseases, including arrhythmias, coronary artery disease, myocardial infarction, and congestive heart failure.[109–113] Those with severe OSA have 3-fold higher risk of fatal cardiovascular events. CPAP therapy reduces cardiovascular risk and mortality in patients with OSA.[112,114–118]

OSA is associated with impaired glucose tolerance and insulin resistance especially in those with the highest apnea-hypopnea index. It has been suggested that OSA causes intermittent hypoxia and recurrent sleep arousals, which in turn stimulate the sympathetic nervous system, hypothalamic-pituitary-adrenal axis, and adipocytes with release of catecholamines, cortisol, and inflammatory cytokines and other vasoactive intermediates, which may mediate the development of glucose intolerance, insulin resistance, and, ultimately, type 2 diabetes.[119–121] Babu and colleagues[122] reported that CPAP improved glycemic control in diabetic patients with OSA.

Up to 40% of people who are morbidly obese have OSA. Obesity is a well-established risk factor for the development of OSA and could be a consequence of OSA.[123] OSA-associated obesity might be due to decreased physical activity secondary to excessive daytime sleepiness and/or higher levels of nonfunctional leptin.[124] Significant weight loss usually results in reduction of OSA severity.[125]

Insomnia

Insomnia is the most commonly reported sleep disorder. Insomnia could be sleep-onset insomnia; difficulty to initiate sleep or sleep maintenance insomnia; or difficulty to maintain sleep. Insomnia could result in daytime consequences, such as tiredness, lack of energy, difficulty concentrating, and/or irritability.[126,127] Insomnia affects between 15% and 20% of adults in the United States. However, prevalence increase was noted recently among young adults, elderly, women, whites, Hispanics, diabetics, and patients with joint pain.[128,129] Family history of insomnia, low socioeconomic status, stressful lifestyles, medical and psychiatric disorders, and shift work are other risk factors for insomnia.[130–134]

Daily experiences of discrimination, workplace harassment and incivilities, and other stressors are significant factors for poor sleep quality and insomnia.[135,136] In a study of 1289 pregnant Latinas, Manber and colleagues[137] found that depression, lack of social support, and low income were significant risk factors for insomnia; however, strong family ties, group identity, and English proficiency were protective factors.

Insomnia is conceptualized as a state of hyperarousal. The exact causes of insomnia are poorly understood. Biological, psychological, and social factors might play a role in insomnia pathogenesis. Adults with insomnia have higher levels of cortisol and adrenocorticotropic hormone, reduced cortisol awakening response, and flattened diurnal cortisol profile. Studies suggest that insomnia might be due to overactivity of multiple neural systems, particularly brainstem, hypothalamus, and basal forebrain. In addition, limbic and paralimbic structures that regulate basic emotions and instinctual behaviors, such as the amygdala, hippocampus, ventromedial prefrontal cortex, and anterior cingulate cortex, have been shown to be abnormally active during sleep in individuals with insomnia.[138–141]

Pain is another major risk factor for insomnia. Bazargan and colleagues[142] found that patients with a level of pain of 5 or higher (on a scale of 0–10) showed a higher level of insomnia. Cognitive factors, such as worry, rumination, and fear of sleeplessness, light exposure, non–regular sleep schedule, and exposure to trauma, increase the odds of insomnia.[105,143] Chronic insomnia is associated with increased risk of cardiovascular diseases, such as acute myocardial infarction, hypertension, arrhythmias, cerebrovascular diseases, diabetes, psychiatric disorders, and all-cause mortality.[144–147]

Circadian Rhythm Disorders

Circadian rhythm sleep disorders are persistent or recurrent patterns of sleep disturbance due to misalignment of the circadian clock in relation to environmental cues and the terrestrial light-dark cycle. They usually cause insomnia, excessive sleepiness, or both and are associated with impairment of social, occupational, or other functions. Delayed sleep phase and advanced sleep phase disorders are the most common circadian rhythm disorders.[148]

Delayed sleep phase syndrome is characterized by sleep onset and wake times that are typically delayed 3 to 6 hours relative to conventional sleep-wake times. On the other hand, advanced sleep phase syndrome is characterized by involuntary bedtimes and awake times that are more than 3 hours earlier than societal means. In both conditions, the amount of sleep is not affected.[149] Circadian rhythm disorders are more prevalent in adolescents and young adults.[150,151] Biological, physiologic, and genetic factors play an important role in pathogenesis of circadian rhythm disorders. Nightshift workers are at higher risk for delayed sleep phase syndrome due to irregular circadian entrainment. Similarly, individuals who live in extreme latitudes and are exposed to extended periods of light may also be at increased risk.[152–156] Polymorphisms in circadian clock genes have been identified in familial delayed and advanced sleep phase syndromes.[157–159] Delayed and advanced sleep phase syndromes impair an individual's job performance and are associated with marital problems and financial difficulty. In adolescents, they are associated with increased daytime irritability, poor school performance, and psychiatric disorders.[150]

Treatment of delayed sleep phase syndrome requires resynchronizing to a more appropriate phase to the 24-hour light-dark cycle. In addition to a structured sleep-wake schedule and good sleep hygiene practices, potential therapies include resetting the circadian pacemaker with bright light, melatonin, or a combination of both.[160] Treatment options for individuals with advanced sleep phase syndrome are limited. Bright light therapy in the evening has been used successfully.[161] It is also hypothesized that administration of low levels of melatonin in the early morning may also be used.[162]

Restless Leg Syndrome

Restless leg syndrome (RLS) is one of the most common movement disorders with a prevalence of 5%. It is more common in older adults and women; however, it may be found in adolescents and teenagers. It is characterized by an irresistible urge to move the legs, which worsens during rest or inactivity, especially in the evening and at night, causing most individuals difficulty falling asleep. It also may affect the arms, trunk, or head and neck. It may also be associated with paresthesias, which individuals describe as creepy-crawly, jittery, itchy, or burning feelings. The symptoms are partially or completely relieved by movement. Individuals with RLS often experience periodic limb movements; however, periodic limb movement disorder is not always associated RLS.[163–167]

RLS affects more than 20% of pregnant women secondary to transient low levels of ferritin and folate; therefore, they typically disappear within 4 weeks after delivery.[168] It may also be associated with attention-deficit hyperactivity disorder (ADHD). Chervin and colleagues[169] reported that ADHD symptoms were almost twice as likely to occur with symptoms of RLS as would be expected by chance alone.

The exact cause of RLS is not completely understood. It likely results from altered dopamine and iron metabolism. RLS commonly occurs in individuals with iron deficiency, including end-stage renal disease, iron-deficiency anemia, pregnancy, and bariatric surgery. Iron is necessary for the synthesis of dopamine and the activity of the D_2 dopamine receptor. In patients with RLS, reduced iron levels were noted in the substantia nigra, which is responsible for controlling voluntary movement through neurons that rely on dopamine as a neurotransmitter. The association between dopamine, iron deficiency, and RLS is further supported by observations that dopamine antagonists cause worsening of RLS symptoms, while dopamine agonists are used to treat RLS. There is strong evidence for genetic predisposition, in which susceptibility gene loci have been identified on chromosomes 12q, 14q, and 9p; however, no genetic markers are currently available.

There is early evidence that RLS is more common in underserved communities, with one recent survey noting RLS symptoms greater than 3 times per week in more than 10% of rural poor respondents.[170] Higher rates have also been seen in older patients, women, those with lower socioeconomic status, those with lower education, and those unemployed, retired, or disabled, and non-Hispanic whites.[170,171] Dopaminergic agents are the primary treatment option for individuals with RLS.[169–184]

In conclusion, the PCP working in underserved areas should be aware of the common sleep disturbances discussed above, their untoward health effects, and their increased incidence among underserved populations. Treatment approaches can be complex and often require multidisciplinary interventions, but the potential rewards in patient well-being, societal benefit, and physician satisfaction make addressing such issues paramount.

OCCUPATIONAL HEALTH IN UNDERSERVED POPULATIONS
Occupational Health Services for Underserved Populations

Historical context

Occupational health and safety is the field pertaining to the health and safety of the workforce and lies at the interface between work and health.[185] Workplace hazards impact one's health status, which in turn impacts one's ability obtain, perform, and tolerate work as well as gain satisfaction from work. Not only is it important for the PCP to know the type of work an individual does but also to be familiar with the workplace and its hazards, whether physical, chemical, biologic, mechanical, or psychosocial, will assist the astute PCP to render optimal care to their working patients. The workplace, home, and social environment, as well as diet and genetics among other factors, work together to affect an individual's health status.[186]

The PCP might overlook work-related causes of injury and illness if an index of suspicion does not exist.[187] The focus may be placed on fitting the presenting signs and symptoms into a nonoccupational cause when the diagnosis may be right at hand if occupation is queried. As such, all patients who present to their PCP should be queried as to their occupation.[188] This simple question is imperative, because many workers may not seek care from an occupational and environmental medicine

(OEM) physician for a work-related injury or illness for several reasons. They may not realize that their injury or illness is work related; they may not have access to an OEM physician; they may not know how to report a work related event, or they may fear reprisal.[189] As many as 25% of visits to PCPs are for work-related conditions.[190] It is in understanding a patient's work that, through educating the patient on preventive measures, future similar injuries may be prevented.[191] Indeed, approximately one-quarter of physicians have no work history recorded in their chart.[192]

Workers' compensation

Workers' compensation insurance covers workers whose injuries or illnesses arise out of work. The oldest form of social insurance in the United States and the third largest source of support for disabled workers after Social Security and Medicare, the Workers' compensation system started during the early part of the twentieth century for the purpose of providing monetary compensation for medical and rehabilitation costs and lost wages to certain workers with work-related injuries or disabilities. The Workers' compensation system can be credited for helping to create a more humane environment for covered workers. Workers' compensation statutes are based on the legal principle of "exclusive remedy" whereby an injured employee can only claim compensation within the system. Workers in effect have given up the right to sue the employer at common law. In return, the injured employee receives total reimbursement for the medical costs incurred as well as full or partial wage replacement during the period during which the employee was unable to work. The United States does not have a unified Workers' compensation law because each state, federal jurisdiction, and territory have individual systems, statutes, and regulations. As such, the PCP may need to be familiar with the law in the area in which they practice.[193]

Some categories of workers are excluded from Workers' compensation protection. This includes workers employed by companies with 5 or fewer employees, agricultural workers, domestic (household) workers, casual laborers, independent contractors, the self-employed, business owners and partners, and state, municipal, and nonprofit institution employees. In addition, Workers' compensation insurance is not compulsory for most private employment in some states.

Health status of underserved workers

Underserved workers have various vulnerabilities. They may not fall under the protection of Workers' compensation[193] and may also have no private medical insurance.[194–196] In the event they are insured under Workers' compensation, they may be unaware of their eligibility of the Workers' compensation laws or they may be in the country illegally and as such may not want to come forward for fear of deportation, even if the injury or illness is work related.[197] The PCP may also be unaware of their patient's eligibility.[198]

In general, underserved workers have an unequal increased burden of chronic disease.[199–202] Chronic disease, if unrecognized and untreated, may delay recovery from a work-related injury[203] or even render a worker more prone to occupational injury or illness.

Often in the Workers' compensation arena, the occupational medicine physician may be the only physician the worker sees for an extended period of time. Given that workers must often work in a job for a minimum period of time before medical insurance is available to them, there may be a financial barrier to timely referral to primary care. On the other hand, a worker may present to the PCP for treatment of an injury that is not recognized as work related. The PCP may focus on the newly diagnosed chronic disease, such as hypertension and diabetes, without taking steps toward educating the worker on how to prevent such an injury or illness form recurring or getting worse.

Burden of occupational injury and illness

The magnitude of occupational disease and injury burden is underestimated but significant.[204] In 2014, private industries in the United States reported nearly 3.0 million nonfatal workplace injuries and illnesses—a rate of 3.2 cases per 100 equivalent full-time workers.[205] The public sector reported 5.7 cases among full-time state and local workers, such as police and firefighters, with almost half the injuries being sprains and strains. The 5 industries reporting the greatest workplace risk are the health care and social assistance sector (8.3/100 workers); transportation and warehousing (5.2/100 workers); arts, entertainment, and recreation (4.8/100 workers); agriculture, forestry, fishing, and hunting (4.8/100 workers); and manufacturing (4.4/100 workers).[206]

Regulations and Regulatory Bodies

The Occupational Safety and Health Administration

The Occupational Safety and Health Act of 1970 (OSH Act) signed into law in 1970 led to the establishment of the Occupational Safety and Health Administration (OSHA) and the National Institute of Occupational Safety and Health (NIOSH). The OSH Act contains the "General Duty Clause," which places a duty on the employer to provide a safe workplace and was created to cover all possible hazards, not just those that could be foreseen at the time. In general, the working environment has become "safer" since OSHA was created; there has been a reduction in workplace injuries and fatalities.[207] However, injury and illness do remain and are undercounted in underserved workers, who routinely work the more hazardous trades and who may not report or seek treatment due to fear of reprisal.[189]

OSHA is the agency of the Department of Labor that enforces the regulatory mandates of the OSH Act by setting standards, rules, and regulations by which covered employers are expected to conduct business. Its purpose is to prevent work-related injuries, illnesses, and occupational fatalities by issuing and enforcing standards for workplace safety and health. However, OSHA has limited resources such that it is unable to inspect every workplace that needs inspection. Priority is given to more dangerous situations or otherwise targeted inspections.[208]

NIOSH, a part of the Centers for Disease Control and Prevention, is the primary federal agency conducting research on the safety and health of the workplace and providing recommendations for the prevention of work-related illnesses and injuries. The National Occupational Research Agenda (NORA) is the research framework for NIOSH and the nation. Based on critical issues in workplace safety and health identified by stakeholders, goals and objectives are developed to address work-related injuries and diseases.[209] NORA places an explicit emphasis on worker populations that have been underserved, such as immigrant workers, health care workers, and hotel workers, among others.[210]

Selected Underserved Worker Populations: Hazards, Injuries, and Illnesses

Health care workers

Health care workers (HCWs) are within the sector with the highest rate of occupational injury (health care and social assistance sector), yet 11% are underserved in they have no health insurance.[211,212] The uninsured HCW is more likely to be young, unmarried, African American or Hispanic, to have lower income, and to work part time, and is less likely to have a college degree. Within this group, home health aides have the highest rate of uninsurance at 23.8%; licensed practical nurses are next at 14.5%, and then registered nurses at 5%. Nursing home workers were more likely to be uninsured than hospital-based workers with a rate of 20% compared with 8.2%.[213]

Despite being among the least insured in this sector, workers at nursing and residential care facilities experience the highest rate of workplace injuries and illnesses, with 8.3 incidents per 100 employees, whereas hospital-based health care workers saw an incidence rate of 7.0 per 100 employees. Ambulatory health care services and social assistance were more in line with the cross-industry average, with incidence rates of 2.8 and 3.5 per 100 employees, respectively.[206]

Injuries in this industry are mostly due to heavy lifting when handling patients[214] and exposure to blood-borne pathogens.[215] Home HCWs (home health aides, personal/home care aides, companions, nursing assistants, or home health nurses), among the least insured and most underserved in this sector, provide hands-on long-term care and personal assistance to clients with disabilities or other chronic conditions in patients' homes and in community-based services such as group homes. They have little control over their work environment, where in addition to encountering hazards, such as blood-borne pathogens, other biological hazards, and ergonomic hazards, may also encounter violence, latex, hostile animals, animal waste, tripping hazards, hazards on the road as they drive from home to home, overexertion, stress, guns and other weapons, illegal drugs, verbal abuse, temperature extremes, unhygienic conditions, lack of water, and otherwise dangerous conditions.[214]

With lack of insurance come delays in seeking care, fewer prevention visits, and poorer health status.[211] As such, if these underserved workers present, the PCP may be able to use this as an opportunity to try to address other issues such as chronic disease[216] and psychological strain,[217] if present. Even with insurance, these HCWs may be less likely to file a Workers' compensation claim.[189] The astute PCP will query appropriately regarding the work relatedness of the injury or illness, thus optimizing the visit and not only treating the injury or illness but also counseling on prevention of further similar work-related injury or illness. The Bureau of Labor Statistics (BLS) projects home health care employment as the fastest growing occupation for this decade.[218] The PCP, being aware of their working conditions, will be better able to serve them.

Hotel workers

The hotel employee is another demographic that is underinsured. Many room attendants are immigrant or minority women, with most being Asian, Latin American, or African American.[219] Migrant and many immigrant workers are not covered by labor legislation and fear losing their jobs and hence livelihood.[189] Immigrants comprise 39.7% of maids and housekeeping cleaners[220] and are less likely to report an injury or illness that occur and also less likely to file a Workers' compensation claim.[206]

Despite this, hotel workers have higher rates of occupational injury and sustain more severe injuries than those in the service sector as a whole[221] with an overall injury rate in housekeepers at ~5.2 injuries per 100 worker-years. The highest rate was found for Hispanic housekeepers (10.6/100) with acute trauma rates highest in kitchen workers (4.0/100). Independently associated risk factors for injury in these workers are older age, female gender, and being Hispanic. In general, Hispanic workers have the highest rate of fatal and nonfatal OSHA-reported injuries in the United States, followed by black non-Hispanic workers.

The workload of hotel housekeepers that results in high injury and illness rates surpassing the national average involves physical hazards such as constant repositioning, changing body postures, including bending, kneeling, lifting, stooping, squatting, twisting, and pushing[221] during room cleaning work, which is physically strenuous. They are also exposed to chemical hazards, such as cleaning products, and biological hazards, such as blood and waste.[222] They are also at risk for psychological distress as they experience conflicts within the workplace.[223] In addition, they often work isolated with little interaction with other housekeepers while on the job,[224] which can contribute to psychosocial stress.

The astute PCP will give optimal care within this context with an eye to prevention, in terms of both chronic disease and work-related injury and illness prevention as well as psychosocial support. The worker may not attribute their symptoms to work for fear of reprisal, in the case of immigration issues, the fear of deportation, for example, and this may affect the amount of information the worker shares with the PCP.[225–227]

International Occupational Health

Burden of occupational injury and illness worldwide
Exposure to occupational hazards results in a significant proportion of the burden of disease and injury worldwide.[228] Much could be prevented using prevention strategies.[229] According to the International Labor Organization (ILO), 6300 people die every day as a result of occupational accidents or work-related diseases: more than 2.3 million deaths per year. There are 317 million accidents on the job annually. Many of these incidents lead to extended absences from work. There is a vast human cost of this daily adversity. Indeed, the economic burden of poor occupational safety and health (OSH) practices is estimated at 4% of global gross domestic product each year.[230] Employers face issues such as costly early retirement, absenteeism, loss of skilled staff, and high insurance premiums, due to work-related accidents and diseases. According to data from the World Health Organization, occupational risk factors are responsible for 8.8% of the global burden of mortality due to unintentional injuries. This is thought to be an underestimate due to underreporting. These global data are inadequate as they do not include intentional injury at work or commuting injury. Known prevention strategies implemented widely would diminish the avoidable burden of injuries in the workplace.[231]

Regulation and enforcement
In 2003, the ILO adopted a Global strategy to improve occupational safety and health (OSH), which included the introduction of a preventive safety and health culture, the promotion and development of relevant instruments, and technical assistance. The ILO Constitution set forth the principle that workers should be protected from sickness, disease, and injury arising from their employment. ILO standards on OSH provide essential tools for governments, employers, and workers to establish such practices and to provide for maximum safety at work because many of these tragedies can be prevented through implementing sound prevention, reporting, and inspection practices. ILO Codes of Practice provide practical guidelines for public authorities, employers, workers, enterprises, and specialized OSH protection bodies. These instruments are not legally binding and are not intended to replace the laws, regulations, or standards in various countries. They provide guidance on safety and health at work.[232] More recently, ILO devised a Plan of Action toward a significant reduction in the unacceptable human suffering and economic losses that are still caused by work-related accidents and illnesses worldwide. ILO affirms the right to "decent, safe and healthy working conditions and environment."[233]

An example of parallel legislation to protect workers in 3 systems are the OSH Act in the United States,[234] legislation in Canada through the Canadian Centre for

Occupational Health and Safety (CCOHS, 2015[235] and the Health and Safety at Work Act of Britain[236]). Other countries may base their legislation on these. The OSH Act passed with the goal to "to assure so far as possible every working man and woman in the Nation safe and healthful working conditions" places the responsibility for eliminating or minimizing hazardous conditions on the employer.[234] The CCOHS stipulates that an employer is to "exercise due diligence to implement a plan to identify possible workplace hazards and carry out corrective action to prevent accidents or injuries arising from these hazards,"[235] whereas The Health and Safety at Work Act of Britain[236] stipulates that "employers are to ensure as far as reasonably practicable, the health, safety and welfare at work of all his employees."

SUMMARY

As employers, governments, and national and international organizations work toward improving the health and safety of all workers, the road toward improved worker health will continue to be made clearer. There are inequities in that some workers are afforded care, whereas others are afforded suboptimal care or no care at all. Poverty and marginalized status in societies play a role. Indeed, in the United States, health insurance and Workers' compensation insurance are usually tethered to full-time employment so this safety net is only available to covered lives. Even so, workers with a real or perceived barrier to seeking care for a related injury or illness, covered or not, will not receive this benefit. Prevention is the optimal way to improve worker health and safety. As the science improves and occupational health and safety becomes more mainstream, PCPs will be increasingly equipped to help workers and worker populations attain high-quality, longer lives free of preventable disease, disability, injury, and premature death.[237]

REFERENCES

1. Deak M, Epstein LJ. History of polysomnography. Sleep Med Clin 2009;4(3): 313–21.
2. Dement WC. History of sleep medicine. Sleep Med Clin 2008;3(2):147–56.
3. Adams CD. The Genuine Works of Hippocrates. 1868. Available at: https://archive.org/stream/genuineworksofhi01hippuoft/genuineworksofhi01hippuoft_djvu.txt. Accessed May 25, 2016.
4. Aristotle. On Sleep and Sleepiness. 350 B.C. Available at: http://classics.mit.edu/Aristotle/sleep.html. Accessed May 25, 2016.
5. Kryger MH. Sleep apnea. From the needles of Dionysius to continuous positive airway pressure. Arch Intern Med 1983;143(12):2301–3.
6. Barbara O'Neill. Sleep and the sleeping in ancient Egypt. 2012. Available at: http://www.egyptological.com/2012/04/sleep-and-the-sleeping-in-ancientegypt-8146. Accessed May 25, 2016.
7. Shakespeare W. "Prince of Denmark." The complete works of William Shakespeare. London: Collins; 1960. p. 1141. Act II, Scene ii.
8. Dickens C. The Posthumous Papers of the Pickwick Club. 1836. Available at: http://charlesdickenspage.com/pickwick.html. Accessed May 25, 2016.
9. Burwell CD, Robin ED, Whaley RD, et al. Extreme obesity associated with alveolar hypoventilation: a Pickwickian syndrome. Am J Med 1956;2:811–8.
10. Loomis AL, Harvey EN, Hobart GA. Cerebral states during sleep as studied by human brain potentials. J Exp Psychol 1937;21:127–44.
11. Aserinsky E, Kleitman N. Regularly occurring periods of eye motility, and concomitant phenomena, during sleep. Science 1953;118(3062):273–4.

12. Dement W, Kleitman N. Cyclic variations in EEG during sleep and their relation to eye movements, body motility, and dreaming. Electroencephalogr Clin Neurophysiol 1957;9(4):673–90.

13. Konopka RJ, Benzer S. Clock mutants of drosophila melanogaster. Proc Natl Acad Sci U S A 1971;68:2112–6.

14. Moore RY, Eichler VB. Loss of a circadian adrenal corticosterone rhythm following suprachiasmatic lesions in the rat. Brain Res 1972;42(1):201–6.

15. Shepard JJW, Buysse DJ, Chesson JAL, et al. History of the development of sleep medicine in the United States. J Clin Sleep Med 2005;1(1):61–82.

16. NHLBI (National Heart, Lung, and Blood Institute). National sleep disorders research plan, 2011. Bethesda (MD): National Institutes of Health; 2011.

17. Centers for Disease Control and Prevention (CDC). Perceived insufficient rest or sleep among adults—United States, 2008. MMWR Morb Mortal Wkly Rep 2009; 58:1179.

18. Centers for Disease Control and Prevention (CDC). Youth risk behavior surveillance—United States, 2009. MMWR Morb Mortal Wkly Rep 2010;59:1.

19. National Sleep Foundation. Sleep in America Poll. 2008. Washington, DC. Available at: http://www.sleepfoundation.org/article/sleep-america-polls/2008-sleep-performanceand-the-workplace. Accessed May 25, 2016.

20. Roth T, Ancoli-Israel S. Daytime consequences and correlates of insomnia in the United States: results of the 1991 National Sleep Foundation survey. II. Sleep 1999;22(suppl 2):S354–8.

21. Healthy people 2020. Department of Health and Human Services; 2010. Office of Disease Prevention and Health Promotion Publication No. B0132.

22. Klauer SG, Dingus TA, Neale VL, et al. The impact of driver inattention on near-crash/crash risk: an analysis using the 100-car naturalistic driving study data. Washington, DC: National Highway Traffic Safety Administration; 2006. p. 1–192. HS810594.

23. Gellis LA, Lichstein KL, Scarinci IC, et al. Socioeconomic status and insomnia. J Abnorm Psychol 2005;114(1):111–8.

24. Moore PJ, Adler NE, Williams DR, et al. Socioeconomic status and health: the role of sleep. Psychosom Med 2002;64(2):337–44.

25. Krueger PM, Friedman EM. Sleep duration in the United States: a cross-sectional population-based study. Am J Epidemiol 2009;169(9):1052–63.

26. Cespedes EM, Dudley KA, Sotres-Alvarez D, et al. Joint associations of insomnia and sleep duration with prevalent diabetes: the Hispanic Community Health Study/Study of Latinos (HCHS/SOL). J Diabetes 2016;8(3):387–97.

27. Grandner MA, Patel NP, Gehrman PR, et al. Who gets the best sleep? Ethnic and socioeconomic factors related to sleep complaints. Sleep Med 2010;11:470–8.

28. Chen X, Wang R, Zee P, et al. Racial/ethnic differences in sleep disturbances: the Multi-Ethnic Study of Atherosclerosis (MESA). Sleep 2015;38(6):877–88.

29. Hale L, Troxel WM, Kravitz HM, et al. Acculturation and sleep among a multi-ethnic sample of women: the Study of Women's Health across the Nation (SWAN). Sleep 2014;37(2):309–17.

30. Ancoli-Israel S, Ayalon L, Salzman C. Sleep in the elderly: normal variations and common sleep disorders. Harv Rev Psychiatry 2008;16:279–86.

31. Clayton J, Kyriacou C, Reppert S. Keeping time with the human genome. Nature 2001;409:829–31.

32. Shanahan T, Czeisler C. Physiological effects of light on the human circadian pacemaker. Semin Perinatol 2000;24:299–320.

33. Mistlberger R, Skene D. Social influences on mammalian circadian rhythms: animal and human studies. Biol Rev Camb Philos Soc 2004;79:533–56.
34. Van Someren E. More than a marker: interaction between the circadian regulation of temperature and sleep, age-related changes, and treatment possibilities. Chronobiol Int 2000;17:313–54.
35. Beersma D, Gordij M. Circadian control of the sleep-wake cycle. Physiol Behav 2007;90:190–5.
36. Åkerstedt T. Altered sleep/wake patterns and mental performance. Physiol Behav 2007;90:209–18.
37. Moore RY. Circadian rhythms: basic neurobiology and clinical applications. Annu Rev Med 1998;48:253–66.
38. Basheer R, Strecker RE, Thakkar MM, et al. Adenosine and sleep-wake regulation. Prog Neurobiol 2004;73:379–96.
39. Blagrove M, Alexander C, Horne JA. The effects of chronic sleep reduction on the performance of cognitive tasks sensitive to sleep deprivation. Appl Cogn Psychol 1995;9:21–40.
40. Bonnet MH, Rosa RR. Sleep and performance in young adults and older normals and insomniacs during acute sleep loss and recovery. Biol Psychol 1987;25:153–72.
41. The Economist. Life in the Fast Lane. Business people are racing to learn from Formula One drivers. Available at: http://www.economist.com/news/business/21699456-business-people-are-racing-learn-formula-one-drivers-life-fast-lane. Accessed June 6, 2016.
42. Zepelin H, Siegel JM, Tobler I. Mammalian sleep. In: Kryger MH, Roth T, Dement WC, editors. Principles and practice of sleep medicine. 4th edition. Philadelphia: Elsevier/Saunders; 2005. p. 91–100.
43. Carskadon M, Dement W. Normal human sleep: an overview. In: Kryger MH, Roth T, Dement WC, editors. Principles and practice of sleep medicine. 4th edition. Philadelphia: Elsevier Saunders; 2005. p. 13–23.
44. Westerman D. The concise sleep medicine handbook. 2nd edition. Atlanta (GA): CreateSpace Independent Publishing Platform; 2013. p. 1–10.
45. Gais S, Molle M, Helms K, et al. Learning-dependent increases in sleep spindle density. J Neurosci 2002;22(15):6830–4.
46. Bader G, Gillberg C, Johnson M, et al. Activity and sleep in children with ADHD. Sleep 2003;26:A136.
47. Crick F, Mitchison G. The function of dream sleep. Nature 1983;304(5922):111–4.
48. Smith C, Lapp L. Increases in number of REMS and REM density in humans following an intensive learning period. Sleep 1991;14(4):325–30.
49. Mirmiran M, Maas Y, Ariagno R. Development of fetal and neonatal sleep and circadian rhythms. Sleep Med Rev 2003;7:321–34.
50. Goessel-Symank R, Grimmer I, Korte J, et al. Actigraphic monitoring of the activity-rest behavior of preterm and full-term infants at 20 months of age. Chronobiol Int 2004;21:661–71.
51. Adair RH, Bauchner H. Sleep problems in childhood. Curr Probl Pediatr 1993;23(4):142, 147–70.
52. Biagioni E, Boldrini A, Giganti F, et al. Distribution of sleep and wakefulness EEG patterns in 24-h recordings of preterm and full-term newborns. Early Hum Dev 2005;81:333–9.
53. Rivkees S. A developing circadian rhythmicity in infants. Pediatrics 2003;112:373–81.

54. Jenni OG, Carskadon MA. Sleep research society. SRS basics of sleep guide. Westchester (IL): Sleep Research Society; 2000. p. 11–9. Normal human sleep at different ages: infants to adolescents.
55. Roffward HP, Muzio JN, Dement WC. Ontogenetic development of the human sleep-dream cycle. Science 1966;152(3722):604–19.
56. Beltramini AU, Hertzig ME. Sleep and bedtime behavior in preschool-aged children. Pediatrics 1983;71(2):153–8.
57. Mercer PW, Merritt SL, Cowell JM. Differences in reported sleep need among adolescents. J Adolesc Health 1998;23(5):259–63.
58. Figueiro M, Rea M. Evening daylight may cause adolescents to sleep less in spring than in winter. Chronobiol Int 2010;27:1242–58.
59. Karacan I, Anch M, Thornby JI, et al. Longitudinal sleep patterns during pubertal growth: four-year follow up. Pediatr Res 1975;9(11):842–6.
60. Dijk DJ, Duffy JF, Czeisler CA. Contribution of circadian physiology and sleep homeostasis to age-related changes in human sleep. Chronobiol Int 2000; 17(3):285–311.
61. Duffy JF, Dijk DJ, Klerman EB, et al. Later endogenous circadian temperature nadir relative to an earlier wake time in older people. Am J Physiol 1998;275(5 Pt 2):R1478–87.
62. Astrom C, Trojaborg W. Relationship of age to power spectrum analysis of EEG during sleep. J Clin Neurophysiol 1992;9(3):424–30.
63. Ancoli-Israel S, Sleep Research Society. SRS basics of sleep guide. Westchester (IL): Sleep Research Society; 2005. p. 21–6. Normal human sleep at different ages: sleep in older adults.
64. Reynolds CF III, Kupfer DJ, Taska LS, et al. Sleep of healthy seniors: a revisit. Sleep 1985;8(1):20–9.
65. Redline S, Kirchner HL, Quan SF, et al. The effects of age, sex, ethnicity, and sleep-disordered breathing on sleep architecture. Arch Intern Med 2004; 164(4):406–18.
66. Monk TH, Buysse DJ, Reynolds CF III, et al. Circadian temperature rhythms of older people. Exp Gerontol 1995;30(5):455–74.
67. Dinges D, Rogers N, Baynard MD. Chronic sleep deprivation. In: Kryger MH, Roth T, Dement WC, editors. Principles and practice of sleep medicine. 4th edition. Philadelphia: Elsevier/Saunders; 2005. p. 67–76.
68. Centers for Disease Control and Prevention (CDC). Effect of short sleep duration on daily activities–United States, 2005-2008. MMWR Morb Mortal Wkly Rep 2011;60(8):239–42.
69. Nunes J, Jean-Louis G, Zizi F, et al. Sleep duration among black and white Americans: results of the National Health Interview Survey. J Natl Med Assoc 2008;100(3):317–22.
70. Hale L, Do DP. Racial differences in self-reports of sleep duration in a population-based study. Sleep 2007;30(9):1096–103.
71. Jackson CL, Redline S, Kawachi I, et al. Racial disparities in short sleep duration by occupation and industry. Am J Epidemiol 2013;178(9):1442–51.
72. Hale L, Rivero-Fuentes E. Negative acculturation in sleep duration among Mexican immigrants and Mexican Americans. J Immigr Minor Health 2011; 13(2):402–7.
73. Patel NP, Grandner MA, Xie D, et al. "Sleep disparity" in the population: poor sleep quality is strongly associated with poverty and ethnicity. BMC Public Health 2010;10:475.

74. Grandner MA, Hale L, Jackson N, et al. Perceived racial discrimination as an independent predictor of sleep disturbance and daytime fatigue. Behav Sleep Med 2012;10(4):235–49.

75. Steffen PR, Bowden M. Sleep disturbance mediates the relationship between perceived racism and depressive symptoms. Ethn Dis 2006;16(1):16–21.

76. Brimah P, Oulds F, Olafiranye O, et al. Sleep duration and reported functional capacity among black and white US adults. J Clin Sleep Med 2013;9(6):605–9.

77. Beihl DA, Liese AD, Haffner SM. Sleep duration as a risk factor for incident type 2 diabetes in a multiethnic cohort. Ann Epidemiol 2009;19(5):351–7.

78. Bidulescu A, Din-Dzietham R, Coverson DL, et al. Interaction of sleep quality and psychosocial stress on obesity in African Americans: the Cardiovascular Health Epidemiology Study (CHES). BMC Public Health 2010;10:581.

79. Owens JF, Buysse DJ, Hall M, et al. Napping, nighttime sleep, and cardiovascular risk factors in mid-life adults. J Clin Sleep Med 2010;6(4):330–5.

80. Spaeth AM, Dinges DF, Goel N. Sex and race differences in caloric intake during sleep restriction in healthy adults. Am J Clin Nutr 2014;100(2):559–66.

81. Hairston KG, Bryer-Ash M, Norris JM, et al. Sleep duration and five-year abdominal fat accumulation in a minority cohort: the IRAS family study. Sleep 2010; 33(3):289–95.

82. Simpson NS, Banks S, Arroyo S, et al. Effects of sleep restriction on adiponectin levels in healthy men and women. Physiol Behav 2010;101(5):693–8.

83. Matthews K, Hall M, Dahl R. Sleep in healthy black and white adolescents. Pediatrics 2014;133(5):e1189–96.

84. Troxel WM, Lee L, Hall M, et al. Single-parent family structure and sleep problems in black and white adolescents. Sleep Med 2014;15(2):255–61.

85. Combs D, Goodwin JL, Quan SF, et al. Longitudinal differences in sleep duration in Hispanic and Caucasian children. Sleep Med 2016;18:61–6.

86. Martinez SM, Tschann JM, Greenspan LC, et al. Is it time for bed? Short sleep duration increases risk of obesity in Mexican American children. Sleep Med 2014;15(12):1484–9.

87. Phillipson EA. Sleep apnea–a major public health problem. N Engl J Med 1993; 328:1271–3.

88. Rosen RC, Zozula R, Jahn EG, et al. Low rates of recognition of sleep disorders in primary care: comparison of a community-based versus clinical academic setting. Sleep Med 2001;2:47–55.

89. White DP. Central sleep apnea. In: Kryger MH, Roth T, Dement WC, editors. Principles and practice of sleep medicine. 4th edition. Philadelphia: Elsevier/Saunders; 2005. p. 969–82.

90. Thorpy MJ. Classification of sleep disorders. In: Kryger MH, Roth T, Dement WC, editors. Principles and practice of sleep medicine. 4th edition. Philadelphia: Elsevier/Saunders; 2005. p. 615–25.

91. Redline S, Tishler PV, Hans MG, et al. Racial differences in sleep-disordered breathing in African-Americans and Caucasians. Am J Respir Crit Care Med 1997;155:186–92.

92. Ancoli-Israel S, Klauber MR, Stepnowsky C, et al. Sleep-disordered breathing in African-American elderly. Am J Respir Crit Care Med 1995;152:1946–9.

93. Kripke DF, Ancoli-Israel S, Klauber MR, et al. Prevalence of sleep disordered breathing in ages 40–64 years: a population-based survey. Sleep 1997;20: 65–76.

94. O'Connor GT, Lind BK, Lee ET, et al, Sleep Heart Health Study Investigators. Variation in symptoms of sleep-disordered breathing with race and ethnicity: the Sleep Heart Health Study. Sleep 2003;26(1):74–9.

95. Friedman M, Bliznikas D, Klein M, et al. Comparison of the incidences of obstructive sleep apnea-hypopnea syndrome in African-Americans versus Caucasian-Americans. Otolaryngol Head Neck Surg 2006;134(4):545–50.

96. Ram S, Seirawan H, Kumar SK, et al. Prevalence and impact of sleep disorders and sleep habits in the United States. Sleep Breath 2010;14(1):63–70.

97. Schmidt-Nowara WW, Coultas DB, Wiggins C, et al. Snoring in a Hispanic-American population. Risk factors and association with hypertension and other morbidity. Arch Intern Med 1990;150:597–601.

98. Goldstein NA, Abramowitz T, Weedon J, et al. Racial/ethnic differences in the prevalence of snoring and sleep disordered breathing in young children. J Clin Sleep Med 2011;7(2):163–71.

99. Bouscoulet LT, Vazquez-Garcia JC, Muino A, et al. Prevalence of sleep related symptoms in four Latin American cities. J Clin Sleep Med 2008;4:579–85.

100. Young T, Palta M, Dempsey J, et al. The occurrence of sleep-disordered breathing among middle-aged adults. N Engl J Med 1993;328:1230–5.

101. Jean-Louis G, Zizi F, Casimir G, et al. Sleep-disordered breathing and hypertension among African Americans. J Hum Hypertens 2005;19(6):485–90.

102. Sjöström C, Lindberg E, Elmasry A, et al. Prevalence of sleep apnoea and snoring in hypertensive men: a population based study. Thorax 2002;57(7):602–7.

103. Lackland DT, Lin Y, Tilley BC, et al. An assessment of racial differences in clinical practices for hypertension at primary care sites for medically underserved patients. J Clin Hypertens (Greenwich) 2004;6:26–31.

104. Meetze K, Gillespie MB, Lee F. Obstructive sleep apnea: a comparison of black and white subjects. Laryngoscope 2002;112:1271–4.

105. Partinen M, Hublin C. Epidemiology of sleep disorders. In: Kryger MH, Roth T, Dement WC, editors. Principles and practice of sleep medicine. 4th edition. Philadelphia: Elsevier/Saunders; 2005. p. 626–47.

106. Faulx MD, Larkin EK, Hoit BD, et al. Sex influences endothelial function in sleep-disordered breathing. Sleep 2004;27(6):1113–20.

107. Nieto FJ, Herrington DM, Redline S, et al. Sleep apnea and markers of vascular endothelial function in a large community sample of older adults. Am J Respir Crit Care Med 2004;169(3):354–60.

108. Robinson GV, Stradling JR, Davies RJ. Sleep 6: Obstructive sleep apnoea/hypopnoea syndrome and hypertension. Thorax 2004b;59(12):1089–94.

109. Young T, Peppard PE, Gottlieb DJ. Epidemiology of obstructive sleep apnea: a population health perspective. Am J Respir Crit Care Med 2002;165(9): 1217–39.

110. Shahar E, Whitney CW, Redline S, et al. Sleep-disordered breathing and cardiovascular disease: cross-sectional results of the Sleep Heart Health Study. Am J Respir Crit Care Med 2001;163(1):19–25.

111. Jennum P, Hein HO, Suadicani P, et al. Risk of ischemic heart disease in self-reported snorers. A prospective study of 2,937 men aged 54 to 74 years: the Copenhagen Male Study. Chest 1995;108(1):138–42.

112. Yaggi HK, Concato J, Kernan WN, et al. Obstructive sleep apnea as a risk factor for stroke and death. N Engl J Med 2005;353(19):2034–41.

113. Bradley TD, Logan AG, Kimoff RJ, et al. Continuous positive airway pressure for central sleep apnea and heart failure. N Engl J Med 2005;353(19):2025–33.

114. Marin JM, Carrizo SJ, Vicente E, et al. Long-term cardiovascular outcomes in men with obstructive sleep apnoea-hypopnoea with or without treatment with continuous positive airway pressure: an observational study. Lancet 2005; 365(9464):1046–53.
115. Doherty LS, Kiely JL, Swan V, et al. Long-term effects of nasal continuous positive airway pressure therapy on cardiovascular outcomes in sleep apnea syndrome. Chest 2005;127(6):2076–84.
116. He J, Kryger MH, Zorick FJ, et al. Mortality and apnea index in obstructive sleep apnea. Experience in 385 male patients. Chest 1988;94(1):9–14.
117. Ancoli-Israel S, Kripke DF, Klauber MR, et al. Morbidity, mortality and sleep-disordered breathing in community dwelling elderly. Sleep 1996;19(4):277–82.
118. Lindberg E, Janson C, Svardsudd K, et al. Increased mortality among sleepy snorers: a prospective population-based study. Thorax 1998;53(8):631–7.
119. Martin BC, Warram JH, Krolewski AS, et al. Role of glucose and insulin resistance in development of type 2 diabetes mellitus: results of a 25-year follow-up study. Lancet 1992;340(8825):925–9.
120. Punjabi NM, Beamer BA. Sleep apnea and metabolic dysfunction. In: Kryger MH, Roth T, Dement WC, editors. Principles and practice of sleep medicine. 4th edition. Philadelphia: Elsevier/Saunders; 2005. p. 1034–42.
121. Al-Delaimy WK, Manson JE, Willett WC, et al. Snoring as a risk factor for type II diabetes mellitus: a prospective study. Am J Epidemiol 2002;155(5):387–93.
122. Babu AR, Herdegen J, Fogelfeld L, et al. Type 2 diabetes, glycemic control, and continuous positive airway pressure in obstructive sleep apnea. Arch Intern Med 2005;165(4):447–52.
123. Phillips BG, Hisel TM, Kato M, et al. Recent weight gain in patients with newly diagnosed obstructive sleep apnea. J Hypertens 1999;17(9):1297–300.
124. Phillips BG, Kato M, Narkiewicz K, et al. Increases in leptin levels, sympathetic drive, and weight gain in obstructive sleep apnea. Am J Physiol Heart Circ Physiol 2000;279(1):H234–7.
125. Kalra M, Inge T, Garcia V, et al. Obstructive sleep apnea in extremely overweight adolescents undergoing bariatric surgery. Obes Res 2005;13(7):1175–9.
126. Ohayon MM. Epidemiology of insomnia: what we know and what we still need to learn. Sleep Med Rev 2002;6(2):97–111.
127. American Psychiatric Association. Diagnostic and statistical manual of mental disorders: DSM-IV.. 4th edition. Washington, DC: American Psychiatric Association; 2000.
128. Ford ES, Cunningham TJ, Giles WH, et al. Trends in insomnia and excessive daytime sleepiness among U.S. adults from 2002 to 2012. Sleep Med 2015; 16(3):372–8.
129. Simon GE, VonKorff M. Prevalence, burden, and treatment of insomnia in primary care. Am J Psychiatry 1997;154(10):1417–23.
130. Ford DE, Kamerow DB. Epidemiologic study of sleep disturbances and psychiatric disorders. An opportunity for prevention? J Am Med Assoc 1989;262(11): 1479–84.
131. Edinger JD, Means MK. Overview of insomnia: definitions, epidemiology, differential diagnosis, and assessment. In: Kryger MH, Roth T, Dement WC, editors. Principles and practice of sleep medicine. 4th edition. Philadelphia: Elsevier/Saunders; 2005. p. 702–13.
132. Petrov ME, Lichstein KL, Baldwin CM. Prevalence of sleep disorders by sex and ethnicity among older adolescents and emerging adults: relations to daytime functioning, working memory and mental health. J Adolesc 2014;37(5):587–97.

133. Roberts RE, Roberts CR, Chan W. Ethnic differences in symptoms of insomnia among adolescents. Sleep 2006;29:359–65.
134. Shafazand S, Wallace DM, Vargas SS, et al. Sleep disordered breathing, insomnia symptoms, and sleep quality in a clinical cohort of US Hispanics in South Florida. J Clin Sleep Med 2012;8(5):507–14.
135. Slopen N, Williams DR. Discrimination, other psychosocial stressors, and self-reported sleep duration and difficulties. Sleep 2014;37(1):147–56.
136. Lewis TT, Troxel WM, Kravitz HM, et al. Chronic exposure to everyday discrimination and sleep in a multiethnic sample of middle-aged women. Health Psychol 2013;32(7):810–9.
137. Manber R, Steidtmann D, Chambers AS, et al. Factors associated with clinically significant insomnia among pregnant low-income Latinas. J Womens Health (Larchmt) 2013;22(8):694–701.
138. Perlis ML, Smith MT, Pigeon WR. Etiology and pathophysiology of insomnia. In: Kryger MH, Roth T, Dement WC, editors. Principles and practice of sleep medicine. 4th edition. Philadelphia: Elsevier/Saunders; 2005. p. 714–25.
139. Vgontzas AN, Bixler EO, Lin HM, et al. Chronic insomnia is associated with nyctohemeral activation of the hypothalamic-pituitary-adrenal axis: clinical implications. J Clin Endocrinol Metab 2001;86(8):3787–94.
140. Hansen AM, Thomsen JF, Kaergaard A, et al. Salivary cortisol and sleep problems among civil servants. Psychoneuroendocrinology 2012;37(7):1086–95.
141. Nofzinger EA, Buysse DJ, Germain A, et al. Alterations in regional cerebral glucose metabolism across waking and non-rapid eye movement sleep in depression. Arch Gen Psychiatry 2005;62(4):387–96.
142. Bazargan M, Yazdanshenas H, Gordon D, et al. Pain in community-dwelling elderly African Americans. J Aging Health 2016;28(3):403–25.
143. Hall Brown TS, Akeeb A, Mellman TA. The role of trauma type in the risk for insomnia. J Clin Sleep Med 2015;11(7):735–9.
144. Laugsand LE, Vatten LJ, Platou C, et al. Insomnia and the risk of acute myocardial infarction: a population study. Circulation 2011;124(19):2073–81.
145. Spiegelhalder K, Scholtes C, Riemann D. The association between insomnia and cardiovascular diseases. Nat Sci Sleep 2010;2:71–8.
146. Fernandez-Mendoza J, Vgontzas AN, Liao D, et al. Insomnia with objective short sleep duration and incident hypertension: the Penn State Cohort. Hypertension 2012;60(4):929–35.
147. Cherniack EP, Ceron-Fuentes J, Florez H, et al. Influence of race and ethnicity on alternative medicine as a self-treatment preference for common medical conditions in a population of multi-ethnic urban elderly. Complement Ther Clin Pract 2008;14:116–23.
148. Reid KJ, Zee PC. Circadian disorders of the sleep-wake cycle. In: Kryger MH, Roth T, Dement WC, editors. Principles and practice of sleep medicine. 4th edition. Philadelphia: Elsevier/Saunders; 2005. p. 691–701.
149. Weitzman ED, Czeisler CA, Coleman RM, et al. Delayed sleep phase syndrome. A chronobiological disorder with sleep-onset insomnia. Arch Gen Psychiatry 1981;38(7):737–46.
150. Regestein QR, Monk TH. Delayed sleep phase syndrome: a review of its clinical aspects. Am J Psychiatry 1995;152(4):602–8.
151. Ando K, Kripke DF, Ancoli-Israel S. Estimated prevalence of delayed and advanced sleep phase syndromes. J Sleep Res 1995;24:509.
152. Santhi N, Duffy JF, Horowitz TS, et al. Scheduling of sleep/darkness affects the circadian phase of night shift workers. Neurosci Lett 2005;384(3):316–20.

153. Pereira DS, Tufik S, Louzada FM, et al. Association of the length polymorphism in the human Per3 gene with the delayed sleep-phase syndrome: does latitude have an influence upon it? Sleep 2005;28(1):29–32.
154. Gronfier C, Wright KP Jr, Kronauer RE, et al. Efficacy of a single sequence of intermittent bright light pulses for delaying circadian phase in humans. Am J Physiol Endocrinol Metab 2004;287(1):174–81.
155. Czeisler CA, Richardson GS, Zimmerman JC, et al. Entrainment of human circadian rhythms by light-dark cycles: a reassessment. Photochem Photobiol 1981; 34(2):239–47.
156. Archer SN, Robilliard DL, Skene DJ, et al. A length polymorphism in the circadian clock gene Per3 is linked to delayed sleep phase syndrome and extreme diurnal preference. Sleep 2003;26(4):413–5.
157. Satoh K, Mishima K, Inoue Y, et al. Two pedigrees of familial advanced sleep phase syndrome in Japan. Sleep 2003;26(4):416–7.
158. Shiino Y, Nakajima S, Ozeki Y, et al. Mutation screening of the human period 2 gene in bipolar disorder. Neurosci Lett 2003;338(1):82–4.
159. Xu Y, Padiath QS, Shapiro RE, et al. Functional consequences of a CKIdelta mutation causing familial advanced sleep phase syndrome. Nature 2005; 434(7033):640–4.
160. Weyerbrock A, Timmer J, Hohagen F, et al. Effects of light and chronotherapy on human circadian rhythms in delayed sleep phase syndrome: cytokines, cortisol, growth hormone, and the sleep-wake cycle. Biol Psychiatry 1996;40(8):794–7.
161. Palmer CR, Kripke DF, Savage HC Jr, et al. Efficacy of enhanced evening light for advanced sleep phase syndrome. Behav Sleep Med 2003;1(4):213–26.
162. Lewy AJ, Ahmed S, Sack RL. Phase shifting the human circadian clock using melatonin. Behav Brain Res 1996;73(1–2):131–4.
163. Michaud M, Chabli A, Lavigne G, et al. Arm restlessness in patients with restless legs syndrome. Mov Disord 2000;15(2):289–93.
164. Montplaisir J, Boucher S, Poirier G, et al. Clinical, polysomnographic, and genetic characteristics of restless legs syndrome: a study of 133 patients diagnosed with new standard criteria. Mov Disord 1997;12(1):61–5.
165. Phillips B, Hening W, Britz P, et al. Prevalence and correlates of restless legs syndrome: 2 results from the 2005 National Sleep Foundation poll. Chest 2006;129(1):76–80.
166. Kryger MH, Otake K, Foerster J. Low body stores of iron and restless legs syndrome: a correctable cause of insomnia in adolescents and teenagers. Sleep Med 2002;3(2):127–32.
167. Nichols DA, Allen RP, Grauke JH, et al. Restless legs syndrome symptoms in primary care: a prevalence study. Arch Intern Med 2002;163(18):2323–9.
168. Lee KA, Zaffke ME, Baratte-Beebe K. Restless legs syndrome and sleep disturbance during pregnancy: the role of folate and iron. J Womens Health Gend Based Med 2001;10(4):335–41.
169. Chervin RD, Hedger AK, Dillon JE, et al. Associations between symptoms of inattention, hyperactivity, restless legs, and periodic leg movements. Sleep 2002;25(2):213–8.
170. Innes KE, Flack KL, Selfe TK, et al. Restless legs syndrome in an Appalachian primary care population: prevalence, demographic and lifestyle correlates, and burden. J Clin Sleep Med 2013;9:1065–75.
171. Szentkiralyi A, Fendrich K, Hoffmann W, et al. Socio-economic risk factors for incident restless legs syndrome in the general population. J Sleep Res 2012; 21:561–8.

172. Allen RP, Picchietti D, Hening WA, et al. Restless legs syndrome: diagnostic criteria, special considerations, and epidemiology. A report from the Restless Legs Syndrome Diagnosis and Epidemiology Workshop at the National Institutes of Health. Sleep Med 2003;4(2):101–19.

173. Winkelmann J, Muller-Myhsok B, Wittchen HU, et al. Complex segregation analysis of restless legs syndrome provides evidence for an autosomal dominant mode of inheritance in early age at onset families. Ann Neurol 2002;52(3):297–302.

174. Desautels A, Turecki G, Montplaisir J, et al. Identification of a major susceptibility locus for restless legs syndrome on chromosome 12q. Am J Hum Genet 2001;69(6):1266–70.

175. Bonati MT, Ferini-Strambi L, Aridon P, et al. Autosomal dominant restless legs syndrome maps on chromosome 14q. Brain 2003;126(6):1485–92.

176. Chen S, Ondo WG, Rao S, et al. Genomewide linkage scan identifies a novel susceptibility locus for restless legs syndrome on chromosome 9p. Am J Hum Genet 2004;74(5):876–85.

177. Silber MH, Richardson JW. Multiple blood donations associated with iron deficiency in patients with restless legs syndrome. Mayo Clin Proc 2003;78(1):52–4.

178. Connor JR, Boyer PJ, Menzies SL, et al. Neuropathological examination suggests impaired brain iron acquisition in restless legs syndrome. Neurology 2003;61(3):304–9.

179. Turjanski N, Lees AJ, Brooks DJ. Striatal dopaminergic function in restless legs syndrome: 18F-dopa and 11C-raclopride PET studies. Neurology 1999;52(5):932–7.

180. Winkelmann J, Schadrack J, Wetter TC, et al. Opioid and dopamine antagonist drug challenges in untreated restless legs syndrome patients. Sleep Med 2001;2(1):57–61.

181. Stiasny K, Wetter TC, Winkelmann J, et al. Long-term effects of pergolide in the treatment of restless legs syndrome. Neurology 2001;56(10):1399–402.

182. Winkelman JW, Chertow GM, Lazarus JM. Restless legs syndrome in end–stage renal disease. Am J Kidney Dis 1996;28(3):372–8.

183. Unruh ML, Levey AS, D'Ambrosio C, et al. Restless legs symptoms among incident dialysis patients: association with lower quality of life and shorter survival. Am J Kidney Dis 2004;43(5):900–9.

184. Hening WA, Allen RP, Earley CJ, et al. Restless legs syndrome task force of the standards of practice committee of the American Academy of Sleep Medicine. An update on the dopaminergic treatment of restless legs syndrome and periodic limb movement disorder. Sleep 2004;27(3):560–83.

185. Gochfeld M. Occupational medicine practice in the United States since the industrial revolution. J Occup Environ Med 2005;47(2):115–31.

186. Healthy People 2020. Social Determinants of Health. Available at: https://www.healthypeople.gov/2020/topics-objectives/topic/social-determinants-of-healthbook. Accessed April 1, 2016.

187. Breyre A, Green-McKenzie J. A case of acute lead toxicity associated with Ayurvedic supplements. British Medical Journal Case Reports, in press. Available at: http://casereports.bmj.com. Accessed May 25, 2016.

188. Jones C, Shofer F, Duran M, et al. Assessment of medical student exposure to occupational and environmental medicine in medical school curriculum. Presented at: American Occupational Health Conference. Chicago (IL), April 11, 2016.

189. Hidden Tragedy: Underreporting of Workplace Injuries and Illnesses. US House of Representatives. Available at: http://www.bls.gov/iif/laborcommreport061908.pdf. Accessed May 15, 2016.

190. Won J, Dembe A. Services provided by family physicians for patients with occupational injuries and illnesses. Ann Fam Med 2006;4(2):138–47.

191. American College of Occupational and Environmental Medicine. The personal physician's role in helping patients with medical conditions stay at work or return to work. Available at: http://www.acoem.org/PhysiciansRole_ReturntoWork.aspx. Accessed November 1, 2012.

192. Politi BJ, Arena VC, Schwerha J, et al. Occupational medical history taking: how are today's physicians doing? A cross-sectional investigation of the frequency of occupational history taking by physicians in a major US teaching center. J Occup Environ Med 2004;46(6):550–5.

193. Kiselica D, Sibson B, Green-McKenzie J. Workers compensation: a historical review and description of a legal and social insurance system. Clin Occup Environ Med 2004;4(2):237–48.

194. Shinkman R. Getting underserved groups to seek health insurance. Med Educ Online 2015. https://doi.org/10.3402/meo.v20.27535.

195. VanderWielen L, Vanderbilt A, Crossman S. Health disparities and underserved populations: a potential solution, medical school partnerships with free clinics to improve curriculum. Med Educ Online 2015;20:27535.

196. Anthony D, El Rayess F, Esquibel AY, et al. Building a workforce of physicians to care for underserved patients. R I Med J (2013) 2014;97(9):31–5.

197. Vanichkachorn G, Roy B, Lopez R, et al. Evaluation and treatment of the acutely injured worker. Am Fam Physician 2014;89(1):17–24.

198. Vanichkachorn G, Green-McKenzie J, Emmett E. Occupational health care. Family medicine: principles & practice. 7th edition. New York: Springer; 2015.

199. Nadkarni M. The double whammy of chronic illness in underserved populations: can we afford not to care? New York: DHHS; 2004. Available at: http://www.modooapc.com/viewarticle/472495. Accessed April 30, 2016.

200. US Department of Health and Human Services. Trends in the Health of Americans. Hyattsville (MD): US Department of Health and Human Services, Centers for Disease Control and Prevention, National Center for Health Statistics Office of Information Services; 2003.

201. Smedley B, Stith A, Nelson A. Unequal treatment. Confronting racial and ethnic disparities in healthcare. Washington, DC: The National Academies Press; 2003.

202. Preventing chronic disease: eliminating the leading preventable causes of premature death and disability in the United States. Available at: http://www.cdc.gov/chronicdisease/pdf/preventing-chronic-disease-508.pdf. Accessed May 25, 2016.

203. Nielson M, Olayiwola J, Grundy P, et al. The Patient-Centered Medical Home's Impact on cost & quality: an annual update of the evidence. Patient Centered Primary Care Collaborative 2012-2013. Available at: http://www.milbank.org/uploads/documents/reports. Accessed May 25, 2016.

204. Schulte P. Characterizing the burden of occupational injury and disease. J Occup Environ Med 2005;47(6):607–22.

205. Numbers: workplace injuries. U.S. Bureau of Labor Statistics. 2013. Available at: http://www.ilo.org/global/standards/subjects-covered-by-international-labour-standards/occupational-safety-and-health/lang–en/index.htm. Accessed March 1, 2016.

206. Corbin K. The 5 Most Injury-Prone Industries. Available at: http://jobs.aol.com/articles/2011/12/08/the-5-most-injury-prone-industries/Schools.com. Accessed May 25, 2016.
207. Walter L. OSHA's role in reducing occupational injuries, fatalities. Available at: http://ehstoday.com/osha/osha-s-role-reducing-occupational-injuries-fatalities-infographic. Accessed May 15, 2016.
208. OSHA fact Sheet. Available at: https://www.osha.gov/OshDoc/data_General_Facts/factsheet-inspections.pdf. Accessed May 15, 2016.
209. National Occupational Safety and Health Administration. About NORA... Partnerships, Research and Practice. Available at: http://www.cdc.gov/niosh/nora/about.html. Accessed May 15, 2016.
210. Centers for Disease Control. National Occupational Safety and Health Administration. NORA Sector Agendas. Available at: http://www.cdc.gov/niosh/nora/comment/agendas/. Accessed May 15, 2016.
211. Chou C-F, Johnson PJ, Ward A, et al. Health care coverage and the health care industry. Am J Public Health 2009;99(12):2282–8.
212. Ward BW, Clarke TC, Freeman G. et al. National Health Interview Survey. Division of Health Interview Statistics, National Center for Health Statistics. Available at: http://www.cdc.gov/nchs/data/nhis/earlyrelease/earlyrelease201506.pdf. Accessed March 30, 2016.
213. Johnson PJ, Blewett LA, Ruggles S, et al. Four decades of population health data: the integrated health interview series. Epidemiology 2008;19:872–5.
214. Occupational Hazards in Home health care. NIOSH Health and Safety Topics. Available at: https://www.osha.gov/SLTC/home_healthcare/#. Accessed March 1, 2016.
215. Green-McKenzie J, McCarthy R, Shofer F. Characterisation of occupational blood and body fluid exposures beyond the Needlestick Safety and Prevention Act. J Infect Prev 2016;17(5):226–32. Available at: http://bji.sagepub.com/content/early/2016/04/29/1757177416645339.abstract. Accessed May 20, 2016.
216. McLellan R, Sherman B, Loeppke R, et al. Optimizing health care delivery by integrating workplaces, homes and communities: how occupational and environmental medicine can serve as a vital connecting link between accountable care organizations and the patient-centered medical home. J Occup Environ Med 2012;54(4):504–12.
217. Ruotsalainen JH, Verbeek JH, Mariné A, et al. Preventing occupational stress in healthcare workers. Cochrane Database Syst Rev 2015;(4). CD002892. Available at: http://www.cochrane.org/CD002892/OCCHEALTH_preventing-occupational-stress-in-healthcare-workers.
218. Occupational Hazards in Home health care. NIOSH health and safety topics. Available at: http://www.cdc.gov/niosh/docs/2010-125/pdfs/2010-125.pdf; https://www.osha.gov/SLTC/home_healthcare/#. Accessed March 1, 2016.
219. Buchanan S, Vossenas P, Krause N, et al. Occupational injury disparities in the US hotel industry. Am J Ind Med 2010;53:116–25.
220. Singer A. Immigrant workers in the U.S. Labor Force. Washington, DC: Brookings; 2012. Available at: http://www.brookings.edu/~/media/research/files/papers/2012/3/15%20immigrant%20workers%20singer/0315_immigrant_workers_singer.pdf.
221. Chou C-F, Johnson PJ, Ward A, et al. Occupational outlook handbook, maids and housekeeping cleaners: pay. Washington, DC: Bureau of Labor Statistics; 2013. Available at: http://www.bls.gov/ooh/building-and-grounds-cleaning/maids-and-housekeeping-cleaners.htm#tab-5.

222. Sanon MA. Agency-hired hotel housekeepers: an at-risk group for adverse health outcomes. Workplace Health Saf 2014;62(2):86.
223. Knox A. Lost in translation: an analysis of temporary work agency employment in hotels. Work Employ Soc 2010;24:449–67.
224. Wells MJ. Unionization and immigrant incorporation in San Francisco hotels. Soc Probl 2000;47:241–65.
225. Underserved Workers Gain Access to UCSF OEM Specialists. Available at: http://coeh.berkeley.edu/bridges/Summer2013/UnderservedWorkers.html. Accessed March 1, 2016.
226. Legal Consciousness of Undocumented Latinos: Fear and Stigma as Barriers to Claims-Making for First- and 1.5-Generation Immigrants. Law and Society Review. Available at: http://plone3.sscnet.ucla.edu:8080/chavez/chavez/people-faculty-and-staff/core-faculty-1/faculty-files/LegalConsciousnessofUndocumentedLatinos.pdf. Accessed May 29, 2016.
227. American College of Occupational and Environmental Medicine Whitepaper. The Health of Immigrant Workers in the US. Available at: https://www.acoem.org/uploadedFiles/About_ACOEM/Components_And_Sections/Section_Home_Pages/White%20Paper%20-%20THE%20HEALTH%20STATUS%20OF%20IMMIGRANT%20WORKERS%20IN%20THE%20US%205-1-2012.pdf. Accessed May 1, 2012.
228. Leigh J, Macaskill P, Kuosma E, et al. Global burden of disease and injury due to occupational factors. Epidemiology 1999;10(5):626–31.
229. Nelson D, Concha-Barrientos M, Driscoll T, et al. The global burden of selected occupational disease and injury risks: methodology and summary. Am J Ind Med 2005;48:400–18.
230. International Labour Standards on Occupational Safety and Health. Available at: http://www.ilo.org/global/standards/subjects-covered-by-international-labour-standards/occupational-safety-and-health/lang–en/index.htm. Accessed March 30, 2016.
231. Concha-Barrientos M, Nelson D, Fingerhut M, et al. Global burden due to occupational injury. Am J Ind Med 2005;48(6):470–81.
232. Global Strategy on Occupational Safety and Health. Conclusions adopted by the International Labor Conference at its 91st Session. International Labour Organization 2994. 2003. Available at: http://www.ilo.org/safework/info/policy-documents/WCMS_107535/lang–en/index.htm. Accessed May 23, 2016.
233. Plan of action (2010-2016) to achieve widespread ratification and effective implementation of the occupational safety and health instruments. Available at: http://www.ilo.org/global/standards/WCMS_125616/lang–en/index.htm. Accessed June 1, 2016.
234. Occupational Safety and Health Administration. 1970. Available at: http://www.osha.gov/pls/oshaweb/owadisp.show_document?p_table=OSHACT&p_id=2743. Accessed May 1, 2016.
235. Canadian Center for Occupational Safety and Health Legislation: Due Diligence. 2015. Available at: http://www.ccohs.ca/topics/legislation/duediligence. Accessed May 1, 2016.
236. UK Legislation, 1974 UK Legislation (1974) Health and Safety at Work etc. Act. c. 37 Part I General duties Section 2. Available at: http://www.legislation.gov.uk/ukpga/1974/37/section/2. Accessed May 1, 2016.
237. Office of Disease Prevention and Health Promotion. Healthy People 2020. Available at: https://www.healthypeople.gov. Accessed April 1, 2016.

Infectious Disease Issues in Underserved Populations

Samuel Neil Grief, MD, FCFP[a],*, John Paul Miller, MD[b]

KEYWORDS

- Infectious disease • Underserved populations • Minorities • Inmates • Homeless
- HIV • Health outcomes • Barriers

KEY POINTS

- Underserved populations are afflicted with infectious diseases at disproportionally higher rates than the general population.
- Underserved populations face many unique barriers to accessing quality health care.
- Although the Affordable Care Act has helped mitigate some of these challenges, significant obstacles remain.
- Primary care physicians are uniquely qualified to deliver high quality, culturally competent care to this important population.

INTRODUCTION

Although underserved populations have many of the same health concerns as the general population, they are disproportionately affected by higher rates of both acute and chronic illness, receive lower quality care, and experience worse health-related outcomes.[1] Although the Affordable Care Act (ACA) has expanded insurance coverage to many Americans, underserved populations continue to face numerous barriers to accessible and quality health care.[2]

Although early identification and treatment of infection have the potential to reduce transmission and improve health outcomes,[3] shortage of primary care physicians; immigration status; difficulties with transportation; communication issues, including health illiteracy, appointment availability, and previous negative experiences with health care, are some of the challenges underserved populations encounter in

This article originally appeared in Primary Care: Clinics in Office Practice, Volume 44, Issue 1, March 2017.
Disclosure Statement: The authors have nothing to disclose.
[a] Department of Family Medicine, University of Illinois at Chicago, 1919 West Taylor Street, Chicago, IL 60612, USA; [b] Bakersfield Memorial Family Medicine Residency Program, Department of Family Medicine, University of California Irvine School of Medicine, 420 34th Street, Bakersfield, CA 93301, USA
* Corresponding author.
E-mail address: sgrief@uic.edu

Physician Assist Clin 4 (2019) 107–125
https://doi.org/10.1016/j.cpha.2018.08.006
2405-7991/19/© 2018 Elsevier Inc. All rights reserved.

navigating the complex health care system.[2] Given these and other obstacles, infectious diseases are much more likely to be diagnosed at a late stage.[4,5]

A comprehensive and integrated patient-centered approach delivered by providers knowledgeable about the specific needs of underserved populations is imperative. In addition, community-based outreach and collaboration with social support services is vital. Primary care physicians are uniquely qualified and positioned to provide essential care to these vulnerable populations.

THE HOMELESS

In the United States, more than 650,000 American men, women, and children of all ages and ethnicities are homeless at any given time.[6] People facing homelessness often lack adequate health insurance coverage, and struggle with substance use, poor nutrition, mental illness, and chronic medical conditions, including infectious diseases.[7] Competing priorities for shelter, food, and safety mean homeless populations often delay seeking health care.[8] These issues contribute to fragmented care that often takes place in crowded emergency departments and requires frequent acute hospitalizations.[8]

Attempts to alleviate an issue may lead to unintended consequences. Although shelters provide protection from the elements, overcrowding may contribute to increased risk of contracting infectious diseases such as pneumonia, tuberculosis (TB), hepatitis A, and skin infestations.[3] Homeless women and youth are particularly vulnerable to contracting infectious diseases because they are more likely to suffer from mental illness, use drugs, and engage in high-risk sexual practices, such as exchanging sex for drugs, shelter, food, or money.[9]

Human Immunodeficiency Virus–Acquired Immunodeficiency Syndrome

An estimated 3.4% of the homeless population is infected with the human immunodeficiency virus (HIV) compared with 0.4% in the general population.[10] Prevalence rates in homeless men who have sex with men (MSM) and injection drug users are much higher at 30% and 8%, respectively.[11] It is also estimated that 50% of persons living with HIV or acquired immunodeficiency syndrome (AIDS) (PLWHA) are at risk for becoming homeless.[12] The lack of affordable housing, high costs of medical care, and job loss due to discrimination are contributing factors.[13] Risky behaviors, such as needle sharing, unprotected sex, and survival sex (exchanging sex for money or drugs), increase transmission risk.[14]

Due to underlying immunosuppression, homeless individuals with HIV/AIDS may be at increased risk of acquiring other infectious diseases. The prevalence of TB in the HIV-positive population is increased 2-fold in those who stay in shelters compared with those who do not.[12] Evidence shows that homeless or marginally housed PLWHA experience delays in HIV diagnosis[15] and entry into care,[16] as well as lower rates of continuity of care.[17] Adherence to treatment is problematic and is complicated in those with underlying depression and/or substance abuse.[18]

Overall, homeless PLWHA have lower CD4 counts, higher viral loads, are less likely to be prescribed or adhere to treatment regimens,[4,19,20] and have higher mortality rates compared with their nonhomeless counterparts.[21] Conversely, stable housing improves access to care, HIV-related outcomes, and reduces the risk of ongoing transmission.[22]

Hepatitis C

Hepatitis C virus (HCV) is the most common chronic blood-borne viral infection in the United States with an estimated prevalence of 2% in the general population.[17]

Prevalence rates in the homeless population were reported as 24% in a recent study[8] and as high as 65% to 69% among those who are HIV-positive.[17] Strikingly, as many as 50% of homeless persons with HCV are unaware that they are infected,[23,24] which puts noninfected contacts at significant risk. Concurrent injection drug use is the strongest risk factor for contracting HCV.[25] Older age, veteran status, having multiple tattoos, and previous incarceration are also risk factors.[26]

Because HCV is asymptomatic until significant complications arise, early screening and detection is paramount.[24] Recent guidelines from the US Preventive Services Task Force and the Centers for Disease Control and Prevention (CDC) recommend routine screening for high-risk individuals.[26,27] The availability of rapid point-of-care testing[28] and more effective, tolerable, and easier to administer treatment regimens hold promise for the future.[29]

Tuberculosis

Despite a declining overall incidence of TB in the United States to a record low,[30] outbreaks of TB in certain populations, including the homeless, continue to be a public health challenge.[3] A prevalence of 6%[31] and incidence 46 times the general population has been estimated for homeless people.[32] Poor nutritional status and concomitant illnesses such as HIV may promote susceptibility to TB and progression to active disease.[33] Poorly ventilated and overcrowded living conditions were responsible for several recent outbreaks.[34]

Early recognition and treatment of disease are imperative to improve health outcomes and limit the spread of TB to others.[33] Unfortunately, issues such as alcohol use, use of illicit drugs, incarceration, and underlying psychiatric illness contribute to difficulties in diagnosis and treatment of TB in the homeless.[30] The transient nature of the homeless population makes contact identification and tracking difficult, and results in delays in diagnosis and treatment.[5] Poor compliance with treatment regimens leads to increased morbidity and mortality compared with the general population.[5]

Interferon-gamma release assays as an alternative to traditional skin testing, chest radiograph screening,[35] incentives,[36] directly observed therapy (DOT),[5] and the use of a simplified 12-dose regimen of isoniazid and rifapentine[37] are some of the strategies used to improve detection and treatment.

Other Infectious Diseases

Scabies and body louse infections are more common in homeless individuals compared with the general population.[38] Transmission occurs through close person-to-person contact or through contaminated clothing or bedding.[38] Louseborne disease caused by *Bartonella quintana* (trench fever) and *Rickettsia prowazekii* (typhus) is also possible.[39] Frequent scratching of pruritic skin can lead to bacterial superinfections.[38]

Community-acquired pneumonia and influenza are common in the homeless population.[40] Overcrowding, smoking and alcohol use, and chronic lung disease increase risk.[41] Vaccination against pneumococcal pneumonia and influenza is underutilized and recommended.[41] Homelessness is also associated with higher rates of tinea pedis, impetigo, and folliculitis.[39]

INJECTION DRUG USERS

Illicit drug use is a common and growing social problem in the United States, with an estimated prevalence of 9.4%.[42] Minorities, including African Americans and Latinos, are disproportionately affected.[43] Persons who inject drugs, also known as injection drug users (IDUs), are at a substantially increased risk of acquiring and transmitting blood-borne viruses such as HIV, hepatitis B virus (HBV), and HCV.[44,45] In addition, illicit drug use is associated with higher rates of TB and sexually transmitted infections (STIs).[46,47]

Factors that facilitate the transmission of infectious disease in drug users include unstable living conditions,[48] inability to access treatment programs,[49] and fear of criminalization and stigmatization,[48] as well as undiagnosed or untreated mental health disorders.[48] In addition, individuals may be asymptomatic and/or unaware they are actively infected, which puts unaffected partners at risk.

Illicit drug use impairs judgment, which can increase disease transmission through risky sexual behavior,[50] needle sharing, and the use of unsterile drug injection equipment (cookers, cotton, and rinse water).[48]

Finally, women IDUs of childbearing age face unique challenges. They often under-utilize family planning and prenatal services.[48] Moreover, actively infected pregnant women who use illicit drugs are at risk of transmitting disease to their children during pregnancy and delivery.[48]

Human Immunodeficiency Virus–Acquired Immunodeficiency Syndrome

Injection drug use is currently the third most common risk factor for contracting HIV and accounted for 8% or 3900 new cases in 2010.[51] HIV transmission also occurs through high-risk sexual behaviors, including but not limited to unprotected sex and engaging in sexual behaviors under the influence of drugs or in exchange for drugs.[52] Coinfection with other infectious diseases, such as HCV and herpes simplex virus (HSV)-2, is common and further increases transmission and progression of disease.[48]

Addressing comorbid conditions, such as mental illness, substance use disorders, and homelessness, improves HIV treatment.[53] Delaying treatment due to concerns about nonadherence is unwarranted,[54] and may contribute to further spread of HIV[55] and lower survival rates.[56] In addition, treatment with antiretroviral therapy (ART) of infected individuals prevents transmission to others.[48] Care should be taken when combining ART with other drugs, such as methadone and buprenorphine, because potentially toxic drug interactions can occur.[57]

Tuberculosis

Similar to other underserved populations, TB prevention, identification, and treatment remain a challenge among illicit drug users.[47] Drug use has been associated with increased prevalence of both latent TB infection (LTBI) and active TB.[58] Several studies report an LTBI prevalence of 10% to 59%.[47] Several factors may contribute to the high prevalence of TB in drug users, including homelessness, prior incarceration,[59] alcohol[60] and tobacco use,[61] and concurrent HIV.[62] Some evidence suggests drug use may have a direct effect on cell-mediated immune response[63,64] but the clinical significance of this remains unclear.[64]

Drug users with TB have higher rates and longer periods of infectivity, which leads to greater likelihood of transmission[65] and extrapulmonary disease.[62] Coinfection with HIV, HBV, and HCV is common.[59] Coinfection with HIV increases progression from latent to active infection[62] and is associated with higher TB-related mortality.[66] Drug users are less likely to get screened or to initiate and complete treatment, resulting in increased transmission, the development of multidrug resistance, and more severe disease.[67]

Hepatitis B and C Viruses

Being an IDU is the most common risk factor in the transmission of HCV in the United States, accounting for 48% of all new infections in 2007.[68] Furthermore, IDUs accounted for 15% of the 43,000 new cases of HBV[68]; 75% to 90% of IDUs are anti-HCV positive.[69] An emerging epidemic of HCV infection is being seen in young adult injection drug users who have transitioned from the use of oral opioids.[70] Coinfection with HBV and HCV is not uncommon.[71] Among HIV-infected persons who inject drugs illicitly, 80% also are infected with HCV.[49] Compared with HIV, HCV is much more infectious[72] and can survive in syringes and on inanimate objects for prolonged periods of time.[73] As a result, environmental contamination and sharing injection preparation equipment are important modes of transmission.[74] Newer, highly effective and tolerated treatment regimens for HCV are available.[29] Administering HCV treatment in concert with medically supervised opioid therapy can increase adherence and treatment success.[29]

Other Infectious Diseases

The reported prevalence rates of STIs among persons who use drugs illicitly are 1% to 6% for syphilis, 1% to 5% for chlamydia, 1% to 3% for gonorrhea, and 38% to 61% for HSV-2 infection.[48] Skin and soft tissue infections, such as cellulitis and abscesses, are common in IDUs and are frequent reasons for hospital admission.[75] Right-sided infective endocarditis, most commonly caused by *Staphylococcus aureus*, can occur.[76] Coinfection with HIV is not infrequent and advanced immunosuppression (CD4 count <200/mm^3) increases mortality.[76] Nonadherence to long inpatient antibiotic treatment regimens is common in IDUs.[76] Shorter courses of antibiotics and the use of oral therapy in the outpatient setting may be appropriate in some cases.[76]

LESBIAN, GAY, BISEXUAL, AND TRANSGENDER

Although some progress has been made in understanding and addressing health disparities in the lesbian, gay, bisexual, and transgender (LGBT) community, it remains a significant national public health issue. LGBT populations, like other marginalized groups, face barriers to culturally competent and quality health care.[77] They are more likely to lack insurance coverage and experience significant societal stigma and discrimination.[77]

Mental illness,[78] substance use,[79] and sexual and physical abuse[80] occur at higher rates compared with the heterosexual population and have negative consequences on general health. In addition to some infectious diseases, studies have found that sexual and gender minorities have more chronic conditions and overall poorer health status.[78] Recent policy and legal changes offering nondiscrimination protections[81] and recognizing same-sex marriage[82,83] may help to mitigate some of these challenges.

Human Immunodeficiency Virus–Acquired Immunodeficiency Syndrome

Although MSM are greatly affected by HIV/AIDS, minority men are disproportionally affected.[77] In 2010, it was estimated that MSM accounted for 56% of all HIV cases and roughly two-thirds of the 50,000 new cases of HIV in the United States.[84] Coinfection with other STIs, including syphilis, among HIV-positive MSM is common.[85]

Transgender women, especially African Americans, are also significantly affected by HIV/AIDS. Prevalence rates of 28% and 56%, respectively, have been reported.[86] However, transgender women are less likely to receive ART[87] and have higher HIV-related morbidity and mortality compared with other populations.[88] Possible interactions between ART and hormone therapy is a concern for many transgender women.[89]

HIV prevalence in transgender men is low (0%–3%)[89] but data are limited.[90] Moreover, although female to female sexual transmission of HIV is rare,[91] lesbian, bisexual, and other women who have sex with women (WSW) are still at risk of HIV primarily through male sexual contact and injection drug use.[92]

Human Papilloma Virus

Transmission of the human papilloma virus (HPV) between female sexual partners is common.[93] Furthermore, most WSW have had sex with men and many continue to do so.[94] Abnormalities have been detected on cervical smear testing, even in women who have not had sex with men,[95] highlighting the importance of adherence to current cervical cancer screening and vaccination guidelines.

The prevalence of HPV is high in MSM, increasing the risk of genital warts and cancers of the penis, oropharynx, and anus.[96] MSM are 17 times more likely to develop anal cancer than heterosexual men,[97] with a much higher rate in those who are coinfected with HIV/AIDS.[98]

Other Infectious Diseases

Primary and secondary syphilis in the United States have continued to increase at an alarming rate in MSM, now accounting for 83% of new cases.[85] MSM transmission accounts for 15% to 25% of all new cases of HBV.[99] In MSM, gonorrheal and chlamydial infections of the rectum and pharynx are common, especially in those with HIV.[100] The prevalence of bacterial vaginosis in WSW is estimated to be nearly 26% compared with 14% in heterosexual populations.[101] The results of several studies suggest female to female sexual transmission is likely.[101,102] Limited data exist on transmission rates of STIs among WSW but probably varies by the type of STI and sexual behavior.[103]

INMATE POPULATION

Individuals who inhabit correctional facilities, both state and federal, are at increased risk for infectious disease.[104] The prevalence of HIV and other infectious diseases is much higher among inmates than among the general population.[104] High-risk sexual behavior and illicit drug use among incarcerated inmates, and a general lack of condoms and sterile needles or syringes, predispose these individuals to greater risk of infectious diseases.[104] The prevalence of ever having an infectious disease among state and federal prisoners and the general population are compared in **Table 1**.[105]

A similar comparison is presented in **Table 2** among jail inmates versus the general population.[105]

Human Immunodeficiency Virus–Acquired Immunodeficiency Syndrome

Contracting HIV for men and women is far more likely in prison.[106] Incarcerated women suffer disproportionately from HIV/AIDS and other infectious diseases.[107] High-risk behavior among prison inmates is likely a significant contributing factor to transmission and acquisition of HIV.[108,109] Unfortunately, prisoners in low- and middle-income countries (LMICs) are at much higher risk for HIV and other infectious diseases. The prisoner prevalence of HIV in 20 LMICs is greater than 10%.[110] Overcrowding, lack of public health initiatives, and inadequate access to clean injecting equipment for intravenous drug users are among the reasons for the continued higher risk for HIV and other infectious diseases among incarcerated prisoners.[111]

Education and enhanced protection from sexually transmitted diseases, along with expanded HIV testing among the US inmate population will likely continue to reduce the rate of HIV among all US incarcerated individuals.[104,112] Awareness of HIV status does affect risk behavior, supporting arguments for increased HIV screening among

Table 1
Prevalence of ever having infectious disease among state and federal prisoners versus general population

	State and Federal Prisoners		General Population	
	Percent (%)	Standard Error	Percent (%)	Standard Error
Ever had an infectious disease[a]	21.0	1.3%	4.8	0.2%
TB	6.0	0.6	0.5	0.1
Hepatitis[b]	10.9	1.0	1.1	0.1
Sexually transmitted diseases[c]	6.0	0.5	3.4	0.1

[a] Excludes HIV or AIDS due to unknown or missing data.
[b] Includes hepatitis B and C for the prison population and all types of hepatitis for the general population.
[c] Excludes HIV or AIDS.
Adapted from The prevalence of ever having an infectious disease among state and federal prisoners and the general population (2011–12). Bureau, National Inmate Survey (NIS), 2011–12; and the Substance Abuse and Mental Health Services Administration, National Survey on Drug Use and Health (NSDUH), 2009–2012.

jail and prison populations.[113] **Fig. 1** reflects the declining rate of HIV or AIDS among US incarcerated individuals.

RACIAL AND ETHNIC MINORITIES

According to the 2010 US Census, approximately 36.3% of the population currently belongs to a racial or ethnic minority group: American Indian or Alaska Native (AI/AN), Asian American, Black or African American, Hispanic or Latino, and Native Hawaiian or other Pacific Islander.[114] Racial and ethnic health disparities are widespread in the United States.[115,116] These disparities are apparent in regard to infectious disease.[117,118] For example, morbidity and mortality rates from HIV/AIDS in the United States are highest among black or African American, Hispanic or Latino, and native Hawaiian or other Pacific Islander racial or ethnic minorities.[119]

Table 2
Prevalence of ever having infectious disease among state and federal jail inmates versus general population

	Jail Inmates		General Population	
	Percent (%)	Standard Error	Percent (%)	Standard Error
Ever had an infectious disease[a]	14.3	0.7%	4.6	0.1%
TB	2.5	0.3	0.4	<0.05
Hepatitis[b]	6.5	0.5	0.9	<0.05
Sexually transmitted diseases[c]	6.1	0.5	3.5	0.1

[a] Excludes HIV or AIDS due to unknown or missing data.
[b] Includes HBV and HCV for the jail population, and all types of hepatitis for the general population.
[c] Excludes HIV or AIDS.
Adapted from The prevalence of ever having an infectious disease among state and federal jail inmates and the general population (2011–12). Bureau, National Inmate Survey (NIS), 2011–12; and the Substance Abuse and Mental Health Services Administration, National Survey on Drug Use and Health (NSDUH), 2009–2012.

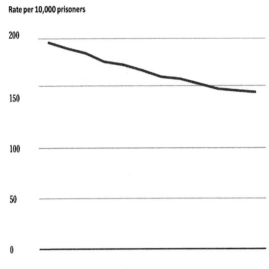

Rate per 10,000 prisoners

2001 2002 2003 2004 2005 2006 2007 2008 2009 2010 2011 2012

Fig. 1. Rate of HIV or AIDS cases among state and federal prisoners, 2001 to 2012. (*Data from* Bureau of Justice Statistics, National Prisoner Statistics Program, 2001–2012. Available at: http://www.bjs.gov/content/pub/pdf/mpsfpji1112.pdf. Accessed March 8, 2016.)

Human Immunodeficiency Virus–Acquired Immunodeficiency Syndrome

The AIDS epidemic disproportionately affects racial and ethnic minorities. In 2007, African Americans made up 13% of the US population but accounted for nearly half of PLWHA. HIV/AIDS rates (cases per 100,000) were 77 among black or African Americans, 35 among Native Hawaiians or other Pacific Islanders, 28 among Hispanics, 13 among AI/AN, 9.2 among whites, and 7.7 among Asian Americans.[120]

Non-Asian racial or ethnic minorities continue to experience higher rates of HIV diagnosis than whites. Compared with whites, a lower percentage of blacks diagnosed with HIV were prescribed ART and a lower percentage of both blacks and Hispanics had suppressed viral loads.[121]

Tuberculosis

TB case rates declined among all racial or ethnic minority groups and among US and foreign-born individuals from 2006 to 2010. However, rates remained higher among racial or ethnic minority groups than among whites in 2010.[122] Case rates of TB in the United States are still highest among the foreign-born who have immigrated from Latin America, Asia, and Africa[122,123] but are also elevated among US born black and AI/AN persons.[124,125] Lower respiratory tract infection morbidity and mortality rates are higher among AI/AN children than US children.[114,126]

There are also substantial racial and ethnic disparities for most, if not all, vaccine-preventable illnesses, most notably including HBV, influenza, and pneumococcal disease.[114] The CDC's Racial and Ethnic Adult Disparities in Immunization Initiative (READII) was a 2-year project aimed to improve immunization rates for influenza and pneumococcal pneumonia among the African-American and Hispanic communities. Results were favorable, and many strategies for bridging the immunization gap were developed and learned.[127,128]

HEALTH LITERACY

Health literacy is the degree to which individuals have the capacity to obtain, process, and understand basic health information and services needed to make appropriate health decisions.[129] Limited health literacy affects all ages, races, incomes, and education levels; however, the impact of limited health literacy disproportionately affects lower socioeconomic and minority groups.[130] It also affects people's ability to search for and use health information, adopt healthy behaviors, and act on important public health alerts. Limited health literacy is also associated with worse health outcomes and higher costs.[131]

Although limited health literacy affects most adults at some point in their lives, there are disparities in prevalence and severity. Some groups are more likely than others to have limited health literacy:

- Adults older than the age of 65 years
- Racial and ethnic groups other than white
- Recent refugees and immigrants
- People with less than a high school or general educational development degree (GED)
- People with incomes at or below the poverty level
- Non-native speakers of English.[132]

Limited health literacy is negatively associated with the use of preventive services (eg, mammograms or flu shots), management of chronic conditions (eg, diabetes, high blood pressure, asthma, and HIV/AIDS), and self-reported health.[132] Recent research has focused on health literacy as one of the critical factors in health disparities.[133–135] The greatest opportunities for reducing health disparities are in empowering individuals and changing the health system to meet their needs.[135] The National Action Plan to Improve Health Literacy, released May 2010 by the US Department of Health and Human Services, seeks to engage organizations, professionals, policymakers, communities, individuals, and families in a linked, multisector effort to improve health literacy.[132] The plan includes 7 broad goals with multiple high-level strategies for various stakeholders and provides a focal point for the field.

What are the 7 Goals in the Plan?

- Goal 1: Develop and disseminate health and safety information that is accurate, accessible, and actionable.
- Goal 2: Promote changes in the health care delivery system that improve information, communication, informed decision-making, and access to health services.
- Goal 3: Incorporate accurate and standards-based health and developmentally appropriate health and science information and curricula into child care and education through the university level.
- Goal 4: Support and expand local efforts to provide adult education, English-language instruction, and culturally and linguistically appropriate health information services in the community.
- Goal 5: Build partnerships, develop guidance, and change policies.
- Goal 6: Increase basic research and the development, implementation, and evaluation of practices and interventions to improve health literacy.
- Goal 7: Increase the dissemination and use of evidence-based health literacy practices and interventions.[132]

BARRIERS TO HEALTH CARE FOR THE UNDERSERVED

The advent of the ACA has made health insurance more accessible for millions of Americans, including underserved populations. It also offers access to preventive services, including screening for HIV, STIs, depression, and substance abuse; the delivery of culturally competent care; coordinated care for chronic conditions; and calls for enhanced data collection and research on health disparities. Despite these advancements, significant barriers to quality medical care still exist (**Box 1**).[47,77,136–141]

DISEASE PREVENTION AND HARM REDUCTION STRATEGIES

Implementing culturally competent public health strategies in a manner that respects the rights of underserved populations is vital for preventing and treating HIV infection, TB, viral hepatitis, STIs, and other infectious diseases.

Box 1
Barriers to heath care

Health care delivery system barriers
- Inadequate number of providers
- Location of clinics and hospitals
- Availability (operating hours and long appointment wait times)
- Limited data or research on issues related to underserved
- Inadequate reimbursement for behavioral health services in primary care setting
- Inadequate education, testing, and counseling services
- Restricted access to substance use treatment, mental health, and specialty care (HIV clinics)
- Increased administrative and infrastructure challenges with Medicaid expansion

Provider barriers
- Lack of cultural competency
- Poor attitudes
- Lack awareness and knowledge of specific health needs of underserved populations
- Bias, unwelcoming environment

Individual or population barriers
- Lack insurance coverage
- Lack of primary care provider
- Low education and health literacy
- Language barriers
- Immigration status
- Lack support system
- Comorbid mental illness and/or substance abuse
- Mistrust of health care system due to previous negative experiences
- Difficulty adhering to treatment or medication regimens
- Concerns about confidentiality
- Sexual and physical violence (LGBT community)
- Lack of documentation, such as an identification card

Health Care Delivery System Improvement Strategies

Although providing comprehensive, integrated, and accessible care in a safe nondiscriminatory environment free from fear of harassment and/or legal intervention is the first priority,[48,66,141,142] the first task may be assessing health care provider's attitudes and knowledge, and providing the necessary training and education.[136]

Targeted counseling, education, and risk assessment (eg, for drug use and STIs) in concert with timely disease-specific testing[48,136,142,143] is fundamental, along with improving the availability and access to condoms[3,48]; vaccination programs[3,48]; evidence-based interventions, such as ART,[136,142] TB, and pre-exposure prophylaxis[142]; and mental health services.[48,136]

Vital for IDUs are access to sterile injection and drug preparation equipment (ie, needle exchange programs),[48,136,140–143] training in overdose prevention and the provision of naloxone,[144] and improving access to substance abuse treatment programs such as medication-assisted therapy (MAT).[48,66,136,141–143]

Prevention and control strategies in shelters include ensuring adequate ventilation[5] and strict enforcement of screening and education programs for all staff and clients.[5,66] Protocols for identifying high-risk clients (eg, those with HIV) and handling and/or referral of symptomatic clients (eg, cough alert logs) are important.[66] Finally, bed systems to position (head to toe) and track potentially infectious clients can be helpful.

Providing multiple services (testing, diagnosis, and treatment) in one location,[48,66] combining treatment services (DOT for TB, MAT for substance abuse,[66] hormone therapy, and ART)[142] and supervised therapy (DOT, MAT)[66] can improve adherence. Adherence reminders, such as beepers, pill boxes and calendars, and providing incentives also may be useful.[48,66,136]

Support Services Improvement Strategies

Community-based outreach programs aim to engage at-risk populations by providing disease-specific and risk reduction education, materials such as condoms and clean needles, and crisis intervention and referrals to essential support services, including drug treatment programs.[48,66,136,137,141]

Despite health insurance becoming more accessible and affordable for many underserved, the enrollment process can be complicated and confusing.[138] Frontline workers, including case managers, are uniquely positioned to help guide individuals through this complex process.[138] In addition, assistance is needed with transportation (eg, bus tickets),[138] housing, employment services, and legal advice.[142]

Confidential notification of partners who may have been exposed to certain infectious diseases (STIs, HIV, and HCV) through high-risk sexual behavior and/or being an IDU is effective in reducing further transmission.[48] Disease-specific testing, counseling, vaccination, and referral for treatment or other needed services may be necessary.[48]

REFERENCES

1. Focus on health care disparities. Disparities in health and health care: five key questions and answers. Menlo park (CA): The Henry J Kaiser Family Foundation; 2012.
2. Kullgren J, McLaughlin C, Mitra N, et al. Nonfinancial barriers and access to care for U.S. adults. Health Serv Res 2011;47(1pt2):462–85.
3. Badiaga S, Raoult D, Brouqui P. Preventing and controlling emerging and reemerging transmissible diseases in the homeless. Emerg Infect Dis 2008;14(9):1353–9.

4. Kidder DP, Wolitski RJ, Campsmith ML, et al. Health status, health care use, medication use, and medication adherence among homeless and housed people living with HIV/AIDS. Am J Public Health 2007;97(12):2238–45.

5. McAdam JM. Combatting tuberculosis and homelessness: recommendations for policy and practice. Nashville (TN): National Health Care for the Homeless Council; 1994.

6. Sermons MW, Witte P. State of homelessness in America. Washington, DC: National Alliance to End Homelessness; 2011.

7. Hwang SW, Henderson MJ. Health care utilization in homeless people: translating research into policy and practice. Agency for Healthcare Research and Quality Working Paper No. 10002. 2010. Available at: http://gold.ahrq.gov. Accessed March 8, 2016.

8. Bharel M, Lin W, Zhang J, et al. Health care utilization patterns of homeless individuals in Boston: Preparing for Medicaid expansion under the Affordable Care Act. Am J Public Health 2013;103(S2):S311–7.

9. Moore J. Unaccompanied and homeless youth: review of literature. Greensboro (NC): National Center for Homeless Education; 1995–2005.

10. HIV/AIDS and homelessness. Washington, DC: National Coalition for the Homeless; 2009.

11. Robertson M, Clark R, Charlebois E, et al. HIV seroprevalence among homeless and marginally housed adults in San Francisco. Am J Public Health 2004;94(7): 1207–17.

12. Fact sheet: homelessness and HIV/AIDS. Washington, DC: National Alliance to End Homelessness; 2006.

13. Tomaszewski EP. Human rights update. HIV/AIDS and homelessness. Washington, DC: National Association of Social Workers; 2011.

14. Marshall B, Shannon K, Kerr T, et al. Survival sex work and increased HIV risk among sexual minority street-involved youth. J Acquir Immune Defic Syndr 2010;53(5):661–4.

15. Aidala A, Cross J, Stall R, et al. Housing status and HIV risk behaviors: Implications for prevention and policy. AIDS Behav 2005;9(3):251–65.

16. Aidala A, Lee G, Abramson D, et al. Housing need, housing assistance, and connection to HIV medical care. AIDS Behav 2007;11(S2):101–15.

17. Chak E, Talal A, Sherman K, et al. Hepatitis C virus infection in USA: An estimate of true prevalence. Liver Int 2011;31(8):1090–101.

18. Royal S, Kidder D, Patrabansh S, et al. Factors associated with adherence to highly active antiretroviral therapy in homeless or unstably housed adults living with HIV. AIDS Care 2009;21(4):448–55.

19. Schwarcz S, Hsu L, Vittinghoff E, et al. Impact of housing on the survival of persons with AIDS. BMC Public Health 2009;9(1):220.

20. Nelson K, Thiede H, Hawes S, et al. Why the wait? Delayed diagnosis among men who have sex with men. J Urban Health 2010;87(4):642–55.

21. Milloy M, Marshall B, Montaner J, et al. Housing status and the health of people living with HIV/AIDS. Curr HIV/AIDS Rep 2012;9(4):364–74.

22. Audain G, Bookhardt-Murray LJ, Fogg CJ, et al, editors. Adapting your practice: treatment and recommendations for unstably housed patients with HIV/AIDS. Nashville (TN): Health Care for the Homeless Clinicians' Network, National Health Care for the Homeless Council, Inc; 2013.

23. Gelberg L, Robertson MJ, Arangua L. Prevalence, distribution, and correlates of Hepatitis C virus infection among homeless adults in Los Angeles. Public Health Rep 2012;127:407–21.

24. Strehlow A, Robertson M, Zerger S, et al. Hepatitis C among clients of health care for the homeless primary care clinics. J Health Care Poor Underserved 2012;23(2):811–33.

25. Hayes B, Briceno A, Asher A, et al. Preference, acceptability and implications of the rapid hepatitis C screening test among high-risk young people who inject drugs. BMC Public Health 2014;14(1):645.

26. Moyer V. Screening for Hepatitis C virus infection in adults: U.S. Preventive Services Task Force recommendation statement. Ann Intern Med 2013;159(5):349.

27. Centers for Disease Control and Prevention. Testing for HCV infection: an update of guidance for clinicians and laboratorians. MMWR Morb Mortal Wkly Rep 2013;62:362–5.

28. Shivkumar S, Peeling R, Jafari Y, et al. Accuracy of rapid and point-of-care screening tests for Hepatitis C. Ann Intern Med 2012;157(8):558.

29. McCance-Katz E, Valdiserri R. Hepatitis C virus treatment and injection drug users: it is time to separate fact from fiction. Ann Intern Med 2015;163(3):224.

30. Centers for Disease Control and Prevention. Trends in Tuberculosis – United States, 2012. MMWR Morb Mortal Wkly Rep 2013;62:201–5.

31. Bamrah S, Yelk Woodruff R, Powell K, et al. Tuberculosis among the homeless, United States, 1994–2010. Int J Tuberc Lung Dis 2013;17(11):1414–9.

32. Beijer U, Wolf A, Fazel S. Prevalence of tuberculosis, hepatitis C virus, and HIV in homeless people: a systematic review and meta-analysis. Lancet Infect Dis 2012;12(11):859–70.

33. Tan de Bibiana J, Rossi C, Rivest P, et al. Tuberculosis and homelessness in Montreal: a retrospective cohort study. BMC Public Health 2011;11(1):833.

34. Centers for Disease Control and Prevention. Reported tuberculosis in the United States, 2013. 2014.

35. Paquette K, Cheng M, Kadatz M, et al. Chest radiography for active tuberculosis case finding in the homeless: a systematic review and meta-analysis. Int J Tuberc Lung Dis 2014;18(10):1231–6.

36. Lutge E, Wiysonge C, Knight S, et al. Material incentives and enablers in the management of tuberculosis. Cochrane Database Syst Rev 2012;(1):CD007952.

37. Sterling T, Villarino M, Borisov A, et al. Three months of rifapentine and isoniazid for latent tuberculosis infection. N Engl J Med 2011;365(23):2155–66.

38. Badiaga S, Menard A, Tissot Dupont H, et al. Prevalence of skin infections in sheltered homeless. Eur J Dermatol 2005;15:382–6.

39. Raoult D, Foucault C, Brouqui P. Infections in the homeless. Lancet Infect Dis 2001;1(2):77–84.

40. Roncarati J, Bernardo J. Community acquired pneumonia. The health care of homeless persons - Part I. In: the health care of homeless persons: a manual of communicable diseases and common problems in shelters and on the streets. Boston: The Boston Health Care for the Homeless Program; 2004.

41. Wrezel O. Respiratory infections in the homeless. UWO Med J 2009;78(2):61–5.

42. National Institute on Drug Abuse. Nationwide trends. Available at: http://www.drugabuse.gov/publications/drugfacts/nationwide-trends. Accessed January 20, 2016.

43. Estrada A. Epidemiology of HIV/AIDS, hepatitis B, hepatitis C, and tuberculosis among minority injection drug users. Public Health Rep 2002;117(Suppl 1): S126–34.

44. Lansky A, Books J, DiNenno E, et al. Epidemiology of HIV in the United States. J Acquir Immune Defic Syndr 2010;55(Suppl 2):S64–8.

45. Nelson P, Mathers B, Cowie B, et al. Global epidemiology of hepatitis B and hepatitis C in people who inject drugs: Results of systematic reviews. Lancet 2011; 378(9791):571–83.

46. Des Jarlais D, Semaan S, Arasteh K. At 30 years: HIV/AIDS and other STDs among persons who use psychoactive drugs. In: Hall B, Hall J, Cockerell C, editors. HIV/AIDS in the post-HAART Era: manifestations, treatment, and epidemiology. Shelton (CT): People's Medical Publishing House; 2011. p. 753–78.

47. Deiss R, Rodwell T, Garfein R. Tuberculosis and illicit drug use: Review and update. Clin Infect Dis 2009;48(1):72–82.

48. Centers for Disease Control and Prevention. Integrated prevention services for HIV infection, viral hepatitis, sexually transmitted diseases, and tuberculosis for persons who use drugs illicitly: summary guidance from CDC and the U.S. Department of Health and Human Services. MMWR Morb Mortal Wkly Rep 2012;61(RR-5):1–46.

49. Tempalski B, Cleland C, Pouget E, et al. Persistence of low drug treatment coverage for injection drug users in large metropolitan areas. Subst Abuse Treat Prev Policy 2010;5:23.

50. Des Jarlais D, Semaan S. HIV and other sexually transmitted infections in injection drug users and crack cocaine smokers. In: Holmes KK, Sparling PF, Stamm WE, et al, editors. Sexually transmitted diseases. 4th edition. New York: McGraw-Hill; 2008. p. 237–55.

51. Centers for Disease Control and Prevention. Estimated HIV incidence in the United States, 2007–2010. HIV Surveillance Supplemental Report 2012;17(4).

52. Kral A, Bluthenthal R, Lorvick J, et al. Sexual transmission of HIV-1 among injection drug users in San Francisco, USA: Risk-factor analysis. Lancet 2001; 357(9266):1397–401.

53. Altice F, Kamarulzaman A, Soriano V, et al. Treatment of medical, psychiatric, and substance-use comorbidities in people infected with HIV who use drugs. Lancet 2010;376(9738):367–87.

54. Malta M, Magnanini M, Strathdee S, et al. Adherence to antiretroviral therapy among HIV-infected drug users: a meta-analysis. AIDS Behav 2008;14(4): 731–47.

55. Cohen M, Chen Y, McCauley M, et al. Prevention of HIV-infection with early antiretroviral therapy. N Engl J Med 2011;365(6):493–505.

56. Kitahata M, Gange S, Abraham A, et al. Effect of early versus deferred antiretroviral therapy for HIV on survival. N Engl J Med 2009;360(18):1815–26.

57. McCance-Katz EF, Sullivan L, Nallani S. Drug Interactions of clinical importance among the opioids, methadone and buprenorphine, and other frequently prescribed medications: a review. Am J Addict 2010;19(1):4–16.

58. Mamani M, Majzoobi M, Torabian S, et al. Latent and active tuberculosis: Evaluation of injecting drug users. Iran Red Crescent Med J 2013;15(9):775–9.

59. Getahun H, Gunneberg C, Sculier D, et al. Tuberculosis and HIV in people who inject drugs: Evidence for action for TB, HIV, prison and harm reduction services. Curr Opin HIV AIDS 2012;7(4):345–53.

60. Getahun H, Baddeley A, Raviglione M. Managing tuberculosis in people who use and inject illicit drugs. Bull World Health Organ 2013;91(2):154–6.

61. Altet-Gomez MN, Alcaide J, Godoy P, et al. Clinical and epidemiological aspects of smoking and tuberculosis: a study of 13,038 cases. Int J Tuberc Lung Dis 2005;9:430–6.

62. Selwyn P, Hartel D, Lewis V, et al. A prospective study of the risk of tuberculosis among intravenous drug users with human immunodeficiency virus infection. N Engl J Med 1989;320(9):545–50.

63. Wei G, Moss J, Yuan C. Opioid-induced immunosuppression: Is it centrally mediated or peripherally mediated? Biochem Pharmacol 2003;65(11):1761–6.

64. Kapadia F, Vlahov D, Donahoe R, et al. The role of substance abuse in HIV disease progression: reconciling differences from laboratory and epidemiologic investigations. Clin Infect Dis 2005;41(7):1027–34.

65. Oeltmann J, Kammerer J, Pevzner E, et al. Tuberculosis and substance abuse in the United States, 1997-2006. Arch Intern Med 2009;169(2):189.

66. World Health Organization (WHO). Policy Guidelines for Collaborative TB and HIV Services for injecting and other drug users an integrated approach. 2008.

67. Golub JE, Bur S, Cronin WA, et al. Delayed tuberculosis diagnosis and tuberculosis transmission. Int J Tuberc Lung Dis 2006;10:24–30.

68. Daniels D, Grytdal S, Wasley A. Surveillance for acute viral hepatitis—United States, 2007. MMWR Surveill Summ 2009;58(SS-3):1–27.

69. Amon J, Garfein R, Ahdieh-Grant L, et al. Prevalence of hepatitis C virus infection among injection drug users in the United States, 1994–2004. Clin Infect Dis 2008;46(12):1852–8.

70. Page K, Morris M, Hahn J, et al. Injection drug use and hepatitis C virus infection in young adult injectors: Using evidence to inform comprehensive prevention. Clin Infect Dis 2013;57(Suppl 2):S32–8.

71. Chu C, Lee S. Hepatitis B virus/hepatitis C virus coinfection: epidemiology, clinical features, viral interactions and treatment. J Gastroenterol Hepatol 2008; 23(4):512–20.

72. Wicker S, Cinatl J, Berger A, et al. Determination of risk of infection with blood-borne pathogens following a needlestick injury in hospital workers. Ann Occup Hyg 2008;52(7):615–22.

73. Doerrbecker J, Friesland M, Ciesek S, et al. Inactivation and survival of hepatitis C virus on inanimate surfaces. J Infect Dis 2011;204(12):1830–8.

74. Pouget E, Hagan H, Des Jarlais D. Meta-analysis of hepatitis C seroconversion in relation to shared syringes and drug preparation equipment. Addiction 2012; 107(6):1057–65.

75. Ebright J, Pieper B. Skin and soft tissue infections in injection drug users. Infect Dis Clin North Am 2002;16(3):697–712.

76. Moss R, Munt B. Injection drug use and right sided endocarditis. Heart 2003; 89(5):577–81.

77. Kates J, Ranji U, Beamesderfer A, et al. Health and access to care and coverage for lesbian, gay, bisexual, and transgender individuals in the US. Menlo Park (CA): The Henry J. Kaiser Family Foundation; 2015. Issue Brief.

78. Lick D, Durso L, Johnson K. Minority stress and physical health among sexual minorities. Perspect Psychol Sci 2013;8(5):521–48.

79. Ostrow D, Stall R. Alcohol, tobacco, and drug use among gay and bisexual men. In: Wolitski R, Stall R, Valdiserri R, editors. Unequal opportunity: health disparities affecting gay and bisexual men in the United States. New York: Oxford University Press; 2008. p. 1–60.

80. Centers for Disease Control and Prevention. The National Intimate Partner and Sexual Violence Survey: 2010 findings on victimization by sexual orientation. 2013.

81. Department of Health and Human Services. Patient Protection and Affordable Care Act; standards related to essential health benefits, actuarial value and accreditation. Final rule. Fed Reg 2013;78(37):12833–72.

82. Supreme Court of the United States, United States v. Windsor, June 26, 2013.

83. Supreme Court of the United States, Obergefell v. Hodges, June 26, 2015.

84. Centers for Disease Control and Prevention. HIV among gay, bisexual, and other men who have sex with men. 2013.

85. Centers for Disease Control and Prevention. Sexually transmitted disease surveillance 2014. Atlanta (GA): U.S. Department of Health and Human Services; 2015.

86. Centers for Disease Control and Prevention. HIV among transgender people. 2013.

87. Melendez R, Pinto R. HIV prevention and primary care for transgender women in a community-based clinic. J Assoc Nurses AIDS Care 2009;20(5):387–97.

88. San Francisco Department of Public Health. HIV/AIDS epidemiology annual report. San Francisco (CA): HIV Epidemiology Section 2010.

89. Sevelius J. Transgender issues in HIV. HIV Specialist December 2013.

90. Bauer G, Redman N, Bradley K, et al. Sexual health of trans men who are gay, bisexual, or who have sex with men: results from Ontario, Canada. Int J Transgend 2013;14(2):66–74.

91. Kwakwa H, Ghobrial M. Female-to-female transmission of human immunodeficiency virus. Clin Infect Dis 2003;36(3):e40–1.

92. Chan S, Lupita R, Thornton K, et al. Likely female-to-female sexual transmission of HIV — Texas, 2012. MMWR Morb Mortal Wkly Rep 2014;63(10):209–12.

93. Marrazzo J, Stine K, Koutsky L. Genital human papillomavirus infection in women who have sex with women: a review. Am J Obstet Gynecol 2000; 183(3):770–4.

94. Diamant A, Schuster M, McGuigan K, et al. Lesbians' sexual history with men. Arch Intern Med 1999;159(22):2730.

95. Marrazzo J, Koutsky L, Kiviat N, et al. Papanicolaou test screening and prevalence of genital human papillomavirus among women who have sex with women. J Low Genit Tract Dis 2002;6(1):61–2.

96. Goldstone S, Palefsky J, Giuliano A, et al. Prevalence of and risk factors for human papillomavirus (HPV) infection among HIV-seronegative men who have sex with men. J Infect Dis 2011;203(1):66–74.

97. Frisch M. Cancer in a population-based cohort of men and women in registered homosexual partnerships. Am J Epidemiol 2003;157(11):966–72.

98. Frisch M. Human papillomavirus-associated cancers in patients with human immunodeficiency virus infection and acquired immunodeficiency syndrome. J Natl Cancer Inst 2000;92(18):1500–10.

99. Centers for Disease Control and Prevention. Viral hepatitis and men who have sex with men. 2012.

100. Scott K, Philip S, Ahrens K, et al. High prevalence of gonococcal and chlamydial infection in men who have sex with men with newly diagnosed HIV infection. J Acquir Immune Defic Syndr 2008;48(1):109–12.

101. Evans A, Scally A, Wellard S, et al. Prevalence of bacterial vaginosis in lesbians and heterosexual women in a community setting. Sex Transm Infect 2007;83(6): 470–5.

102. Vodstrcil L, Walker S, Hocking J, et al. Incident bacterial vaginosis (BV) in women who have sex with women is associated with behaviors that suggest sexual transmission of BV. Clin Infect Dis 2015;60(7):1042–53.

103. Fethers K. Sexually transmitted infections and risk behaviours in women who have sex with women. Sex Transm Infect 2000;76(5):345–9.

104. Hammett TM. HIV/AIDS and other infectious diseases among correctional facilities: Transmission, burden, and an appropriate response. Am J Public Health 2006;96(6):974–8.

105. Bureau, National Inmate Survey (NIS), 2011-12; and the Substance Abuse and Mental Health Services Administration, National Survey on Drug Use and Health (NSDUH). The prevalence of ever having an infectious disease among state and federal prisoners and the general population (2011-12). 2009-2012.

106. Chandler C. Death and dying in America: The prison industrial complex's impact on women's health. Berkeley Womens Law J 2003;18:40–60.

107. Acoca L. Defusing the time bomb: understanding and meeting the growing health care needs of incarcerated women in America. Crime & Delinquency. Sage Publications 1998;49–69. Available at: http://cad.sagepub.com/content/44/1/49.Crime & Delinquency 44.1.

108. Choopanya K, Des Jarlais DC, Vanichseni S, et al. Incarceration and risk for HIV infection among injection drug users in Bangkok. J Acquir Immune Defic Syndr 2002;29:86–94.

109. Buavirat A, Page-Shaffer K, van Griensven GJP, et al. Risk of prevalent HIV infection associated with incarceration among injecting drug users in Bangkok: case-control study. BMJ 2003;326:308.

110. Dolan K, Kite B, Black E, et al. HIV in prison in low-income and middle-income countries. Lancet Infect Dis 2007;7:32–41.

111. Simooya OO. Infections in prison in low and middle income countries: Prevalence and prevention strategies. Open Infect Dis J 2010;4:33–7.

112. Gough E, Kempf MC, Graham L, et al. HIV and hepatitis B and C incidence rates in U.S. correctional populations and high risk groups: A systematic review and meta-analysis. BMC Public Health 2010;10:777.

113. Marks G, Crepaz N, Senterfitt JW, et al. Meta-analysis of high-risk sexual behavior in persons aware and unaware they are infected with HIV in the United States. J Acquir Immune Defic Syndr 2005;39:446–53.

114. National Foundation for Infectious Diseases and the National Coalition for Adult Immunization. A report on reaching underserved ethnic and minority populations to improve adolescent and adult immunization rates. October 2002.

115. Braveman PA, Cubbin C, Egerter S, et al. Socioeconomic disparities in health in the United States: What the patterns tell us. Am J Public Health 2010;100(Suppl 1):S186–96.

116. Richardus JH, Kunst AE. Black-white differences in infectious disease mortality in the United States. Am J Public Health 2001;91(8):1251–3.

117. Adekoya N. Medicaid/state children's health insurance program patients and infectious diseases treated in emergency departments: U.S., 2003. Public Health Rep 2007;122(4):513–20. Available at: http://www.ncbi.nlm.nih.gov/pubmed/17639655. Accessed January 19, 2016.

118. Centers for Disease Control and Prevention. HIV surveillance report. Diagnosis of HIV Infection and AIDS in the United States and Dependent Areas. 2009.

119. Available at: https://report.nih.gov/nihfactsheets/viewfactsheet.aspx?csid=124. Accessed January 29, 2016.

120. Available at: http://stacks.cdc.gov/view/cdc/20865/cdc_20865_DS1.pdf. Accessed January 29, 2016.

121. Cain KP, Benoit SR, Winston CA, et al. Tuberculosis among foreign-born persons in the United States. JAMA 2008;300(4):405–12.

122. Cain KP, Haley CA, Armstrong LR, et al. Tuberculosis among foreign-born persons in the United States: achieving tuberculosis elimination. Am J Respir Crit Care Med 2007;175(1):75–9.
123. Bloss E, Holtz TH, Jereb J, et al. Tuberculosis in indigenous peoples in the U.S., 2003-2008. Public Health Rep 2011;126(5):677–89. Centers for Disease Control and Prevention, 2012. Available at: http://www.ncbi.nlm.nih.gov/pubmed/21886328. Accessed February 3, 2016.
124. Centers for Disease Control and Prevention (CDC). Trends in tuberculosis - United States, 2011. MMWR Morb Mortal Wkly Rep 2012;61(11):181–5. Available at: http://www.ncbi.nlm.nih.gov/pubmed/22437911. Accessed January 12, 2016.
125. Peck AJ, Holman RC, Curns AT, et al. Lower respiratory tract infections among American Indian and Alaska native children and the general population of U.S. Children. Pediatr Infect Dis J 2005;24(4):342–51.
126. Singleton RJ, Holman RC, Folkema AM, et al. Trends in lower respiratory tract infection hospitalizations among American Indian/Alaska native children and the general U.S. child population. J Pediatr 2012;161(2):296–302.e2.
127. Kicera TJ, Douglas M, Guerra FA. Best-practice models that work: The CDC's Racial and Ethnic Adult Disparities Immunization Initiative (READII) Programs. Ethn Dis 2005;15(2 Suppl 3). S3-17–20.
128. Morita J. Addressing racial and ethnic disparities in adult immunization, Chicago. J Public Health Manag Pract 2006;12(4):321–9.
129. U.S. Department of Health and Human Services. Healthy People 2010 (2nd ed.) [with understanding and improving health (vol. 1) and objectives for improving health (vol. 2)]. Washington, DC: U.S. Government Printing Office; 2000.
130. Kutner M, Greenberg E, Jin Y, et al. The health literacy of America's adults: results from the 2003 National Assessment of Adult Literacy (NCES 2006-483). Washington, DC: U.S. Department of Education, National Center for Education Statistics; 2006.
131. Berkman ND, DeWalt DA, Pignone MP, et al. Literacy and health outcomes (AHRQ Publication No. 04-E007-2). Rockville (MD): Agency for Healthcare Research and Quality; 2004.
132. Available at: http://health.gov/communication/hlactionplan/pdf/Health_Literacy_Action_Plan.pdf. Accessed February 2, 2016.
133. Kelly PA, Haidet P. Physician overestimation of patient literacy: A potential source of health care disparities. Patient Educ Couns 2007;66(1):119–22.
134. Osborn CY, Paasche-Orlow MK, Davis TC, et al. Health literacy: an overlooked factor in understanding HIV health disparities. Am J Prev Med 2007;33(5):374–8.
135. Sentell TL, Halpin HA. Importance of adult literacy in understanding health disparities. J Gen Intern Med 2006;21(8):862–6.
136. Song J. HIV/AIDS and homelessness: recommendations for clinical practice and public policy. Nashville (TN): National Health Care for the Homeless Council, Health Care for the Homeless Clinician's Network; 1999. p. 14. Available at: www.nhchc.org/Publications/HIV.pdf.
137. Zlotnick C, Zerger S, Wolfe P. Health care for the homeless: what we have learned in the past 30 years and what's next. Am J Public Health 2013;103(S2):S199–205.
138. Medicaid and the uninsured. Medicaid coverage and care for the homeless population: key lessons to consider for the 2014 Medicaid expansion. Washington, DC: The Henry J Kaiser Family Foundation; 2012.

139. Rabiner M, Weiner A. Health care for homeless and unstably housed: Overcoming barriers. Mt Sinai J Med 2012;79(5):586–92.
140. Inungu J, Beach E, Skeel R. Challenges facing health professionals caring for HIV-infected drug users. AIDS Patient Care STDs 2003;17(7):333–43.
141. Comprehensive HIV prevention for people who inject drugs, Revised guidance. Washington, DC: The U.S. President's Emergency Plan for AIDS Relief (PEPFAR); 2010.
142. Poteat T, Keatley J. Transgender people and HIV: policy brief. Geneva (Switzerland): World Health Organization (WHO); 2015.
143. Valdiserri R, Khalsa J, Dan C, et al. Confronting the emerging epidemic of HCV infection among young injection drug users. Am J Public Health 2014;104(5): 816–21.
144. Piper T, Rudenstine S, Stancliff S, et al. Overdose prevention for injection drug users: Lessons learned from naloxone training and distribution programs in New York City. Harm Reduct J 2007;4:3.

Psychological Issues in Medically Underserved Patients

Mathew Devine, DO[a,b,]*, Lauren DeCaporale-Ryan, PhD[c,d,e],
Magdalene Lim, PsyD[f,g], Juliana Berenyi, DO[h]

KEYWORDS

- Underserved • Psychosocial • Mental health • Depression • Primary care • Suicide

KEY POINTS

- Multiple populations in the United States face increased social and environmental stressors. These populations often seek mental health care from their primary care physician. Recommendations are outlined to improve their care experience.
- Recognize that subgroups of underserved populations that face additional stigma are at increased risked psychosocially (eg, based on race, age, and SES). Culturally sensitive programs help patients feel supported by their treatment team.
- Increase comfort using behavioral screening tools, such as Patient Health Questionnaire–9, to assess for mood disorders in underserved populations to more effectively identify and provide help for mental health conditions.
- Identify ways to support engagement in behavioral health (eg, having colocated care, ability to conduct a warm hand-off).
- Identify a team member who can support practical needs (eg, completion of paperwork, referrals to community resources), such as a social worker or care manager.

This article originally appeared in Primary Care: Clinics in Office Practice, Volume 44, Issue 1, March 2017.

Disclosure: The authors of this article report no direct financial interest in the subject matter or any material discussed in this article.

[a] Department of Family Medicine, University of Rochester, 777 South Clinton Avenue, Rochester, NY 14620, USA; [b] Accountable Health Partners, 135 Corporate Woods Suite 320, Rochester, NY 14623, USA; [c] Department of Psychiatry, University of Rochester Medical Center, 300 Crittenden Boulevard, Box Psych, Rochester, NY 14642, USA; [d] Department of Medicine, University of Rochester Medical Center, 300 Crittenden Boulevard, Box Psych, Rochester, NY 14642, USA; [e] Department of Surgery, University of Rochester Medical Center, 300 Crittenden Boulevard, Box Psych, Rochester, NY 14642, USA; [f] Department of Psychiatry, University of Rochester Medical Center, 300 Crittenden Boulevard, Rochester, NY 14642, USA; [g] Department of Medicine, University of Rochester Medical Center, 300 Crittenden Boulevard, Rochester, NY 14642, USA; [h] Department of Family Medicine, University of Rochester Family Medicine Resident, 777 South Clinton Avenue, Rochester, NY 14620, USA

* Corresponding author.

E-mail address: Mathew_devine@urmc.rochester.edu

INTRODUCTION

Improving the health of underserved populations is an ongoing focus of many medical industries including the US government. One critical problem with underserved populations is their potential for increased suffering from psychosocial stressors/mental health disorders. Practicing family physicians have many day-to-day interactions with psychosocial issues as part of their primary care practice workload. It has been identified that about half of the care for common mental disorders is delivered in general medical settings, leading Nordquist and Regier[1] to describe general medical settings as the "de facto mental health care system" in the United States. This article describes categories of underserved populations, including racially and culturally diverse; pediatric; geriatric; refugee; rural; and lesbian, gay, bisexual, or transgender (LGBT) individuals. Each section defines the population is being presented, identifies the mental health problems each is likely to encounter, explores the barriers that prevent access to care, and identifies potential methods to minimize such barriers. The following sections differentiate the ways in which psychiatric issues vary in underserved settings compared with the general population. Recommendations are offered for primary care physicians (PCP) to support improved recognition and management of psychosocial stressors and psychiatric illness among the underserved, who frequently present to primary care settings for such care.

Prevalence of Mental Health Diagnoses Identified in Primary Care

Recent analyses suggest that approximately 8% of adults in the United States suffer from current depressive symptoms. Prevalence rates for a lifetime diagnosis of depression suggest that nearly 16% of adults have suffered from depressive symptoms. Additionally, 4% endorse having suffered from a lifetime diagnosis of anxiety without evidence of depressive symptoms.[2] These rates are significantly influenced by patient demographic factors, including age, sex, race and ethnicity, education, employment status, and place of living. It is in this context that understanding the unique needs of the underserved is important to best care for the populations described next.

UNDERSERVED POPULATIONS IN THE UNITED STATES
Racially and Culturally Diverse Individuals

Racial minorities in the United States include Hispanics (12.5%), African Americans (12.3%), and Asians (3.6%), and account for one-third of the US population.[3] Racial minorities often suffer from poorer health and are overrepresented in drug-induced death, infant mortality, preterm birth, homicide rates, periodontitis, tuberculosis, obesity, and human immunodeficiency virus.[4] Racial health disparities are influenced by several other factors, including cultural identity, psychosocial stressors (eg, poverty), environmental factors (eg, violence), and unmet health needs.[5,6] The higher prevalence of mental health problems among racial minority individuals is largely accounted for by social determinants.[5]

Research to create and improve effective therapeutic interventions for racial minatory groups emphasizes understanding mental health stigma and the impact of perceived discrimination among these individuals.[7,8] Each individual has a different life experience rooted in culture and history, and different perceptions of his or her care needs. For example, barriers to care include "self-reliance and self-silence" coping among African American women,[9] and low perceived need despite significant psychosocial trauma among subgroups of immigrant Latinos.[10] Research on racial matching and culturally sensitive treatments highlights the need to consider how racial and cultural experiences influence interest and engagement in care.[11]

Individuals with Deprived Socioeconomic Status

More than 46 million people live below the poverty line in the United States.[12] Lower socioeconomic status (SES) frequently places people in unsafe environments and vulnerable positions.[13] Lower SES results in food insecurity, and reduced access to education, employment, and community resources.[14] Chronic adversity, exposure to trauma and loss, and discrimination[15,16] attribute to higher rates of homelessness, crime, incarceration, and substance abuse. Such predisposing vulnerabilities increase risk for poor health behaviors, chronic disease, and psychiatric disorders,[13] and limit personal resources, such as mastery and coping strategies.[17]

Diagnoses of depression, anxiety, posttraumatic stress disorder (PTSD), substance abuse, and schizophrenia have all been shown to have higher prevalence in impoverished, urban neighborhoods.[17–20] These patients tend to receive less specialty care for mental health. Instead, patients rely on acute hospital care[21] for medical and psychiatric needs, especially schizophrenia and substance abuse.[19] Multiple obstacles prevent those with low SES from engaging in specialty care including long wait times for service, limited health insurance benefits, limited clinicians willing or able to provide services at lower rates of reimbursement, and multicultural barriers (perceived bias, cultural mistrust).[13]

A case example (**Fig. 1**) is presented demonstrating how psychosocial barriers preclude patients from adequately accessing care. This case outlines the experience of a 25-year-old African American woman, and the adversity she faced from an early age Recommendations for interventions outlined in the case are also included in **Fig. 1**.

Children and Adolescents

Children younger than age 18 experiencing psychosocial stressors sometimes create increased challenges for families as a result of their dependence on their parent or guardian. The leading mental health burdens for children younger than 10 and their families are developmental disabilities, emotional disorders, and disruptive behavioral disorders.[22] Pediatric behavioral health specialists are in an even smaller supply than those working with the adult population. However, there are school-based services and community programs that can offer some assistance to this population.

In the United States, barriers to care in the underserved pediatric population include cost of care, inconvenience of access, poorly integrated systems of care, and inadequate insurance coverage.[22] Through the use of developmental and mental health screening tools and general screenings, PCPs can help to identify and work with school-based and behavioral health teams for ongoing treatment. Because of the shortage of specialty care it is important that PCPs are well educated and trained to work with minor to moderate psychosocial disturbances in children. For severe needs it is important that there is appropriate access for consultation and assistance because rectifying these problems early on provides health benefits throughout that child's life and development. According to the Centers for Disease Control and Prevention's National Health and Nutrition Examination Survey, which includes prevalence data for children ages 8 to 15, the three most prevalent mental health issues for children are (1) attention-deficit/hyperactivity disorder, (2) mood disorders, and (3) major depression disorders. Screening for these mental health conditions should be considered during outpatient visits including sports physical and well child visits (**Table 1** for screening details).[23]

Older Adults

Older adults have unique clinical needs and face multiple transitions. Estimates suggest that about 6 to 8 million (nearly 1 in 5) of those older than 65 have a mental health

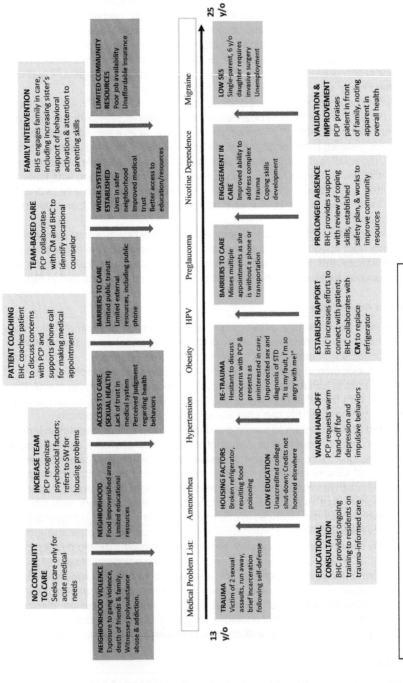

Figure Key: ▮ Community Level Factors   ▮ Patient Level Factors   ▮ Medical Team Response

or substance use disorder, and as the population doubles by 2030, so too will the number who suffer from such diagnoses.[24] Older adults with mental health conditions often experience poorer health behaviors and outcomes, and account for a disproportionate amount of health care costs.[25] Despite such prevalence rates, older adults less frequently engage in behavioral health care because of limited financial resources, difficulty accessing care due to chronic medical illness, lack of transportation, and the perceived stigma associated with treatment.[25] These limiting factors are further exacerbated by a significant shortage of specialty-trained workforce; currently, there is less than one geriatric psychiatrist per every 6000 older adults in need.[24,25]

Subsequently, care is most often sought in brief visits with PCPs, who are less likely to screen for mood symptoms and to refer older adults to specialty mental health care.[25,26] Anxiety and mood disorders are often undetected, as is suicide risk. Older adults account for nearly 18% of completed suicides in the United States,[27] with an average of 58% having seen their PCP within the month before their death.[28] Diagnosis of behavioral health concerns and risk of self-harm is often complicated by patients' presentation of somatic complaints and the complexity of differentiating between mood symptoms, medical problems, and dementia processes.[29] Moreover, PCPs generally have insufficient time to provide the necessary follow-up for improved outcomes (see **Table 1** for screening details).[30]

Refugee Individuals and Families

Refugees are given legal status and entry into the United States based on demonstration that they have been persecuted or have fear of persecution because of race, religion, nationality, political opinion, or membership in a particular social group.[31] In 2014, approximately 70,000 refugees entered the United States primarily hailing from Afghanistan, Iraq, Somali, Democratic Republic of Congo, Myanmar, Colombia, Sudan, Vietnam, Eritrea, China, and Syria.[32]

Leaving one's home and resettling in a new place creates significant distress and places refugees at risk for a variety of mental health concerns. Experiences of fleeing one's home are most often traumatic. Refugees suffer hardships, such as imprisonment, torture, loss of property, malnutrition, physical and sexual assault, and separation from family. These traumatic experiences can lead to PTSD, anxiety, and depressive disorders, such as major depression and adjustment disorder. The prevalence of these conditions in refugee populations varies greatly and can range anywhere from 4% to 86% for PTSD and 5% to 31% for depression.[33] The manifestations of these diseases differ on a case-by-case basis, with acute and chronic presentation, and symptoms may include psychosis and somatization.

Once refugees resettle in a new country, although their lives are often safer, the stress they experience is great. Frequently their family and friends remain in the countries they have fled or are still fleeing and the worry for their well-being can be extreme.

◄───

Fig. 1. Timeline depicting the experiences of a 25-year-old, underserved African American woman, single parent to 6-year-old daughter, and victim of domestic violence, referred to a psychologist for management of depression and anxiety. Timelines, developed collaboratively with patients can help clinicians understand the patient-level factors and sociocultural/environmental context that influence overall health. By working with an integrated team, the environmental factors, although still troublesome, are mitigated and patients are able to begin pursuing improved health and meet other personal goals for a more optimal lifestyle. BHC, Behavioral Health Clinician; CM, Care Manager; HPV, human papilloma virus; PCP, Primary Care Physician; STD, sexually transmitted disease; SW, Social Worker.

Table 1
Point of care screening tools for PCPs

Patient Population	Modify Direct Patient Experience	Collaborate with Others About	Seek Continued Education About
To improve access to care, PCPs can…			
All	Use tools, such as a timeline and/or genogram, to understand psychosocial experiences and their impact on health	Seek supportive consultation and consider warm hand-off to improve patient comfort with specialty care	Please review specific education examples below
Racially/ethnically diverse	Inquire about and understand an individual's perception regarding mental health treatment, rooted in family and cultural history, including their past experiences with the mental health system and experiences of stigma and discrimination Communicate respect to patients regarding their cultural perspective of illness and value their partnership throughout the treatment process Offer patient education materials tailored to race, education level, and language	Patient culture-specific concerns (eg, stigma about mental health treatment)	Diversity training, and training for Trauma-Informed Medical Care[51] for clinicians and staff
Low SES individuals/ families	Address patients' functional needs using supportive inquiry focused on patients' safety, including: • Whether their basic needs of food, shelter, and utilities are met, • What exposure to risk and violence they encounter, and • What types of relationships (supportive and deleterious) exist Ensure availability of transportation, eliminating potential barriers to care	Identify ways to support engagement in behavioral health (eg, having co-located care, ability to conduct a warm hand-off) Identify a team member who can support practical needs (eg, completion of paperwork, referrals to community resources), such as a social worker or care manager	Community resources (eg, churches, local organizations) that support access to housing, clothing, food, and hygiene products

Pediatrics	Screen for risk of abuse or neglect and make appropriate referrals to reduce risk of harm Be able to screen for development, and intellectual disabilities and behavioral health disorders	If case is severe to identify specialty care clinicians for medication management and therapeutic interventions	Be informed about alternative means of care, including home visits and tele health services Unique presentation of clinical symptoms and how to work best with parents/guardians and school-based professionals
Older adults	Screen all older adults for depression and risk of suicide Recognize the family as "patient," attending to caregiver needs Screen for risk of abuse or neglect and make appropriate referrals to reduce risk of harm	Identify specialty care clinicians for medication management and therapeutic interventions Work with depression care managers to facilitate access to and use of interventions	Unique presentation of clinical symptoms Community resources, such as churches, respite programs, and support groups for patients and caregivers Be informed about alternative means of care, including home visits and tele health services
Refugees	Use of screening tools (eg, Harvard Trauma Questionnaire, Resettlement Stressor Scale, War Trauma Scale) to help initiate dialogue about trauma experiences while overcoming some of the cultural and communication barriers that exist[52] Because of their traumatic experiences, refugees can be fearful and hesitant to provide the truth Extra care and awareness must be given in assessing this population	Ensure collaboration with social work/care management for maintenance of insurance benefits Consider interpreter services available	Understand how language can be stigmatizing (eg, "depression" or "mental health" may have negative connotations") Learn how to frame questions (eg, do not ask, "Are you depressed?" but instead ask "How are you sleeping?" Be informed about community resources available for resettlement

(continued on next page)

Table 1
(continued)

Patient Population	Modify Direct Patient Experience	Collaborate with Others About	Seek Continued Education About
Rural populations	Use behavioral screening tools, such as Patient Health Questionnaire-9, to access for depression in rural populations specifically farmers to identify and provide help for mental health conditions Improve access to medical centers with improved communication methods (telemedicine, and/or geographic location)		Increase in trained community workers/personnel to come to the homes of this population
LGBT individuals	Create a safe environment that allows patients to trust clinicians and staff, thereby building rapport and opportunity for information sharing about sexual orientation and psychosocial experiences Routinely screen critical health behaviors, including substance use and safe sex practices, and of mood disorders, risk for suicide and self-harm behaviors Allow time for discussion about patients' coming out experience and/or plans to do so; provide support and resources available in your community		Subgroups of this population and the additional stigma they face because of increased risked psychosocially (eg, based on race, age, and SES) Culturally sensitive programs help patients feel supported by their treatment team

Family and friends abroad depend financially on refugees. More than $1 billion in remittance was sent from the United States in 2012, making up a significant percent of the household income of recipients.[34] Refugees often must restart their careers, because professional degrees do not transfer; former professionals are forced to work in manual labor or minimum wage jobs. Assimilating into a new culture and learning a new language also has challenges and feelings of isolation, confusion, and frustration are common. These stressors not only put refugees at higher risk for mental health concerns but can also exacerbate existing chronic medical conditions.

Rural Populations

Multiple studies have evaluated the prevalence of mental health conditions in urban versus rural environments. These studies conclude that in general the prevalence of overall mental health disorders seems higher in urban settings. Despite the lower prevalence in rural communities there is an appreciable decrease in access to mental health services. Moreover, there is some evidence that certain conditions, such as functional psychosis and manic-depressive psychosis, are higher in rural areas.[35]

Additionally, there is an increased rate of suicides in rural populations specifically among farmers (which is just under twice the rate of the US adult suicide rate).[36] The rates of suicide in most rural communities are 17.14 per 100,000 versus 11.51 per 100,000 in most urban areas.[37] Studies also show suicide rates are higher with those individuals taking antidepressant medications.[37]

To bridge this gap, Federally Qualified Health Centers (CHCs) continue to grow as a delivery medical network in rural communities. A recent study identified that treatment of mental health and substance abuse are some of the most common reasons that individuals visit CHCs. These centers use a treatment model that includes housing other specialties to work within these practices to increase access to all forms of medical care not just from their PCPs. However, with the visit demand high for addressing mental health needs there is a shortage of behavioral health specialists to provide this care even though most centers have rooms to have them working in their facilities. Based on this shortage only 6.5% of these encounters are with on-site behavioral health specialists at rural CHCs. The lack of these services again identifies that the opportunities for having mental health professionals directly involved with care in rural communities is less than urban communities.

Lesbian/Gay/Bisexual/Transgender Individuals

Estimates suggest that 3.5% of individuals identify as LGBT in the United States.[38] LGBT individuals face multiple stressors: discrimination, disproportionate poverty rates compared with the general population,[39] and increased chronic medical conditions. Subgroups of the LGBT population encounter higher rates of asthma, headaches, allergies, osteoarthritis, gastrointestinal problems, and human immunodeficiency virus/AIDS.[40] Lesbians, gay men, and bisexual individuals are more likely to smoke than heterosexual peers. Tobacco, alcohol, and illicit drug use vary significantly as a result of age, affiliation with LGBT culture, stressful life events, and emotional regulation.[41]

Often, LGBT individuals face rejection by their communities, resulting in inequality in the workplace and in access to medical care,[40] and increased exposure to physical and sexual violence.[42] Individuals frequently report a lack of familial support, which correlates to increased rates of mental illness and substance abuse.[43] Discrimination and higher levels of day-to-day stress create greater risk for psychiatric disease. A study of women found that lesbians had higher frequency of depression, PTSD, and phobias compared with heterosexual women.[44] Similarly, gay men tend to experience higher rates of depression and anxiety.[45] Research supports that similar mood disturbances are common among bisexual and transgender individuals; however, data pertaining to the mental health needs among these groups are presently limited.[46]

LGBT individuals are at increased risk of suicidal ideation. Bisexuals are more likely to report higher levels of self-harm, thoughts of suicide, and suicidal attempts compared with heterosexual, gay men, and lesbians; rates increase for lesbian and bisexual women who are not "out."[47] Research indicates that among transgender individuals, suicidal ideation has been reported from 38% to 65% of the time; 16% to 32% of transgender patients have reported a history of suicide attempt.[48]

Despite the need for medical and mental health intervention, in 2011, the Institute of Medicine noted that LGBT patients face barriers to care because of a lack of understanding about their treatment needs. Studies show that lesbian and bisexual women frequently consult PCPs for emotional support if their PCP is aware of their sexual orientation; however, not all want or choose to disclose this information.

METHODS TO RESOLUTION AND IMPROVING MENTAL HEALTH CARE IN THE UNDERSERVED

Meeting the mental health needs of the underserved requires many changes be made to improve access to care. Establishing a system to improve accessibility to trained PCPs or specialty providers is critical. This section focuses on the methods (previously evaluated or currently under consideration) in various settings across the United States to improve mental health care for the general population and the underserved. **Table 2** provides information on how to maximize care in the various underserved populations discussed previously.

Because of the ongoing shortage of PCPs and behavior health service (BHS) providers emerging technologies may increase flexibility to reaching the underserved, although research on efficacy of such technology use is still needed. Health information technologies, such as smart phones, smart televisions, handheld apps, and desktop software, and the Internet can improve patient education and access to care for those previously underserved populations.[49] These technologies offer a wide range of possibilities for treatment remotely of underserved populations. Because of the early stages of these technologies data on their usefulness are limited. Such technology requires upfront costs to practices and patients (eg, having necessary devices). However, technology offers flexibility of coding, allowing for customizable software that adapts for different languages and visual technologies for the consumer. Mass screenings can be done using online forms, which can be scored and delivered to health professionals to identify high-risk patients in need of care. Video capabilities can link mental health and PCPs to patients from far distances to save on travel and compensate for barriers (eg, chronic illness, inability to drive). Such interventions do not currently have as much oversight, and the efficacy, and ethical nature of these interventions are still being evaluated.[49] In our opinion the oversight of this sector will certainly help to improve evaluation and dissemination of these well-intentioned efforts.

Increased education and specialty training should be offered by health systems or medical educators for mental health providers and physicians to recognize symptoms and know when and how to treat and when to refer. These ongoing issues can better be addressed if practices are able have designated BHS providers involved in underserved primary care practices. Because there are not enough BHS professionals, many rural practices have begun to use evidence-based community partnerships models. These models are still being researched and they are used to provide remote

Table 2
How to maximize care provided for populations of the underserved

	Depression and Mood Disorders	Anxiety	Substance Use	Other
Children and adolescents	• Beck Depression Inventory for Youth • Children's Depression Inventory • Center for Epidemiologic Studies–Depression Scale for Children • Reynolds Child Depression Scale • Reynolds Adolescent Depression Scale	• Beck Anxiety Inventory for Youth • Multidimensional Anxiety Scale for Children	• CRAFFT Screener • Drug Abuse Screen Test –10 (for older youth) • Teen Addiction Severity Index	• Autism Behavior Checklist • Child Behavior Checklist • Conners' Rating Scales–Revised • Vanderbilt ADHD Rating Scales
Adults	• Beck Depression Inventory–II • Beck Depression Inventory–Primary Care[a] • Center for Epidemiologic Studies Depression • Center for Epidemiologic Studies–Depression Revised • Mood Disorder Questionnaire (Bipolar Disorder) • Patient Health Questionnaire–2/9	• Abbreviated PTSD Checklist–Civilian[a] • Generalized Anxiety Disorder–7[a] • Harvard Trauma Questionnaire • Primary Care–PTSD[a] • Life Event Checklist • War Trauma Scale	• Alcohol Use Disorders Identification Test • Alcohol Use Disorders Identification Test–PC[a] • CAGE AID • Drug Abuse Screen Test-10	• Resettlement Stressor Scale
Older adults	• Cornell Scale for Depression in Dementia[a] • Geriatric Depression Scale[a] • Geriatric Depression Scale–Short • Hamilton Depression Scale (see "Adults" section)	• Geriatric Anxiety Inventory • Geriatric Anxiety Scale	• CAGE AID • T-ACE	• Katz Index of Independence in Activities of Daily Living • Lawton Instrumental Activities of Daily Living

Screening should be an ongoing process and means of assessing symptom severity, effectiveness of intervention.
These are designed to be brief and can be implemented in primary care settings.
[a] Denotes measures specifically assessed for use in primary care settings.

training and mental health education and screening for primary care offices.[50] This quality improvement initiative gives clinicians opportunities to provide point-of-care tools to their patients that can help with their treatment. These initiatives are still being studied and if effective these community-based partnerships can be used across the country to help underserved communities improve access to their patients.

SUMMARY

The underserved have a significantly greater prevalence of mental health problems and face significantly greater barriers to care. PCPs serve on the front line in their roles with the underserved populations. They need to continue to be aware of the needs of those with mental health conditions, and to know how to address them until the barriers have been solved with future promising interventions.

REFERENCES

1. Norquist GS, Regier DA. The epidemiology of psychiatric disorders and the de facto mental health care system 1. Annu Rev Med 1996;47:473–9.
2. Strine TW, Mokdad AH, Balluz LS, et al. Depression and anxiety in the United States: findings from the 2006 behavioral risk factor surveillance system. Psychiatr Serv 2008;59:1383–90.
3. Centers for Disease Control and Prevention. Disparities analytics. 2013. Available at: http://www.cdc.gov/disparitiesanalytics/. Accessed February 10, 2016.
4. U.S. Census Bureau. 2010 census redistricting data (Public Law 94-171) summary file. Available at: http://www.census.gov/prod/cen2010/doc/pl94-171.pdf. Accessed June 1, 2016.
5. Chang TE, Weiss AP, Marques L, et al. Race/ethnicity and other social determinants of psychological well-being and functioning in mental health clinics. J Health Care Poor Underserved 2014;25:1418–31.
6. Parrish MM, Miller L, Peltekof B. Addressing depression and accumulated trauma in urban primary care: challenges and opportunities. J Health Care Poor Underserved 2011;22(4):1292–301.
7. Barry CL, McGinty EE, Pescosolido BA, et al. Stigma, discrimination, treatment effectiveness, and policy: public views about drug addiction and mental illness. Psychiatr Serv 2014;65(10):1269–72.
8. Pedersen ER, Paves AP. Comparing perceived public stigma and personal stigma of mental health treatment seeking in a young adult sample. Psychiatry Res 2014;219(1):143–50.
9. Watson NN, Hunter CD. Anxiety and depression among African American women: the costs of strength and negative attitudes toward psychological help-seeking. Cultur Divers Ethnic Minor Psychol 2015;21(4):604.
10. Fortuna LR, Porche MV, Alegria M. Political violence, psychosocial trauma, and the context of mental health services use among immigrant Latinos in the united states. Ethn Health 2008;13(5):435–63.
11. Chen FM, Fryer GE Jr, Phillips RL Jr, et al. Patients' beliefs about racism, preferences for physician race, and satisfaction with care. Ann Fam Med 2005;3(2):138–43.
12. DeNavas-Walt C, Proctor BD. U.S. Census Bureau, current population reports, P60–252, Income and poverty in the United States: 2014. 2015.
13. Groh C. Poverty, mental health, and women: implications for psychiatric nurses in primary care settings. J Am Psychiatr Nurses Assoc 2007;13(5):267–74.

14. Stafford M, Marmot M. Neighbourhood deprivation and health: does it affect us all equally? Int J Epidemiol 2003;32(3):357–66.
15. Myers HF, Wyatt GE, Ullman JB, et al. Cumulative burden of lifetime adversities: trauma and mental health in low-SES African Americans and Latino/as. Psychol Trauma 2015;7(3):243–51.
16. Glover DA, Williams JK, Kissler KA. Using novel methods to examine stress among HIV-positive African American men who have sex with men and women. J Behav Med 2012;36:283–94.
17. Lorant V, Deliège D, Eaton W, et al. Socioeconomic inequalities in depression: a meta-analysis. Am J Epidemiol 2003;157(2):98–112.
18. Chow JC, Jaffee K, Snowden L. Racial/ethnic disparities in the use of mental health services in poverty areas. Am J Public Health 2003;93(5):792–7.
19. Curtis S, Copeland A, Fagg J, et al. The ecological relationship between deprivation, social isolation and rates of hospital admission for acute psychiatric care: a comparison of London and New York city. Health Place 2006;12(1):19–37.
20. Fryers T, Melzer D, Jenkins R. Social inequalities and the common mental disorders: a systematic review of the evidence. Soc Psychiatry Psychiatr Epidemiol 2003;38(5):229–37.
21. Kangovi S, Barg F, Carter T, et al. Understanding why patients of low socioeconomic status prefer hospitals over ambulatory care. Health Aff 2013;32(7):1196–203.
22. Patel V, Kieling C, Maulik PK, et al. Improving access to care for children with mental disorders: a global perspective. Arch Dis Child 2013;98(5):323–7.
23. National Institute of Mental Health. Any disorder among children. Available at: http://www.nimh.nih.gov/health/statistics/prevalence/any-disorder-among-children.shtml. 2016. Accessed June 2, 2016.
24. Committee on the Mental Health Workforce for Geriatric Populations. In: Eden J, Maslow K, Le M, Board on Health Care Services, Institute of Medicine, et al, editors. The mental health and substance use workforce for older adults: in whose hands? Washington, DC: National Academies; 2012.
25. Bartels SJ, Gill L, Naslund JA. The affordable care act, accountable care organizations, and mental health care for older adults: implications and opportunities. Harv Rev Psychiatry 2015;23(5):304–19.
26. Klap R, Unroe KT, Unützer J. Caring for mental illness in the United States: a focus on older adults. Am J Geriatr Psychiatry 2003;11:517–24.
27. Drapeau CW, McIntosh JL. U.S.A. suicide: 2013 official final data. 2015. Available at: http://www.suicidology.org/Portals/14/docs/Resources/FactSheet. Accessed December 12, 2015.
28. Luoma JB, Martin CE, Pearson JL. Contact with mental health and primary care providers before suicide: a review of the evidence. Am J Psychiatry 2002;159(6):909–16.
29. Unützer J, Schoenbaum M, Druss BG, et al. Transforming mental health care at the interface with general medicine: report for the president's commission. Psychiatr Serv 2006;57(1):37–47.
30. Arean PA, Ayalon L, Hunkeler E, et al. Improving depression care for older, minority patients in primary care. Med Care 2005;43(4):381–90.
31. US Citizenship & Immigration Services. Refugees. 2015. Available at: http://www.uscis.gov/humanitarian/refugees-asylum/refugees. Accessed February 10, 2016.
32. Centers for Disease Control and Prevention. About refugees. 2012. Available at: www.cdc.gov/immigrantrefugeehealth/about-refugees.html. Accessed February 10, 2016.

33. Hollifield M, Warner TD, Lian N, et al. Measuring trauma and health status in refugees: a critical review. JAMA 2002;288(5):611–21.
34. Pew Research Center. Remittance flows worldwide in 2012. 2014. Available at: http://www.pewsocialtrends.org/2014/02/20/remittance-map/. Accessed February 10, 2016.
35. Peen J, Schoevers RA, Beekman AT, et al. The current status of urban-rural differences in psychiatric disorders. Acta Psychiatr Scand 2010;121:84–93.
36. Spoont M, Minneapolis V. Rural vs. urban ambulatory health care: a systematic review. Minneapolis (MN): Department of Veterans Affairs Health Services Research & Development Service; 2011.
37. Gregoire A. The mental health of farmers. Occup Med (Lond) 2002;52(8):471–6.
38. Gallup Politics. Special report: 3.4% of U.S. adults identify as LGBT. 2012. Available at: http://www.gallup.com/poll/158066/special-report-adults-identify-lgbt.aspx. Accessed January 6, 2016.
39. Badgett M, Durso L, Schneebaum A. New patterns of poverty in the lesbian, gay, and bisexual community. Los Angeles (CA): The Williams Institute; 2013.
40. Ranji U, Beamesderfer A, Kates J, et al. Health and access to care and coverage for lesbian, gay, bisexual, and transgender individuals in the US. Menlo Park (CA): Kaiser Foundation Issue Brief; 2015.
41. Centers for Disease Control and Prevention. CDC fact sheet, substance abuse among gay and bisexual men. Atlanta (GA): Author; 2010.
42. Lick D, Durso L, Johnson K. Minority stress and physical health among sexual minorities. Perspect Psychol Sci 2013;8(5):521–48.
43. Ryan C, Huebner D, Diaz RM, et al. Family rejection as a predictor of negative health outcomes in white and Latino lesbian, gay, and bisexual young adults. Pediatrics 2009;23(1):346–52.
44. Gilman SE, Cochran SD, Mays VM, et al. Risk of psychiatric disorders among individuals reporting same-sex sexual partners in the national comorbidity survey. Am J Public Health 2001;91:933–9.
45. Berg MB, Mimiaga MJ, Safren SA. Mental health concerns of gay and bisexual men seeking mental health services. J Homosex 2008;54(3):293–306.
46. Institute of Medicine. The health of lesbian, gay, bisexual, and transgender people: building a foundation for better understanding. Washington, DC: National Academies Press; 2011.
47. Koh AS, Ross LK. Mental health issues: a comparison of lesbian, bisexual and heterosexual women. J Homosex 2006;51(1):33–57.
48. Clements-Nolle K, Marx R, Katz M. Attempted suicide among transgender persons: the influence of gender-based discrimination and victimization. J Homosex 2006;51(3):53–69.
49. Clarke G, Yarborough BJ. Evaluating the promise of health IT to enhance/expand the reach of mental health services. Gen Hosp Psychiatry 2013;35(4):339–44.
50. Hunt JB, Curran G, Kramer T, et al. Partnership for implementation of evidence-based mental health practices in rural federally qualified health centers: theory and methods. Prog Community Health Partnersh 2012;6(3):389–98.
51. Green BL, Saunders PA, Power E, et al. Trauma-informed medical care: CME communication training for primary care providers. Fam Med 2015;47(1):7–14.
52. Bolton E. PTSD in refugees. 2015. Available at: http://www.ptsd.va.gov/professional/trauma/other/ptsd-refugees.asp. Accessed February 10, 2016.

Substance Use Issues Among the Underserved

United States and International Perspectives

Alicia Ann Kowalchuk, DO*, Sandra J. Gonzalez, PhD,
Roger J. Zoorob, MD, MPH

KEYWORDS

- Alcohol • Drugs • Illicit drugs • Substance use • Substance use disorders
- Substance abuse • Tobacco

KEY POINTS

- Substance use and substance use disorders (SUDs) have a disproportionate impact on the underserved, with tobacco use most prevalent worldwide and causing the greatest morbidity and mortality.
- Trauma, which has a disproportionate impact on underserved populations, is a strong risk factor for the development of SUDs.
- Integration of substance use screening and SUD treatment into primary care is a promising solution for increasing access and engagement in care.

GLOBAL SCOPE OF SUBSTANCE USE

The most commonly used substance worldwide Is tobacco: 21% of the world's population 15 years old and older smokes tobacco products. Approximately 80% of the world's 1 billion smokers live in low-income and middle-income countries. Tobacco kills approximately half its users and 6 million people globally every year, 90% of whom are direct users; 10% of these deaths are due to second-hand exposure. Rates of use vary by country and region and are inversely related to education level attainment, socioeconomic status, and the consumer price of tobacco products, which is strongly tied to tax rates. Tobacco use rates are directly related to the marketing of tobacco products in a society. Globally, tobacco smoking prevalence rates are 5 times higher in men (37%) than women (7%), with that gap narrowest in Europe, where approximately 20% of women smoke tobacco products.[1]

This article is an update of an article that originally appeared in *Primary Care: Clinics in Office Practice*, Volume 44, Issue 1, March 2017.
Department of Family and Community Medicine, Baylor College of Medicine, 3701 Kirby Drive, Suite 600, Houston, TX 77098, USA
* Corresponding author.
E-mail address: aliciak@bcm.edu

Alcohol, the second most commonly used substance, is the third leading cause of disability and disease worldwide and the leading cause in middle-income countries, although per capita alcohol consumption and binge drinking are highest among high-income countries. Alcohol consumption causes more than 3 million deaths worldwide annually. Although the highest rates of alcohol abstinence are found in the lowest socioeconomic strata in societies around the world, the burdens of alcohol-related disability, disease, and mortality are disproportionately borne by those of lower socioeconomic status and less developed countries. This discrepancy has been attributed to a variety of factors, including poorer access to health care; smaller support networks to help individuals address their alcohol problems; higher rates of manual labor employment (in which on-the-job alcohol impairment injuries are more likely); poorly maintained roads and less safe and reliable vehicles, contributing to higher alcohol-impaired driving fatalities; and nutritional deficiencies. There are also substantial gender differences in alcohol consumption and associated mortality, with male drinkers consuming on average approximately 2.5 times more alcohol than female drinkers worldwide and suffering approximately double the mortality rate of alcohol-attributable deaths.[2]

Worldwide, drug use rates have remained stable since 2010; however, up to 7%, or 300 million, of the world's population between 15 and 64 years of age have used an illicit drug in the past year. It is estimated that 16 to 39 million people are regular users and/or have an SUD, and 12.7 million inject drugs. Annually, there are 183,000 drug-related deaths, accounting for a mortality rate of 40 deaths per million. Cannabis, used by 2.5% of the world's population, is the most widely used substance after tobacco and alcohol and is associated with the most arrests for drug offenses globally. Opiates are used by 0.2% of the global population yet are responsible for the largest disease burden and highest number of drug-related deaths worldwide, primarily from injection drug use–related infectious diseases, such as HIV and hepatitis C virus, and overdoses. Cocaine is also consumed by 0.2% of the world's population, although, unlike tobacco, alcohol, cannabis, and opiates, cocaine use is less widespread, concentrated primarily in the Americas and Europe. As seen with tobacco and alcohol, illicit drug use is more prevalent in men than women.[3]

SCOPE OF SUBSTANCE USE IN THE UNITED STATES

Among US adults, 18% use tobacco products, a decrease of more than 50% in the past 50 years. Despite this public health achievement, tobacco products kill half a million US adults annually, and tobacco use remains the leading preventable cause of premature disability and death. Tobacco use is not evenly distributed across US society. As seen globally, tobacco use rates are inversely related to educational level attainment and socioeconomic status. The tobacco smoking rate in the Medicaid population is double that of the general population, with tobacco-related diseases accounting for 15%, or $40 billion, of total Medicaid spending. Geographically, tobacco use is highest in the southern and western states and lowest in the west coast and northeastern states. Of all US ethnic and racial groups, non-Latino whites and Native Americans have the highest tobacco use rates. The gender gap for tobacco use is small in the United States, with female tobacco use rates approximately 80% of male tobacco use rates. Persons with mental illness are a group particularly vulnerable to tobacco use effects in the United States due to high prevalence of use and low rates of successful quit attempts. The picture for the general US population is brighter, with former tobacco users now outnumbering current tobacco users.[4]

Among US adults, 88% report consuming alcohol during their lifetime, with 72% reporting use within the past year and 57% within the past month. Past-month binge drinking (5 or more drinks on any 1 occasion) prevalence is 25%, and 7% of US adults report heavy drinking (5 or more binge drinking episodes) in the past month. Among US adults, 7% have an alcohol use disorder (AUD).[5] Alcohol use is the third leading preventable cause of death in the United States, after tobacco use and obesity, with approximately 88,000 deaths from alcohol-related causes reported annually.[6] Alcohol is involved in approximately a third of all motor vehicle accident fatalities, and alcohol misuse costs are estimated at more than $224 billion annually, primarily due to binge drinking.[7,8] As with tobacco use, alcohol consumption is unevenly distributed across US society, with binge drinking rates highest in Alaska, the upper Midwest, and New England states.[9] Although AUD rates are highest in non-Latino whites and Native Americans, African Americans and Latinos have higher rates of persistent and recurrent AUDs, and the consequences of alcohol misuse remain greater for African Americans, Latinos, and Native Americans compared with Asian Americans and non-Latino whites, which is at least partially attributable to socioeconomic disparities.[10]

Barriers to care, such as lack of access to and availability of treatment in underserved areas, lack of transportation and/or child care, being uninsured or underinsured, and stigma, are all associated with poor engagement and retention in AUD treatment. Minority groups may be less likely to seek or receive specialty care, making the primary care encounter vitally important in the early identification of problematic alcohol consumption in underserved communities.[11] Avoiding stigmatizing language in their practices can be an easy and low-cost practice change intervention for decreasing that barrier to care across underserved populations with SUDs. Stigmatizing language has been eliminated in the *Diagnostic and Statistical Manual of Mental Disorders* (Fifth Edition), and addiction medicine experts are encouraging rapid adoption of this newer terminology.[12–14]

Approximately half (49%) of the US population age 12 and older has used an illicit drug in their lifetime, 17% in the past year, and 10% in the past month. As seen globally, cannabis use accounts for most illicit drug use, with nonmedical use of prescription drugs a distant second.[5] Unintentional prescription drug overdose, however, primarily involving opioids, has become the leading cause of accidental death in US working age adults since 2011.[15] From 1997 to 2007, the milligram-per-person use of prescription opioids in the United States increased 402%, and retail pharmacies dispensed 48% more opiate prescriptions in 2009 than in 2000.[16,17] The rates of opiate prescribing and nonmedical use of prescription opiates have leveled off since 2012, but opiate overdose deaths have continued to increase, and heroin use is on the rise. The rate of overdose deaths involving synthetic opioids doubled in the US from 2015 to 2016 primarily driven by illicit fentanyl.[18] Unlike increasing opioid related overdose death rates, which have been seen across geographic, racial, ethnic and age groups, increasing rates of cocaine related overdose deaths in the US have been concentrated in urban, poor communities of color, and remain largely unaddressed at the national public health policy level.[18] Rates of other illicit drug use, except cannabis (which has been increasing), have been stable or declining.[19] As with tobacco and alcohol, illicit drug use is unevenly distributed across US society. Prevalence of use of an illicit substance in a community is directly tied to its availability in that community, which is linked primarily to routes of distribution of the illicit drug trade. Overall, most underserved populations in the United States, including adolescents and children, the elderly, minority racial and ethnic groups, and those in the lower socioeconomic strata, have lower rates of illicit drug use than the general population.[17] The homeless and incarcerated populations, however, have higher rates. Women use fewer illicit drugs overall and across all drug classes compared with men except for sedative-hypnotics, such as benzodiazepines and zolpidem.[19]

EFFECTS/COSTS TO FAMILIES/SOCIETY

The economic and societal costs of substance use are astounding. In the United States, more than $700 billion per year in costs related to health care, lost work productivity, and crime can be attributed to the misuse of alcohol, tobacco, and illicit drugs.[20] Risky alcohol use alone cost the country $249 billion in 2010.[21] SUDs have been noted to significantly increase the health care costs in Medicaid beneficiaries with coexisting mental or physical illnesses.[22] Based on global prevalence rates, it is estimated that $250 billion (or approximately 0.3%–0.4% of the world's gross domestic product) would be needed to treat individuals for conditions related to the use of substances, placing a significant financial burden on families and society as a whole.[23]

Although the economic costs associated with substance use are substantial, it is also important to note the societal and personal costs to families. The effects of SUDs are experienced by every member of a family. In addition to higher prevalence of abuse, emotional and physical neglect, legal problems, and difficulties with attachment, children growing up in the care of an adult or adults with SUDs are also at an increased risk of developing an SUD themselves.[24] According to the Substance Abuse and Mental Health Services Administration, 2 in 5 children (40%) live with at least 1 adult with an SUD during their childhood/adolescence and 1 in 4 is exposed to alcohol problems in their family.[25]

Worldwide, the burden for families is great, particularly for those who are socioeconomically disadvantaged. In many countries, when the primary income earner is unable to work or maintain employment due to substance use, the responsibility of ensuring that the family's needs are met falls solely on the nonusing adult partner.[26]

ACCESS TO TREATMENT — GLOBAL PERSPECTIVE

Studies in the United States and other countries have shown that SUD treatment is cost effective, saving a society 7 times the cost of the treatment provided.[27] Globally, although 66% of countries have a government unit or official responsible for SUD treatment services, less than half have a dedicated budget for SUD treatment. Consequently, there is a median of 1.7 beds for SUD treatment per 100,000 people worldwide, illustrating the discrepancy between treatment need and available resources. Inpatient detoxification is the most prevalent acute treatment service available; however, longer-term, longitudinal care of this chronic medical illness is less prevalent. Treatment access within a society is most limited for the underserved of a given society.[27] Retention in SUD treatment has been consistently linked to improved outcomes; however, access to the continuum of care is often limited.

Evidence-based pharmacologic treatment of SUDs, also called medication management or medication-assisted treatment (MAT), is available primarily for alcohol and opiate use disorders (OUDs). Medication managed withdrawal from alcohol or alcohol detoxification is the most widely available MAT worldwide, and benzodiazepines remain the most commonly used medication for that indication and are considered the safest and most effective medications for alcohol withdrawal.[28] There are worrisomely high rates of use of chlorpromazine use in lower-income countries for alcohol withdrawal, because chlorpromazine, which lowers seizure threshold, is not recommended for treatment of alcohol withdrawal.[29] Other MATs for AUD focus on relapse prevention and include acamprosate, naltrexone, and gabapentin, which are all used most frequently in higher-income countries.[30–32]

Three primary medications are available for MAT of OUDs: buprenorphine, methadone, and naltrexone. Buprenorphine and methadone, used as partial and full agonist maintenance medications, respectively, have been shown to decrease injection drug use, increase retention in treatment, and decrease relapse rates in individuals with OUD.[33] Naltrexone, an opioid receptor blocker, has shown the most success in relapse prevention of OUD in populations and societies in which full or partial agonist medications are not available, such as in Russia, where agonist treatment of OUD remains illegal.[34] Methadone is the most widely available MAT for OUD worldwide, with buprenorphine access essentially limited to high income countries.[27]

Although not formally considered an SUD treatment, mutual aid societies or self-help groups, such as Alcoholics Anonymous and Narcotics Anonymous, are active sources of support for individuals with SUDs in approximately 3 of 4 countries worldwide with larger presence in higher income countries. Nongovernmental organizations provide a significant amount of SUD treatment in many countries, with involvement of traditional healers and peers in recovery in formal SUD treatment settings common, especially in lower-income countries and lower-resourced areas. Engagement in helping peers has been shown to have a positive impact on individuals in recovery from SUDs.[27]

ACCESS TO TREATMENT IN THE UNITED STATES

Only 1 in 9 of the more than 23 million people with an SUD enter treatment in the United States. More than 90% of those not entering treatment do not actively seek out treatment because they do not feel they need it. Stigma associated with SUDs and SUD treatment remains a significant barrier as does the lack of knowledge, understanding, and acceptance of the SUD as a chronic disease.[35] Approximately all medications available around the globe for SUD treatment are also available in the United States; however, access to MAT for SUDs is limited by health insurance status and coverage. Mutual aid societies and peer recovery–based services remain widely used resources for underserved persons with SUDs in this country.[36]

TRAUMA AND SUBSTANCE USE

A trauma is an upsetting and frightening event that an individual experiences or witnesses in which there is a threat to the safety of themselves or someone else. The experience of trauma is common throughout the globe, with exposure estimated higher in lower-income countries compared with higher-income countries.[37] It is estimated that approximately 60% of men and 50% of women experience a traumatic event at least once in their lives.[38] In the United States, the lifetime prevalence rate of posttraumatic stress disorder (PTSD) is estimated to be between 6.8% and 8.0%. Among the underserved, however, the rate is at least triple.[39] Risk factors, such as poverty, low levels of social support, and low social capital, are associated with greater rates of PTSD in urban communities.[39,40] Primary care providers practicing in these areas are likely to encounter individuals with PTSD and posttraumatic stress symptoms, making the primary care setting ideal for identification and treatment.[41] Unfortunately, PTSD and posttraumatic stress symptoms often go unrecognized, contributing to greater health care costs and poorer outcomes.[42,43] Adopting a trauma-informed approach, as discussed later, is one method by which providers can better address the impact of trauma in their patients.

The relationship between trauma and substance use is well established in the literature.[39] PTSD and SUDs are often comorbid and associated with increased chronic medical conditions, poor social and occupational functioning, more legal troubles, and higher incidences of intimate partner violence and suicide.[44–46] Sexual assault has been shown associated with a higher risk of drug use and risky drinking in women.[47]

Adverse childhood experiences, such as abuse and neglect, have been shown to increase the risk of developing SUDs in adulthood.[48] Traumatized persons, especially those with childhood trauma, are higher utilizers of health care services but may be less likely to effectively engage in care plans because they can be more distrustful of institutions of care and perceived authority figures such as medical providers.[40,49]

The rates of comorbid SUD and PTSD among veterans are also significant. In a study of 456,502 Iraq and Afghanistan veterans, researchers found that 82% to 93% of soldiers with a diagnosis of either AUD or other SUD also had a comorbid mental health disorder. Of these disorders, PTSD was the most commonly diagnosed in Veterans Affairs health care centers and accounted for up to a 4-fold increase in the diagnosis of AUD and a 3-fold increase in the diagnosis of other SUDs.[50]

AUD prevalence rates are much lower in foreign-born individuals than in US-born adolescents and adults. The risk of developing an SUD after the experience of a traumatic event, however, was higher for foreign-born than for US-born individuals.[51]

WOMEN AS AN UNDERSERVED POPULATION (SEE LUZ M. FERNANDEZ AND JONATHAN A. BECKER'S ARTICLE, "WOMEN'S SELECT HEALTH ISSUES IN UNDERSERVED POPULATIONS," IN THIS ISSUE)

Overall, global prevalence rates show that women use substances at a much lower rate than their male counterparts. In developed countries, where there is greater gender equality and more fluidity when it comes to gender roles, particularly in the workforce, attention is paid to the diminishing difference in drinking patterns between men and women.[52] Among women in the US, alcohol use, high risk drinking and prevalence of AUDs continue to increase toward gender parity.[53] Additionally, although SUDs are more prevalent in men, the gender gap in rates of SUDs has narrowed over the past 30 years.[54] When examining gender differences, women experience the progression from first use to development of an SUD at a much faster rate and may exhibit more severe symptoms than men even though they may have used for a shorter period of time or used less of the substance.[55,56] Women are initiating alcohol use at a much younger age than in the past and their drinking patterns and rates of SUDs are becoming more similar to those of men.[57]

In 2014, 15.8 million women reported that they used illicit drugs in the past year and an additional 4.6 million women reported misuse of prescription drugs. Given the high rate of unplanned pregnancies, the use of substances for women of childbearing age poses an additional concern. Substance use during pregnancy has many short-term and long-term effects for women and their children. Women of childbearing age who drink and are not using effective and consistent contraception may be at risk for an alcohol-exposed pregnancy.[58] If a woman uses substances on a regular basis during pregnancy, her baby may experience withdrawal symptoms at birth, a condition known as neonatal abstinence syndrome, which can occur if a woman uses caffeine, alcohol, opioids, or sedatives.[59] In the US, the incidence of NAS increased 400% between 2000 and 2012, primarily driven by increased maternal opioid exposure.[60] Recently published data from the Behavioral Risk Factor Surveillance System describe drinking patterns in both pregnant and nonpregnant women from 2011 to 2013. Among nonpregnant women, 53.6% reported any use in the past 30 days whereas approximately 1 in 5 women (18.2%) reported binge drinking. Among pregnant women, 1 in 10 reported drinking alcohol in the past 30 days and 3.1% reported binge drinking in the past 30 days.[61] Alcohol consumption during pregnancy has been associated with the development of fetal alcohol spectrum disorders, a group of conditions that may produce physical and neurodevelopmental problems in children whose mothers drank while pregnant.[62]

A particularly vulnerable group of women are those who are engaged in commercial sex work. In the United States and worldwide, commercial sex workers use illicit drugs at a much higher rate compared with women in the general population, placing this group at high risk of HIV infection, sexually transmitted infections, and violence.[63–65] Primary care providers working in underserved communities where commercial sex work may be more prevalent can provide more effective care if they are aware of the complex needs of these women, including the relationship between trauma and substance use.

RACIAL AND ETHNIC MINORITIES

In 2014, it was estimated that 10.2% of the US population had used an illicit drug in the past month. Rates were 12.4% among African Americans ages 12 and up; 14.9% for American Indians and Alaska Natives; 4.1% for Asian Americans; 15.6% among Native Hawaiians or Pacific Islanders; 8.9% for Hispanics/Latinos; and 10.4% for non-Latino whites.[66] Rates of heavy alcohol use tend to be higher among Native Americans compared with other groups.[10]

Underserved populations, including some racial and ethnic groups, often experience greater negative health effects from substance use than other groups.[67,68] African Americans and Latinos are at a greater risk of developing alcohol-related liver disease than whites and have higher rates of deaths from alcohol-related illnesses, including cirrhosis. This may be, in part, attributable to the drinking patterns of those considered heavy drinkers. Among all heavy drinkers, Hispanics and African Americans drink larger quantities of alcohol over a longer period of time than non-Latino whites.[69] Diverse communities often disproportionately experience the weight of SUDs due to cultural and socioeconomic factors, including environmental stress and poor access to or quality of medical care.[70] Once in treatment, studies have shown that African Americans and Latinos are less likely to complete treatment as a result of socioeconomic factors.[71,72] It is important for primary care providers to be aware of the impact of these and other social determinants of health when working with underserved communities.

OLDER ADULTS AS AN UNDERSERVED POPULATION

Historically, the prevalence of illicit drug use by older adults has been significantly lower than that of younger age groups. Moreover, the lifetime rates of drug use for people ages 65 and up are approximately half compared with all other age groups, from 19 to 64.[66] Recent studies, however, point to an increase in SUDs among older adults in the United States and Europe.[73] Of particular public health interest is the impact of the large baby-boomer generation (Americans born between 1946 and 1964), whose substance use is higher than previous cohorts. Researchers recently projected that past-year SUD in adults ages 50 to 59 will increase from 1.9 million in 2002 to 2006 to 3.1 million in 2020 whereas those ages 60 to 69 will increase from 0.6 million to 1.9 million.[74]

ADOLESCENTS

Substance use remains a significant contributor to the death and disease burden of adolescents in many societies.[75] In 2014, 5% of all US adolescents had an SUD.[66] Risk factors, such as increased availability of drugs and alcohol, parental substance use, exposure to violence and trauma, and poverty, all contribute to the incidence of drug and AUDs by adolescents. Overall rates of past-month illicit drug use by adolescents (youth ages 12–17) decreased from 11.6% in 2002 to 8.8% in 2013. The most commonly used substance was cannabis (7.1%) followed by psychotherapeutics, such as benzodiazepines and amphetamines (2.2%), hallucinogens (0.6%), inhalants (0.5%), cocaine (0.2%), and heroin (0.1%). Compared with 2002, past-month alcohol use declined from 28.8% to 22.7% and binge drinking declined from 19.3% to 14.2% in 2013. Although the rates of tobacco use have significantly decreased over the past decade (13.0% in 2002 to 5.6% in 2013), there has been an increase in the use of nicotine products, such as e-cigarettes.[5] Worldwide, there seems to be a discrepancy in the use patterns when it comes to cannabis. A recent study in 30 European and North American countries found that the use of cannabis by adolescents seems to be decreasing in Western Europe and the United States and increasing in Eastern European countries.[76]

RESOURCES AND SOLUTIONS

Several innovative solutions to substance use and SUD problems in the underserved have been developed. Housing First is one such solution and focuses on homeless individuals with co-occurring mental health disorders and SUDs. In the more traditional, treatment-first, stepped approach to housing of the homeless, homeless individuals qualify for increasingly stable and independent housing options as they engage in treatment services. Engagement in treatment, substance use abstinence, and mental health stability are required to move from shelter-based group housing to individual, independent-living housing units. Housing First provides independent living units first, with on-site robust social services and sometimes mental health care, SUD treatment, and health care services on site as well. Housing First residents are encouraged to engage these services but are not required to do so to remain in their homes. Housing First initiatives, pioneered in inner cities across the United States and now being implemented in Canada, Australia, and Europe, have reduced homelessness in the chronically homeless population with co-occurring mental health disorders and SUDs while increasing linkages to care and decreasing substance use.[77]

A second solution also increasingly promoted to increase SUD treatment access and engagement in the United States and around the globe is integration of SUD treatment and primary care services in a chronic care model.[27,35,78] These efforts recognize and address several barriers to SUD treatment, including too few SUD treatment providers, the stigma associated with engaging with traditional SUD treatment settings, and lack of insight by individuals with SUDs that they have an SUD and need treatment.[35] For primary care providers in underserved communities who are working with persons affected by SUDs, more information on chronic care models may be found at http://www.ihi.org/Pages/default.aspx.

Addressing risky substance use behaviors with all preadolescent and adult patients is essential to providing comprehensive care to the underserved. Primary care screening for tobacco use and risky alcohol use in adults and offering a brief intervention are grade B recommendations from the US Preventive Services Task Force.[79] There are numerous resources available for incorporating tobacco screening and cessation counseling as well as alcohol screening and brief intervention into primary care practices.[80]

Beyond screening and brief intervention for alcohol and tobacco use, OUD treatment integration into primary care settings is one of the primary desired outcomes of the US Drug Addiction Treatment Act of 2000 (DATA 2000), which allows physicians to prescribe Food and Drug Administration (FDA)–approved schedule III, IV, or V medications for the treatment of OUDs outside of a licensed methadone facility.[81] Currently, buprenorphine and buprenorphine/naloxone products are the only schedule III medications FDA approved for OUD treatment. Primary care physicians may prescribe buprenorphine products to their patients with OUDs by obtaining a DATA 2000 waiver from the Drug Enforcement Administration after completing 8 hours of training on buprenorphine and OUD treatment and ensuring ability to refer their patients to counseling services.[81] More than 32,000 US physicians have obtained a DATA 2000 waiver, and more than a quarter of waivered physicians are also approved to treat more than 30 patients for OUDs with buprenorphine medications in their practice.[82] Further access to OUD treatment is critical to stemming the ongoing opiate overdose crisis in the United States and many resources are available to help primary care physicians incorporate OUD treatment into their practices.[83]

A third solution to increase SUD treatment retention and effectiveness specifically for traumatized individuals is trauma-informed care. In addition to evidence-based counseling interventions, including Addiction and Trauma Recovery Integration Model and Seeking Safety, which are often delivered in specialized SUD treatment settings, the National Center for Trauma Informed Care lists 4 central themes that any individual, organization, or system can embrace to provide a trauma-informed approach to service delivery:

1. Understand the widespread impact of trauma and paths toward recovery.
2. Recognize signs and symptoms of trauma in clients/patients/consumers, families, and staff/providers.
3. Respond with full integration of knowledge of trauma in policies, procedures, and practices.
4. Actively avoid retraumatization.

Six principles (safety, trustworthiness and transparency, peer support, collaboration, empowerment, and cultural and gender relevancy) underpin these themes. Following these general principles, trauma-informed care can be applied in many settings, including primary care.[82]

REFERENCES

1. World Health Organization. WHO global report on trends in prevalence of tobacco smoking 2015. Geneva (Switzerland): World Health Organization; 2015.
2. World Health Organization. Global status report on alcohol and health, 2014. Geneva (Switzerland): World Health Organization; 2014.
3. United Nations Office on Drugs and Crime. World Drug Report 2014. Available at: http://www.unodc.org/wdr2014/. Accessed February 22, 2016.
4. US Department of Health and Human Services. The health consequences of smoking—50 years of progress: a report of the Surgeon General. Atlanta (GA): US Department of Health and Human Services; Centers for Disease Control and Prevention; National Center for Chronic Disease Prevention and Health Promotion; Office on Smoking and Health; 2014. p. 17.
5. Substance Abuse and Mental Health Services Administration, results from the 2013 National Survey on Drug Use and Health: summary of national findings, NSDUH Series H-48, HHS Publication No. (SMA) 14-4863. Rockville (MD): Substance Abuse and Mental Health Services Administration; 2014.
6. US Centers for Disease Control and Prevention. Alcohol use and health. Available at: http://www.cdc.gov/alcohol/fact-sheets/alcohol-use.htm. Accessed February 22, 2016.
7. National Highway Traffic Safety Administration. 2013 motor vehicle crashes: Overview.

8. Centers for Disease Control and Prevention. Excessive drinking costs U.S. $223.5 billion. Available at: http://www.cdc.gov/features/alcoholconsumption/. Accessed February 12, 2016.
9. US Centers for Disease Control and Prevention. Behavioral Risk Factor Surveillance System. survey data. Atlanta (GA): US Department of Health and Human Services, Centers for Disease Control and Prevention; 2014.
10. Chartier K, Caetano R. Ethnicity and health disparities in alcohol research. Alcohol Res Health 2010;33(1–2):152–60.
11. Schmidt L, Greenfield T, Mulia N. Unequal treatment: racial and ethnic disparities in alcoholism treatment services. Alcohol Res Health 2006;29(1):49.
12. American Psychiatric Association. Diagnostic and statistical manual of mental disorders (DSM-5®). Arlington (VA): American Psychiatric Pub; 2013.
13. Saitz R. Things that Work, Things that Don't Work, and Things that Matter—Including Words. J Addict Med 2015;9(6):429–30.
14. Saitz R. International Statement Recommending Against the Use of Terminology That Can Stigmatize People. J Addict Med 2016;10(1):1–2.
15. National Safety Council Injury Facts Book. 2014.
16. Laxmaiah Manchikanti M, Bert Fellows M, Hary Ailinani M. Therapeutic use, abuse, and nonmedical use of opioids: a ten-year perspective. Pain Physician 2010;13:401–35.
17. United States Food and Drug Administration. Joint Meeting of the anesthetic and life support drugs advisory committee and the drug safety and risk management advisory committee. 2010. Available at: http://www.fda.gov/downloads/AdvisoryCommittees/CommitteesMeetingMaterials/Drugs/AnestheticAndLifeSupport%20DrugsAdvisoryCommittee/UCM217510.pdf. Accessed March 29, 2016.
18. Seth P, Scholl L, Rudd RA, et al. Overdose Deaths Involving Opioids, Cocaine, and Psychostimulants — United States, 2015–2016. MMWR Morb Mortal Wkly Rep 2018;67:349–58.
19. Center for Behavioral Health Statistics and Quality. Behavioral health trends in the United States: results from the 2014 National Survey on Drug Use and Health (HHS Publication No. SMA 15–4927, NSDUH Series H-50). 2015. Available at: http://www.samhsa.gov/data/. Accessed January 29, 2016.
20. National Institute on Drug Abuse. Costs of Substance Abuse. Available at: https://www.drugabuse.gov/related-topics/trends-statistics. Accessed February 29, 2016.
21. Sacks JJ, Gonzales KR, Bouchery EE, et al. 2010 national and state costs of excessive alcohol consumption. Am J Prev Med 2015;49(5):e73–9.
22. Clark RE, Samnaliev M, McGovern MP. Impact of substance disorders on medical expenditures for medicaid beneficiaries with behavioral health disorders. Psychiatr Serv 2009;60(1):35–42.
23. Murray CJ, Lopez AD. Measuring the global burden of disease. N Engl J Med 2013;369(5):448–57.
24. Lander L, Howsare J, Byrne M. The Impact of Substance Use Disorders on Families and Children: From Theory to Practice. Soc Work Public Health 2013;28(3–4):194–205.
25. Substance Abuse and Mental Health Services Administration. Data Spotlight: Over 7 million children live with a parent with alcohol problems. 2012. Available at: http://media.samhsa.gov/data/spotlight/Spot061ChildrenOfAlcoholics2012.pdf. Accessed March 29, 2016.
26. World Health Organization. Global status report on alcohol 2004. Geneva (Switzerland): World Health Organization; 2004.

27. World Health Organization. Atlas on substance use (2010): resources for the prevention and treatment of substance use disorders. Geneva (Switzerland): World Health Organization; 2010.

28. Amato L, Minozzi S, Vecchi S, et al. Benzodiazepines for alcohol withdrawal. Cochrane Database Syst Rev 2010;(3):CD005063.

29. Hedges D, Jeppson K, Whitehead P. Antipsychotic medication and seizures: a review. Drugs Today (Barc) 2003;39(7):551–7.

30. Mason BJ, Goodman AM, Chabac S, et al. Effect of oral acamprosate on abstinence in patients with alcohol dependence in a double-blind, placebo-controlled trial: The role of patient motivation. J Psychiatr Res 2006;40(5):383–93.

31. Garbutt JC, Kranzler HR, O'Malley SS, et al. Efficacy and tolerability of long-acting injectable naltrexone for alcohol dependence: a randomized controlled trial. JAMA 2005;293(13):1617–25.

32. Furieri FA, Nakamura-Palacios EM. Gabapentin reduces alcohol consumption and craving: a randomized, double-blind, placebo-controlled trial. J Clin Psychiatry 2007;68(11):1691–700.

33. Soyka M, Zingg C, Koller G, et al. Retention rate and substance use in methadone and buprenorphine maintenance therapy and predictors of outcome: results from a randomized study. Int J Neuropsychopharmacol 2008;11(5):641–53.

34. Krupitsky E, Zvartau E, Woody G. Use of Naltrexone to Treat Opioid Addiction in a Country in Which Methadone and Buprenorphine Are Not Available. Curr Psychiatry Rep 2010;12(5):448–53.

35. Padwa H, Urada D, Antonini VP, et al. Integrating substance use disorder services with primary care: The experience in California. J Psychoactive Drugs 2012;44(4):299–306.

36. Huebner RB, Kantor LW. Advances in alcoholism treatment. Alcohol Res Health 2011;33(4):295–9.

37. Atwoli L, Stein DJ, Koenen KC, et al. Epidemiology of posttraumatic stress disorder: prevalence, correlates and consequences. Curr Opin Psychiatry 2015;28(4):307.

38. Gradus JL. Epidemiology of PTSD. Washington, DC: National Center for PTSD (United States Department of Veterans Affairs); 2007.

39. Liebschutz J, Saitz R, Brower V, et al. PTSD in urban primary care: high prevalence and low physician recognition. J Gen Intern Med 2007;22(6):719–26.

40. Gapen M, Cross D, Ortigo K, et al. Perceived neighborhood disorder, community cohesion, and PTSD symptoms among low-income African Americans in an urban health setting. Am J Orthopsychiatry 2011;81(1):31–7.

41. Erickson LD, Hedges DW, Call VR, et al. Prevalence of and factors associated with subclinical posttraumatic stress symptoms and PTSD in urban and rural areas of Montana: a cross-sectional study. J Rural Health 2013;29(4):403–12.

42. Klassen BJ, Porcerelli JH, Markova T. The effects of PTSD symptoms on health care resource utilization in a low-income, urban primary care setting. J Trauma Stress 2013;26(5):636–9.

43. Hall Brown T, Mellman TA. The influence of PTSD, sleep fears, and neighborhood stress on insomnia and short sleep duration in urban, young adult, African Americans. Behav Sleep Med 2014;12(3):198–206.

44. Smith PH, Homish GG, Leonard KE, et al. Intimate partner violence and specific substance use disorders: findings from the National Epidemiologic Survey on Alcohol and Related Conditions. Psychol Addict Behav 2012;26(2):236–45.

45. Devries KM, Child JC, Bacchus LJ, et al. Intimate partner violence victimization and alcohol consumption in women: a systematic review and meta-analysis. Addiction 2014;109(3):379–91.
46. Kartha A, Brower V, Saitz R, et al. The impact of trauma exposure and post-traumatic stress disorder on healthcare utilization among primary care patients. Med Care 2008;46(4):388–93.
47. Ullman SE, Starzynski LL, Long SM, et al. Exploring the relationships of women's sexual assault disclosure, social reactions, and problem drinking. J Interpers Violence 2008;23(9):1235–57.
48. Khoury L, Tang YL, Bradley B, et al. Substance use, childhood traumatic experience, and Posttraumatic Stress Disorder in an urban civilian population. Depress Anxiety 2010;27(12):1077–86.
49. Chartier MJ, Walker JR, Naimark B. Separate and cumulative effects of adverse childhood experiences in predicting adult health and health care utilization. Child Abuse Negl 2010;34(6):454–64.
50. Seal KH, Cohen G, Waldrop A, et al. Substance use disorders in Iraq and Afghanistan veterans in VA healthcare, 2001–2010: Implications for screening, diagnosis and treatment. Drug Alcohol Depend 2011;116(1–3):93–101.
51. Szaflarski M, Cubbins LA, Ying J. Epidemiology of alcohol abuse among US immigrant populations. J immigrant Minor Health 2011;13(4):647–58.
52. Obot IS, Room R. Alcohol, gender and drinking problems: perspectives from low and middle income countries. Geneva (Switzerland): World Health Organization; 2005.
53. Grant BF, Chou SP, Saha TD, et al. Prevalence of 12-Month Alcohol Use, High-Risk Drinking, and DSM-IV Alcohol Use Disorder in the United States, 2001-2002 to 2012-2013 Results From the National Epidemiologic Survey on Alcohol and Related Conditions. JAMA Psychiatry 2017;74(9):911–93.
54. Greenfield SF, Back SE, Lawson K, et al. Substance abuse in women. Psychiatr Clin North Am 2010;33(2):339–55.
55. Greenfield SF, Brooks AJ, Gordon SM, et al. Substance abuse treatment entry, retention, and outcome in women: a review of the literature. Drug Alcohol Depend 2007;86(1):1–21.
56. Hernandez-Avila CA, Rounsaville BJ, Kranzler HR. Opioid-, cannabis- and alcohol-dependent women show more rapid progression to substance abuse treatment. Drug Alcohol Depend 2004;74(3):265–72.
57. Keyes KM, Martins SS, Blanco C, et al. Telescoping and gender differences in alcohol dependence: new evidence from two national surveys. Am J Psychiatry 2010;167(8):969–76.
58. Floyd RL, Sobell M, Velasquez MM, et al. Preventing alcohol-exposed pregnancies: a randomized controlled trial. Am J Prev Med 2007;32(1):1–10.
59. Muhuri PK, Gfroerer JC. Substance use among women: associations with pregnancy, parenting, and race/ethnicity. Matern Child Health J 2008;13(3):376–85.
60. Ko JY, Wolicki S, Barfield WD, et al. CDC Grand Rounds: Public Health Strategies to Prevent Neonatal Abstinence Syndrome. MMWR Morb Mortal Wkly Rep 2017; 66:242–5.
61. Tan CH, Denny CH, Cheal NE, et al. Alcohol use and binge drinking among women of childbearing age-United States, 2011-2013. MMWR Morb Mortal Wkly Rep 2015;64(37):1042–6.
62. US Centers for Disease Control and Prevention. Fetal alcohol spectrum disorders (FASDs). Available at: https://www.cdc.gov/ncbddd/fasd/facts.html. Accessed February 12, 2016.

63. Shannon K, Kerr T, Strathdee SA, et al. Prevalence and structural correlates of gender based violence among a prospective cohort of female sex workers. BMJ 2009;339:b2939.
64. Strathdee SA, Philbin MM, Semple SJ, et al. Correlates of injection drug use among female sex workers in two Mexico–U.S. border cities. Drug Alcohol Depend 2008;92(1–3):132–40.
65. Wechsberg WM, Luseno WK, Lam WK, et al. Substance use, sexual risk, and violence: HIV prevention intervention with sex workers in Pretoria. AIDS Behav 2006;10(2):131–7.
66. Substance Abuse and Mental Health Services Administration, results from the 2011 national survey on drug use and health: summary of national findings, NSDUH Series H-44, HHS Publication No (SMA) 12-4713. Rockville (MD): Substance Abuse and Mental Health Services Administration; 2012.
67. Alegria M, Carson NJ, Goncalves M, et al. Disparities in treatment for substance use disorders and co-occurring disorders for ethnic/racial minority youth. J Am Acad Child Adolesc Psychiatry 2011;50(1):22–31.
68. Breslau J, Kendler KS, Su M, et al. Lifetime risk and persistence of psychiatric disorders across ethnic groups in the United States. Psychol Med 2005;35(3): 317–27.
69. Carrion AF, Ghanta R, Carrasquillo O, et al. Chronic liver disease in the Hispanic population of the United States. Clin Gastroenterol Hepatol 2011;9(10):834–41 [quiz: e109–10].
70. Buka SL. Disparities in health status and substance use: ethnicity and socioeconomic factors. Public Health Rep 2002;117(Suppl 1):S118–25.
71. Cook BL, Alegria M. Racial-ethnic disparities in substance abuse treatment: the role of criminal history and socioeconomic status. Psychiatr Serv 2011;62(11): 1273–81.
72. Daley MC. Race, managed care, and the quality of substance abuse treatment. Adm Policy Ment Health 2005;32(4):457–76.
73. Wang Y-P, Andrade LH. Epidemiology of alcohol and drug use in the elderly. Curr Opin Psychiatry 2013;26(4):343–8.
74. Han B, Gfroerer JC, Colliver JD, et al. Substance use disorder among older adults in the United States in 2020. Addiction 2009;104(1):88–96.
75. Toumbourou JW, Stockwell T, Neighbors C, et al. Interventions to reduce harm associated with adolescent substance use. Lancet 2007;369(9570):1391–401.
76. ter Bogt TFM, de Looze M, Molcho M, et al. Do societal wealth, family affluence and gender account for trends in adolescent cannabis use? A 30 country cross-national study. Addiction 2014;109(2):273–83.
77. Padgett DK, Stanhope V, Henwood BF, et al. Substance use outcomes among homeless clients with serious mental illness: comparing housing first with treatment first programs. Community Ment Health J 2011;47(2):227–32.
78. McLellan AT, Starrels JL, Tai B, et al. Can substance use disorders be managed using the chronic care model? Review and recommendations from a NIDA Consensus Group. Public Health Rev 2014;35(2):1–12.
79. United States Preventive Services Task Force. Published Recommendations. Available at: http://www.uspreventiveservicestaskforce.org/BrowseRec/Index. Accessed March 11, 2016.
80. National Institute on Drug Abuse. NIDA/SAMHSA Blending Initiative. Available at: https://www.drugabuse.gov/nidasamhsa-blending-initiative. Accessed March 11, 2016.

81. Public Law 106-310-106th Congress-An Act. Drug Addiction Treatment Act of 2000.

82. Substance Abuse and Mental Health Services Administration. Trauma-informed approach and trauma-specific interventions. Available at: www.samhsa.gov/nctic/trauma-interventions. Accessed March 11, 2016.

83. Substance Abuse and Mental Health Services Administration. TIP 40: clinical guidelines for the use of Buprenorphine in the treatment of opioid addiction. 2004. Available at: http://store.samhsa.gov/product/TIP-40-Clinical-Guidelines-for-the-Use-of-Buprenorphine-in-the-Treatment-of-Opioid-Addiction/SMA07-3939. Accessed March 11, 2016.

Diet and Obesity Issues in the Underserved

Maria C. Mejia de Grubb, MD, MPH*, Robert S. Levine, MD, Roger J. Zoorob, MD, MPH

KEYWORDS

- Obesity • Diet • Underserved populations • Epidemic • Healthy lifestyle
- Socioeconomically vulnerable • Primary care

KEY POINTS

- The obesity epidemic remains an unchecked threat to the health of the United States and the world, particularly among socioeconomically vulnerable communities.
- Identifying successful models that integrate primary care, public health, and community-based efforts is important for accelerating progress in preventing and treating obesity.
- Primary care providers can help, not only as clinicians but also as role models, educators, and leaders of community-based interventions.

INTRODUCTION

The goal of this article is to inform new directions for addressing inequalities associated with obesity by reviewing current issues about diet and obesity among socioeconomically vulnerable and underserved populations. It highlights recent interventions in selected high-risk populations, as well as gaps in the knowledge base. It then identifies future directions in policy and programmatic interventions to expand the role of primary care providers, with an emphasis on those aimed at preventing obesity and promoting healthy weight. Except as noted, obesity among adults in this article is defined as a body mass index (BMI) of greater than 30.0 and overweight as a BMI of 25.0 to 29.0.[1] For children and teens, overweight is defined as a BMI at or above the 85th percentile and below the 95th percentile for children and teens of the same age and sex. Obesity is defined as a BMI at or above the 95th percentile for children and teens of the same age and sex.[2]

This article is an update of an article that originally appeared in *Primary Care: Clinics in Office Practice*, Volume 44, Issue 1, March 2017.

The authors have nothing to disclose.

Department of Family and Community Medicine, Baylor College of Medicine, 3701 Kirby Drive, Suite 600, Houston, TX 77098, USA

* Corresponding author.

E-mail address: Maria.Mejiadegrubb@bcm.edu

EPIDEMIOLOGY IN THE GENERAL POPULATION
Childhood and Adolescence: United States

Estimates from the US National Health and Examination Survey (NHANES) for 2015 to 2016 showed that the prevalence of obesity among US youth ages 2 to 19 years was 18.5%.[3] This was indicative of the significant positive linear trend from 1999 to 2000, when 13.9% of youth were obese.[3] The prevalence of obesity among adolescents (12–19 years of age) was 20.6% in 2015 to 2016, 18.4% among school-age children (6–11 years), and 13.9% among preschool children (2–5 years). Adolescent (20.2%) and school-age boys (20.4%) had similar levels, and both values were higher than those of preschool boys (14.3%). Values for girls increased from 13.5% (preschool), to 16.3% (school age) and 20.9% (adolescents).[3] Differences by sex and age were not statistically significant, however.[3]

Adulthood: United States

Estimates of obesity among US adults vary somewhat between different national samples. NHANES (2015–2016) found that overall, 39.8% of US adults (ages 20 years and older) were obese. This represents an estimated 95,487,194 people.[4]

The 2016 Gallup and Healthways State of American Well-Being report included self-reported data from a national sample of 177,192 telephone interviews with US adults across all 50 states and the District of Columbia, conducted from January 2 to December 30, 2016.[5] The percentage of people aged 18 years and older who were obese was 28.4%, or approximately 3 percentage points higher than results from a similar survey taken in 2008.[5] The United Health Foundation's survey (America's Health Rankings), which is also based on self-reports, estimated 29.9% adult obesity for 2017.[6]

The Effect of Race, Ethnicity, Gender, and Socioeconomic Status: United States

According to NHANES (2015–2016), 11.0% of non-Hispanic Asian youth (2–19 years of age), were obese, as compared with 22.0% of non-Hispanic black, 25.8% of Hispanic, and 14.1% of non-Hispanic white youth.[3]

Among adults (NHANES 2015–2016), 12.7% of non-Hispanic Asian, 46.8% of non-Hispanic black, 47.0% of Hispanic, and 37.9% of non-Hispanic white adults, were found to be obese.[3] Among men, non-Hispanic Asian adults (10.1%) had a lower prevalence of obesity than non-Hispanic white (37.9%), non-Hispanic black (36.9%), and Hispanic (43.1%) men, with the difference between non-Hispanic Asian and non-Hispanic white men being statistically significant, but that between non-Hispanic black and white men not reaching statistical significance.[3] Non-Hispanic Asian women (14.8%), non-Hispanic black women (54.8%), and non-Hispanic white women (50.6%) all had higher prevalence than their male counterparts.[3]

Among non-Hispanic black and Mexican-American men, those with higher incomes were more likely to be obese than those with low incomes.[7] The same was true for Mexican-American men; however, among non-Hispanic white men, no statistically significant relationship was found with poverty.[8] In contrast, women with higher incomes were less likely to be obese than women with lower incomes, be they non-Hispanic white, non-Hispanic black, or Mexican-American.[8] These trends only reached statistical significance, however, for non-Hispanic white women. Such variations reflect the complex nature of relationships between socioeconomic status (SES) and obesity. Low-income and food-insecure populations in the United States, for example, face a multitude of barriers that may direct purchases toward inexpensive, energy-dense, nutritionally poor food. These populations may also be subject to cycles of food deprivation and overeating; high levels of stress, anxiety, or depression; have fewer opportunities for physical activity; and be subject to greater exposure to the marketing of obesity-promoting products.[9] Still, as previously noted,[8] obesity is not universally associated with low SES. A full understanding has not been reached, nor is this likely to happen without a better understanding of differences in motivations and the meaning of excess weight in different socioeconomic groups.[10] The role of education also seems to be different between men and women. Some observers have found no statistically significant relationship between obesity and education among men and an inverse relationship (lower obesity with a college education) among women.[8] Although longitudinal data linking community context to health are sparse, researchers using data from electronic health records of 163,473 children ages 3 to 18 years residing in 1288 communities in Pennsylvania whose weight and height were measured longitudinally observed that social deprivation at birth was associated with higher BMI at 10.7 years of age and with more rapid growth of BMI over time.[11] Children born into the poorest communities displayed sustained and accelerated BMI growth. Community-level deprivation remained associated with BMI trajectories after adjustment for household socioeconomic deprivation. By way of explanation, the investigators hypothesized that the effect of community socioeconomic deprivation on BMI growth may be mediated by parental behaviors related to food purchases and physical activity.[11] They concluded that individual-level intervention programs that ignore the effect of community context may be less efficient.[11]

Obesity in Special Populations

Incarcerated

Rising obesity rates in the United States may affect the imprisoned population, thereby increasing the prevalence of obesity-related diseases and the cost and performance of correctional health care. Leddy and colleagues[12] note that as rates of obesity increased in the United States so did the US prison population, which nearly tripled between 1987 and 2007, and judged that the frequencies of obesity-related comorbidities are comparable among inmates the general US population. For example, hypertension is 18.3% among inmates and 24.5% for the general US population, respiratory illness is at 8.5% for inmates and 7.8% for the general US population, and diabetes is at 4.8% among inmates and 7.0% for the general US population. They predict that the combination of rising rates of obesity and imprisonment may, therefore, increase the number and proportion of obese inmates.[12] A recent meta-analysis found that average weight gain increased by 0.43 pounds per week during incarceration,[13] although a second meta-analysis restricted to male prisons was inconclusive.[14]

Some research has found women prisoners to be particularly vulnerable to weight gain, although higher average weekly gains were reported for those incarcerated for 2 weeks or less at the time of study enrollment than those incarcerated longer than 2 weeks (1.7 pounds vs 0.8 pounds).[15] Evidence from Japan suggests that restricted diets and enforced physical activity can improve inmate health.[15]

Homeless

Researchers have noted a food insecurity–obesity paradox, whereby food insecurity, often associated with insufficient resources to purchase food, is associated with overconsumption of food and consequent obesity.[16] Many theories have been proposed to explain this correlation, including the low cost of energy-dense foods, binge-eating habits as an adaptive physiologic response to food scarcity, and childhood poverty leading to obesity in adulthood.[16] In a study of 436 chronically homeless adults across 11 US cities, 57% were found to be overweight or obese, with the prevalence being highest among women and Hispanic individuals.[16] The investigators concluded that there was a greater need for attention to obesity in chronically homeless adults and for a better understanding of the seeming paradox of relationships among food insecurity, poverty, and obesity. Recent evidence from a population of sheltered, homeless men corroborated high rates of overweight/obesity,[17] and a small randomized, controlled trial among such a group was optimistic about the potential for tailored intervention.[18]

Military

The US military has long been concerned that increased obesity and poor physical fitness among civilian youth may tend to produce soldiers who are, in the words of some worried military retirees, "Too fat to fight."[19] Military organizations were quicker to respond to the burgeoning US epidemic than their civilian counterparts, implementing an upgraded Physical Fitness and Weight Control Program (Army Regulation 600–9) in 1976.[20] Millions of Americans have been able to maintain a healthy weight and meet physical performance requirements while in military service and, even though it has been found that weight gain is associated with return to civilian life, there is evidence that the health consequences of obesity may be partly mitigated by those who maintain physical fitness.[20] The prevalence of obesity among military veterans as a whole has been estimated as 25.1% (based on the 2004 Behavioral Risk Factor Survey)[21] but estimates within the Veterans Health Administration (VHA) have been higher,[22] In a nationally representative survey of 3122 US veterans taken from October to December 2011, it was observed that 38.0% of those for whom the VHA was the main source of health care were obese.[22]

Global and International Issues

The World Health Organization (WHO) estimates that at least 2.8 million people die globally each year from being overweight or obese.[23] Moreover, the worldwide prevalence more than doubled between 1980 and 2016, at which point 11% of men and 15% of women in the world 18 years of age and older were obese (as defined by a BMI of >30 kg/m^2) versus 5% of men and 8% of women in 1980.[23,24] The higher prevalence among women was found in all WHO regions, translating to obesity among more than 650 million people.[23,24] Significantly, in 2016, 41 million children younger than 5 years worldwide were also obese or overweight (defined as a BMI >25) as well as 340 million children ages 5 to 19 years.[24] Global obesity presents a double burden of disease, in part, because it is now emerging as a problem in lower and middle-income countries, especially in urban centers.[24]

Coexistence of Food Insecurity and Obesity

In addition to the homeless, food insecurity and obesity may coexist in other disadvantaged populations. Food-insecure households are defined as those which, at some or all times during a year, are uncertain of having or unable to acquire enough food to meet the needs of all their members because they had insufficient money or other resources for food.[25] Current research into this association has resulted in mixed findings.[26–29] The Food Research and Action Center, however, has detailed at least 18 reasons why low income and food insecurity may be related to poor nutrition and obesity.[30] And recently, a preliminary study has suggested that food-insecure individuals may be more susceptible to increasing snack food intake in response to experimentally mediated scarcity.[31]

Both food insecurity and obesity may be independent consequences of low income and the resulting lack of access and/or utilization of enough nutritious food (eg, fresh, frozen, canned, in prepared sauces or dishes), stresses of poverty, and a sedentary lifestyle. The ability to afford healthy food and get the right amount of exercise, the 2 factors critical to maintaining a healthy weight, can be challenging for people living in low-income communities. According to the US Department of Agriculture (USDA), 12.3% (15.6 million) of US households were food insecure at some time during 2016.[32] Families with limited resources may select lower-quality diets, including high-calorie, energy-dense foods to maintain adequate energy intake. These foods are traditionally the least expensive, are easy to overconsume, have been shown to promote weight gain, and have been found to be more prevalent in low-income communities compared with healthier food options.[29] Research suggests that low-income, minority, and rural communities have fewer supermarkets compared with more affluent areas.[33] The lack of convenient access to supermarkets and full-service grocery stores that offer a larger selection of healthy and more affordable food (eg, fruits and vegetables) in both urban and rural low-income neighborhoods is an obstacle for attaining a healthy diet.

In addition, low-income communities have greater availability of fast-food restaurants, especially near schools.[29] Fast-food consumption is associated with a diet high in calories and low in nutrients, and frequent consumption may lead to weight gain.[27] Interestingly, McDermott and Stephens[34] found that, on a per-calorie basis, a fast-food, or convenience diet for a single parent raising 1 child in Baltimore, MD, without government support was more expensive than a diet based on generic brand or frozen foods, even though dairy and vegetables cost more than other food groups. They concluded that, "It is difficult to meet current dietary recommendations without income assistance."[34] Programs that currently help low-income families (incomes <185% of the poverty line) include the Women, Infant, and Children (WIC) Program, the Free and Reduced Meal (FARM) program, or the Commodity Supplemental Food Program (CSFP).[34]

Food Deserts

The USDA defines a food desert as a census tract in a low-income community in which at least one-third of the population lives more than 1 mile from the nearest large supermarket or grocery store in an urban area, and more than 10 miles in a rural area (low-access communities).[35] Food equity is achieved only when the residents of a neighborhood have easy access to affordable nutritious food. The location of the store in relationship to the resident, individual travel pattern characteristics (eg, income, car ownership, disability status), and neighborhood characteristics (eg, the availability of public transportation, availability of sidewalks, crime patterns in the area) are key factors to ensure equitable access to affordable, healthy foods.[35]

Higher Exposure to Marketing of Less Nutritious Foods and Media Influences

Research suggests that minority and low-income populations have poor nutrition that is not simply due to independent personal choice. Instead, food-marketing influences the preferences and consumption of unhealthy food choices.[36,37] Targeted marketing has influenced the increased availability and lower cost of processed, high-calorie foods relative to healthier options, increased portion sizes, food advertising, and fast-food promotion, which are all contributors to the obesity epidemic.[38]

In the United States, it has been suggested that future policy recommendations should include setting standards to limit the amount of advertising of foods and beverages of low nutritional value, particularly advertising targeting socioeconomically vulnerable children, via television, radio, new digital and social media, outdoor advertisement, and point-of-sale product placements.[39] This is also an international issue, with persuasive marketing of unhealthy food and beverage products to children in particular emerging as an important and explicitly recognized threat to rights to food and health in human rights instruments.[40]

Limited Access to Safe Places to Be Physically Active

Many low-income neighborhoods offer inadequate opportunities for safe exercise, and they lack community recreation areas with free or low-cost access. This limited access is associated with decreased physical activity and increased obesity rates.[41] In fact, communities with lower and medium SES often display fewer public resources, such as parks, trails, and playgrounds, compared with communities with higher SES.[42,43] Data show that improving certain features of the built environment supports physical activity, especially among underserved populations.[43] Recommended implementation strategies include improved access to places for physical activity, such as recreation areas and parks,[44] improved infrastructure to support bicycling and walking, locating schools closer to residential areas to encourage nonmotorized travel to and from school, zoning to allow mixed-use areas that combine residential with commercial and institutional uses, improving access to public transportation, and improving personal and traffic safety in areas in which persons are or could be physically active.[42–44]

High Levels of Stress and Poor Mental Health

Associations among food insecurity, stress, and poor mental health (eg, depression, psychological distress, anxiety) have been reported.[45,46] The financial and emotional burden of food insecurity, in addition to other socioeconomic factors, such as low-wage employment, lack of access to health care, inadequate transportation, poor housing, and neighborhood violence, pose additional constraints in underserved populations. Stress and poor mental health may lead to weight gain through stress-induced hormonal and metabolic changes, as well as unhealthy eating behaviors and physical inactivity.[47] Specifically, chronic stress can promote visceral fat accumulation by dysregulating the hypothalamic-pituitary-adrenal (HPA) axis. Reciprocally, obesity may promote a state of systemic low-grade inflammation mediated by increased adipokine secretion, which can also chronically stimulate and disturb the HPA axis, leading to a vicious cycle with multiple adverse health effects.[48] The pathophysiology of these interactions is exceedingly complex and is reviewed elsewhere.[48–50]

HEALTH CONSEQUENCES

Higher body weights are associated with higher incidence of many other health problems, including type 2 diabetes, cardiovascular disease, stroke, nonalcoholic fatty liver disease, gallstones, osteoarthritis, asthma, obstructive sleep apnea, female infertility, and increased risk of disability.[51–54] In addition, certain cancers have been linked to obesity, including colon, gall bladder, female breast (postmenopausal), endometrium, renal cell carcinoma, and adenocarcinoma of the esophagus. Higher body weight is also associated with social stigmatization and mental illness.[54]

A review of literature pertaining to psychosocial factors and childhood obesity noted the possibility of a bidirectional relationship with depression and anxiety, suggesting that it is possible that depression is both a cause and a consequence of obesity; a linear relationship between BMI and low body self-esteem in girls, in contrast to a U-shaped relationship in boys; unhealthy weight control behaviors (eg, unhealthy diets); and eating disorder symptoms, including binge-eating episodes, a drive for thinness, and impulse regulation.[53] Weight-based stigmatization and teasing, and weight and shape concerns, were 2 important mediating factors. Specifically, obesity is considered to be a particularly stigmatizing and socially unacceptable condition of childhood, with long-lasting effects related to lower levels of education and family income, higher poverty, and lower marriage rates in later young adulthood.[55,56]

INTERVENTIONS IN SELECTED HIGH-RISK POPULATIONS

The importance of cultural influences is key for many high-risk populations. Caprio and colleagues[57] summarized investigations pertaining to various cultures as part of a consensus statement for Shaping America's Health and the Obesity Society. Regarding body size, they noted that Latinas tend to favor a thin figure for themselves and a plumper figure for their children, whereas African American women and men were more likely to prefer a large body size for women. Feeding practices also have cultural determinants based in part on "Affordability, availability of foods and ingredients, palatability, familiarity, and perceived healthfulness prompt immigrant families to retain or discard certain traditional foods and to adopt novel foods associated with the mainstream culture."[57] Children from immigrant Mexican households, for example, may resist parental efforts to promote lower-calorie traditional foods prepared at home in favor of higher-calorie foods and favor the higher-calorie foods, beverages, and snacks from the mainstream culture.[57] Cultural patterns may also determine the types of foods considered to be healthy or unhealthy. Among Hmong immigrants in California, frozen or canned foods, as well as school meals, are considered unhealthy, in part, because they are not considered to be fresh.[57] The scientific literature pertaining to these topics is vast and growing. A current National Library of Medicine PubMed search for "obesity and culture" (June 2018) revealed more than 12,000 citations. The following examples provide a snapshot of interventions in selected high-risk groups.

Black and African American Communities

Researchers have noted the importance of community context in setting the agenda for African American obesity interventions.[58,59] Employment, safety, academic advancement, substance use disorders, incarceration, dysfunctional social networks, and violence may not only be of more immediate concern than calorie intake or physical activity, they may also play important roles in mediating unhealthy eating.[58,59] Additional mediating environmental factors include availability and access to high-quality foods, and physical activity resources.[59]

   Biologic factors that may contribute to difficulties in weight management among African Americans include lower energy expenditures when sleeping, exercising, or resting; increased propensity for fat storage; higher steady-state ghrelin levels, leading to increased hunger; lower peptide tyrosine production after meals, leading to lower satiety; and decreased energy cost of activity after diet-induced weight loss.[58] Inclusion of a formal maintenance program was associated with lower percentage of regained weight for African American (as well as white) women and there is some evidence that including cultural adaptations may improve outcomes among African American women.[58] The exact composition of effective cultural adaptations, however, seems to be poorly differentiated in the literature.[58] Multidimensional approaches are recommended for future efforts.[58]

US Immigrant Populations

A recent review identified only 20 of 684 potentially relevant articles that met selection criteria for evaluation.[60] Selection criteria were as follows: (1) the intervention targeted an immigrant population in the United States, (2) the intervention objective was the prevention or control of obesity, (3) the study examined measured (vs self-reported) outcomes related to obesity, (4) the findings were published in a peer-reviewed journal, and (5) the article was written in English.[60] Most of the interventions targeted Latinos, predominantly of Mexican origin, and their emphasis was on multiple activities, including diet, physical activity, sleep, and screen time. Successful interventions were characterized by community engagement and/or participation that included placement within community structures and settings, and leveraging community resources to achieve a cultural focus, without which the interventions generally did not work.[60] Child interventions that incorporated parenting practices and promoted a healthy home environment were also effective.[60] A key problem has been that the possible moderating role of acculturation on obesity-related outcomes is rarely considered, even though immigrant weight gain has been overwhelmingly linked to their level of acculturation.[60] The investigators concluded that, notwithstanding the paucity of data on effective interventions, novel obesity prevention strategies to reduce migration-related obesity inequalities are warranted to help inform health policies and programs.[60]

American Indian Communities

"Healthy Children, Strong Families" provides an example of obesity interventions targeted specifically for American Indians.[61] As part of community engagement efforts, it was noted that recognition of obesity was low despite evidence of a high prevalence of both being overweight and obesity. It was also noted that the views of holistic health in the American Indian community might make interventions focused on defining a particular disease ineffective. Investigators were pleasantly surprised at the effective-ness of mailed lessons; however, home visits by mentors, although appreciated, did not seem to make a difference in outcomes. For the future, investigators emphasized the importance of intergenerational inclusion; the availability of fun, easy, interactive learning materials; inclusion of health-related children's books; and a focus on reducing family and environmental barriers to change. Although work specific to American Indian groups is in its infancy, efforts such as this emphasize the common themes, which speak to the importance of community engagement and attention to contextual influences on the family.

Native Hawaiian and Pacific Islander Communities

The PILI 'Ohana project presents an example of obesity prevention efforts among native Hawaiian and Pacific Islander communities.[62] Once again, community context was identified as a key factor. Elements unique to Native Hawaiians and Pacific Islander individuals included a preference for ethnocultural activities as a form of exercise, such as hula for native Hawaiian individuals and ballroom dancing for Filipino individuals. Socially derived eating expectations were important to Pacific Islander individuals, including social pressures from within their own culture to eat and/or prepare large servings of calorie-dense food, such as dishes with Spam, canned corned beef, and side dishes with high-fat mayonnaise. Through 8 years of community-based work, researchers were able to mobilize communities to improve food sovereignty and organic and traditional Hawaiian farming.[62]

Rural Appalachia

The Behavioral Risk Factor Surveillance Survey has identified Rural Appalachia as being at the epicenter of the national obesity epidemic.[63] Because unhealthy behaviors, such as smoking, failure to meet recommendations for fruit and vegetable consumption, and low levels of physical activity are entrenched in the region,[63] innovative methods are needed so that families can acquire new knowledge. Adolescents, particularly disadvantaged and minority students, are targeted as primary family change agents, with the program building on an existing network of 76 science clubs organized in collaboration between communities in West Virginia and West Virginia University's Health Science and Technology Academy.[63] Club members are encouraged to enroll in and graduate from college. They are taught the science that underlies health care, including new knowledge about the importance and implications of lifestyle choices. Cognitive learning is emphasized as a prerequisite for changing behavior. Teachers and students are trained in the conduct of community-based participatory research.[63] Formal research projects are developed, sent through an approved Institutional Review Board, and implemented. From September 2011 to May 2012 there were 744 students in the program and 400 projects in place, 224 of which were related to obesity.[63] As of this writing, this is still a work in progress, so ultimate effectiveness remains to be determined. However, its unique design offers insights into new ideas for community collaboration in an environment in which changing behaviors for health has been an elusive goal.[63]

INTERNATIONAL PERSPECTIVES

According to WHO, a rising global epidemic of overweight and obesity, so-called globesity, is spreading across the world. Once considered a problem only for industrialized and high-income countries, worldwide obesity has more than doubled since 1980 and is now also prevalent in low-income and middle-income countries.[20,23,24] Despite that infectious diseases and undernutrition remain a challenge, low-income and middle-income countries are experiencing a rapid rise in noncommunicable disease risk factors, such as obesity and overweight, especially among urban communities.[24] In fact, 65% of the world's population lives in a country in which overweight and obesity-related mortality is much higher than underweight-related mortality.

Globalization forces, including free trade, economic growth, and urbanization, seem also to be driving the global obesity epidemic, especially in low-income and middle-income countries. These macrolevel mechanisms can promote nutrition transition, a term for the obesity-inducing shift from traditional to Western diets that accompanies modernization and wealth, by changing food and built environments and spreading new technologies.[64]

There is some evidence that the global public health community is taking the rise in obesity seriously (eg, increasing surveillance).[65] However, the obesity epidemic is not only increasing but no country has also reported decreased rates in the past 3 decades.[58–64] Although obesity may be a global issue, the challenges all begin at local levels, considering that dietary, economic, cultural, and lifestyle factors are so widely varied across countries. WHO's action plan to fight the global obesity epidemic recommends a population-based multisector, multidisciplinary, and culturally relevant approach. Changes must be multilateral to meet the complexity of cultural traditions and dietary norms of the world's many ethnic groups. It is important to continue surveillance and monitoring obesity trends and tailor public health intervention toward specific population groups. By working with local communities, stakeholders can better develop strategies that address both nutrition and physical activity to reduce obesity prevalence.[65]

POLICY RECOMMENDATIONS AND PRIMARY CARE

Several scientific organizations have published recommendations and guidelines for primary care providers to address obesity prevention and treatment. The Institute of Medicine (IOM) in its most recent report, "Accelerating Progress in Obesity Prevention,"[66] recommends 4 strategies to expand the role of health care providers and to encourage them to support and advocate publicly for several policy changes:

1. Provide standardized care and advocate for healthy community environments. Disseminate healthy lifestyle recommendations and materials as part of primary prevention efforts in the primary care setting. Physician counseling is effective in promoting healthy behavior. Data show that adults with high BMI who report that their doctors have told them they are overweight are more likely to have accurate perceptions of their own weight.[60–67] They are also more likely to be interested in losing weight and to have tried losing weight. Yet a third of obese patients say their doctors did not tell them they were overweight.[60–67]
2. Ensure coverage of, access to, and incentives for routine obesity prevention, screening, diagnosis, and treatment. The US Preventive Services Task Force recommends screening all adults for obesity and that clinicians offer or refer patients with a BMI greater than 30 kg/m^2 to intensive, multicomponent behavioral interventions. Implementation of capacity building within the primary care setting, such as improvements to organizational systems or care models used by providers, are key for effective practices.
3. Encourage active living and healthy eating at work. The IOM suggests that providers use a multifaceted approach to patient education, recognizing that patients may have different learning styles, needs, and preferences.
4. Encourage healthy weight gain during pregnancy and breastfeeding and promote breastfeeding-friendly environments.

FUTURE DIRECTIONS IN PRIMARY CARE

Primary care providers commonly evaluate and treat obesity and health-related conditions. Nonetheless, there is a recognized need to expand their role to include advocacy, modeling healthy lifestyle behaviors in the community, and counseling individuals and families about obesity prevention.[66]

Research

There is a significant need to identify safe and effective methods of providing weight management to patients with unhealthy weight encountered in primary care practices.[68] Obesity is a chronic condition on which the social determinants of health have considerable impact. Sharing responsibility and resources for the management of obesity has considerable promise. However, additional research and tools to facilitate primary care providers and their practices to locate community resources to partner with are warranted to improve obesity rates in their communities.[68]

Practice

Patients with complex health conditions, particularly among underserved communities, are not easily addressed in a typical physician-directed office visit of 15-minutes' or 20-minutes' duration. Nonetheless, the high prevalence of overweight and obesity in the United States suggests that a patient's weight status should always be addressed and placed at the center of his or her overall health care. Providers can also actively promote the prevention and treatment of obesity through efforts in community settings. Moreover, practice recommendations, such as weight status assessment and monitoring, healthy lifestyle promotion through motivational interviewing, treatment, clinician skill development, clinic infrastructure development, community program referrals, community health education, multisector community initiatives, and policy advocacy, are among the necessary steps for effective interventions. Unfortunately, data show that only 12% of physician office visits of all child or adult patients included counseling about nutrition or diet.[66] Lack of time to obtain relevant information from individual and family contexts may be a major impediment to addressing healthy weight. Additional barriers include a provider's lack of awareness of the issue, lack of comfort or skill counseling families on the issue, need for organizational prompts, and lack of familiarity with available community resources for lifestyle counseling or obesity prevention programs.[69]

SUMMARY

Identifying successful models that integrate primary care, public health, and community-based efforts is important to obesity prevention, particularly among underserved populations. Primary care providers play an important role in obesity interventions, consistent with current recommendations from scientific and professional organizations.

Outside of their clinical role, primary care providers also can serve as role models, educators, and promoters of healthy lifestyle practices, and serve as leaders in community-based obesity prevention initiatives.

REFERENCES

1. US Centers for Disease Control and Prevention. Defining adult overweight and obesity. Available at: https://www.cdc.gov/obesity/adult/defining.html. Accessed June 14, 2018.
2. US Centers for Disease Control and Prevention. Physical activity and health. Available at: https://www.cdc.gov/physicalactivity/basics/pa-health/index.htm. Accessed June 14, 2018.
3. Hales CM, Carroll MD, Fryar CD, et al. Prevalence of obesity among adults and youth: United States, 2015–2016. NCHS data brief, no 288. Hyattsville (MD): National Center for Health Statistics; 2017.
4. Centers for Disease Control and Prevention, National Center for Health Statistics. Compressed Mortality File 1999-2016 on CDC WONDER Online Database, released December 2017. Data are from the Compressed Mortality File 1999-2016 Series 20 No. 2V, 2017, as compiled from data provided by the 57 vital statistics jurisdictions through the Vital Statistics Cooperative Program. Available at: http://wonder.cdc.gov/cmf-icd10.html. Accessed June 14, 2018.
5. Gallup and Healthways. State of American well-being. Available at: http://info.healthways.com/hubfs/Gallup-Healthways%20State%20of%20American%20Well-Being_2016%20State%20Rankings%20vFINAL.pdf. Accessed June 14, 2018.
6. America's Health Rankings. 2017. Available at: https://assets.americashealthrankings.org/app/uploads/ahrannual17_complete-121817.pdf. Accessed June 13, 2018.
7. Wang Y, Beydoun MA. The obesity epidemic in the United States–gender, age, socioeconomic, racial/ethnic, and geographic characteristics: a systematic review and meta-regression analysis. Epidemiol Rev 2007;29:6–28.
8. US Centers for Disease Control and Prevention. Adult obesity facts. 2015. Available at: http://www.cdc.gov/obesity/data/adult.html. Accessed January 13, 2016.

9. Food Research and Action Center (FRAC). Why low-income and food insecure people are vulnerable to obesity. Available at: http://frac.org/obesity-health/low-income-food-insecure-people-vulnerable-poor-nutrition-obesity. Accessed June 14, 2018.

10. Pampel FC, Denney JT, Krueger PM. Obesity, SES, and economic development: a test of the reversal hypothesis. Soc Sci Med 2012;74(7):1073–81.

11. Nau C, Schwartz BS, Bandeen-Roche K, et al. Community socioeconomic deprivation and obesity trajectories in children using electronic health records. Obesity (Silver Spring) 2015;23(1):207–12.

12. Leddy MA, Schulkin J, Power ML. Consequences of high incarceration rate and high obesity prevalence on the prison system. J Correct Health Care 2009;15(4):318–27.

13. Gebremariam MK, Nanogo RA, Arah OA. Weight gain during incarceration: systematic review and meta-analysis. Obes Rev 2018;19(1):98–110.

14. Choudhry K, Armstrong D, Dregan A. Systematic review into obesity and weight gain within male prisons. Obes Res Clin Pract 2018;12(4):327–35.

15. Clarke JG, Waring ME. Overweight, obesity, and weight change among incarcerated women. J Correct Health Care 2012;18(4):285–92.

16. Tsai J, Rosenheck RA. Obesity among chronically homeless adults: is it a problem? Public Health Rep 2013;128(1):29–36.

17. Taylor EM, Kendzor DE, Reitzel LR, et al. Health risk factors and desire to change among homeless adults. Am J Health Behav 2016;40(4):455–60.

18. Kendzor DE, Allicock M, Businelle MS, et al. Evaluation of a shelter-based diet and physical activity intervention for homeless adults. J Phys Act Health 2017;14(2):88–97.

19. Christeson W, Taggart AD, Messner-Zidell S. Too fat to fight: retired military leaders want junk foods out of America's schools. New York: Mission Readyness; 2010.

20. Levine RS, Kilbourne BJ, Kihlberg CH, et al. Military and civilian approaches to the U.S. obesity epidemic [Chapter: 9]. In: Brennan VM, Kumanyika SK, Zambrana RE, editors. Obesity interventions in underserved communities. Baltimore (MD): Johns Hopkins University Press; 2014. p. 176–92.

21. Almond N, Kahwati L, Kinsinger L, et al. Prevalence of overweight and obesity among U.S. military veterans. Mil Med 2008;173(6):544–9.

22. Stefanovics EA, Potenza MN, Pietrzak RH. The physical and mental health burden of obesity in U.S. veterans: results from the National Health and Resilience in Veterans Study. J Psychiatr Res 2018;103:112–9.

23. World Health Organization Global Health Observatory (GHO) data. Obesity. Available at: http://www.who.int/gho/ncd/risk_factors/obesity_text/en/. Accessed June 14, 2018.

24. World Health Organization. Obesity and overweight. Available at: http://www.who.int/news-room/fact-sheets/detail/obesity-and-overweight. Accessed June 14, 2018.

25. Coleman-Jensen A, Rabbitt MP, Gregory CA, et al. Household food security in the United States in 2016. Economic Research Report No. (ERR-237). U.S. Department of Agriculture, Economic Research Service. 2017. p. 44.

26. Institute of Medicine. Hunger and obesity: understanding a food insecurity paradigm: workshop summary. Washington, DC: National Academies Press; 2011.

27. Larson NI, Story MT. Food insecurity and weight status among U.S. children and families: a review of the literature. Am J Prev Med 2011;40(2):166–73.

28. Frongillo EA, Bernal J. Understanding the coexistence of food insecurity and obesity. Curr Pediatr Rep 2014;2(4):284–90.

29. Hartline-Grafton H, Dean O. The impact of poverty, food insecurity, and poor nutrition on health and well-being. Washington, DC: Food Research & Action Center; 2017.

30. Food Research & Action Center. Why low-income and food-insecure people are vulnerable to poor nutrition and obesity. Available at: http://frac.org/obesity-health/low-income-food-insecure-people-vulnerable-poor-nutrition-obesity. Accessed June 14, 2018

31. Crandall AK, Temple JL. Experimental scarcity increases the relative reinforcing value of food in food insecure adults. Appetite 2018;128:106–15.

32. US Department of Agriculture, Economic Research Service. Food security status of U.S. households in 2016. Available at: https://www.ers.usda.gov/topics/food-nutrition-assistance/food-security-in-the-us/key-statistics-graphics.aspx. Accessed June 14, 2018.

33. Larson NI, Story MT, Nelson MC. Neighborhood environments: disparities in access to healthy foods in the U.S. Am J Prev Med 2009;36(1):74–81.

34. McDermott AJ, Stephens MB. Cost of eating: whole foods versus convenience foods in a low-income model. Fam Med 2010;42(4):280–4.

35. Economic Research Service, US Department of Agriculture. Access to affordable and nutritious food. Measuring and understanding food deserts and their consequences: report to congress. Washington, DC: USDA Administrative Publication No. (AP-036); 2009. p. 160.

36. Williams JD, Crockett D, Harrison RL, et al. The role of food culture and marketing activity in health disparities. Prev Med 2012;55(5):382–6.

37. Grier SA, Kumanyika SK. The context for choice: health implications of targeted food and beverage marketing to African Americans. Am J Public Health 2008; 98(9):1616–29.

38. McGinnis JM, Gootman JA, Kraak VI. Food marketing to children and youth: threat or opportunity? Washington, DC: National Academies Press; 2006.

39. The State of Obesity. A project of the Trust for America's Health and the Robert Wood Johnson Foundation special report: racial and ethnic disparities in obesity. Policy recommendations. 2016. Available at: http://stateofobesity.org/disparities/. Accessed January 12, 2016.

40. Granheim SI, Vandevijvere S, Torheim LE. The potential of a human rights approach for accelerating the implementation of comprehensive restrictions on the marketing of unhealthy foods and non-alcoholic beverages to children. Health Promot Int 2018. https://doi.org/10.1093/heapro/dax100.

41. National Recreation and Parks Association. Parks and recreation in underserved areas: a public health perspective. Ashburn (VA): National Recreation and Parks Association. Available at: http://www.nrpa.org/uploadedFiles/nrpa.org/Publications_and_Research/Research/Papers/Parks-Rec-Underserved-Areas.pdf. Accessed January 15, 2016.

42. Gordon-Larsen P, Nelson MC, Page P, et al. Inequality in the built environment underlies key health disparities in physical activity and obesity. Pediatrics 2006; 117(2):417–24.

43. Barrett MA, Miller D, Frumkin H. Parks and health: aligning incentives to create innovations in chronic disease prevention. Prev Chronic Dis 2014;11:E63.

44. Khan LK, Sobush K, Keener D, et al. Recommended community strategies and measurements to prevent obesity in the United States. MMWR Recomm Rep 2009;58(RR-7):1–26.

45. Leung CW, Epel ES, Willett WC, et al. Household food insecurity is positively associated with depression among low-income supplemental nutrition assistance

program participants and income-eligible nonparticipants. J Nutr 2015;145(3): 622–7.

46. Liu Y, Njai RS, Greenlund KJ, et al. Relationships between housing and food insecurity, frequent mental distress, and insufficient sleep among adults in 12 US States, 2009. Prev Chronic Dis 2014;11:E37.

47. Paredes S, Ribeiro L. Cortisol: the villain in metabolic syndrome. Rev Assoc Med Bras 2014;60(1):84–92.

48. Miller WL, Auchus RJ. The molecular biology, biochemistry, and physiology of human steroidogenesis and its disorders. Endocr Rev 2011;32(1):81–151.

49. McAllister EJ, Dhurandhar NV, Keith SW, et al. Ten putative contributors to the obesity epidemic. Crit Rev Food Sci Nutr 2009;49(10):868–913.

50. Block JP, He Y, Zaslavsky AM, et al. Psychosocial stress and change in weight among US adults. Am J Epidemiol 2009;170(2):181–92.

51. Calle EE, Thun MJ. Obesity and cancer. Oncogene 2004;23(38):6365–78.

52. Brennan VM, Kumanyika SK, Zambrana RE. Introduction: advancing a new conversation about obesity in the underserved. Obesity interventions in underserved communities: evidence and directions. Baltimore (MD): Johns Hopkins University Press; 2014. p. 1–21.

53. Russell-Mayhew S, McVey G, Bardick A, et al. Mental health, wellness, and childhood overweight/obesity. J Obes 2012;2012:281801.

54. Pont SJ, Puhl R, Cook SR, et al, Section on Obesity, Obesity Society. Stigma experienced by children and adolescents with obesity. Pediatrics 2017;140(6) [pii:e20173034].

55. Ogden CL, Carroll MD, Fryar CD, et al. Prevalence of obesity among adults and youth: United States, 2011-2014. NCHS Data Brief 2015;(219):1–8.

56. Ogden CL, Carroll MD, Kit BK, et al. Prevalence of childhood and adult obesity in the United States, 2011-2012. JAMA 2014;311(8):806–14.

57. Caprio S, Daniels SR, Drewnowski A, et al. Influence of race, ethnicity, and culture on childhood obesity: implications for prevention and treatment: a consensus statement of Shaping America's Health and the Obesity Society. Diabetes Care 2008;31(11):2211–21.

58. Kumanyika SK, Prewitt TE, Banks J, et al. In the way or on the way?. In: Brennan VM, Kumanyika SK, Zambrana RE, editors. Obesity interventions in underserved communities: evidence and directions. Baltimore (MD): Johns Hopkins University Press; 2014. p. 151–61.

59. Tussing-Humphreys LM, Fitzgibbon ML, Kong A, et al. Weight loss maintenance in African American women: a systematic review of the behavioral lifestyle intervention literature. J Obes 2013;2013:437369.

60. Tovar A, Renzaho AM, Guerrero AD, et al. A systematic review of obesity prevention intervention studies among immigrant populations in the US. Curr Obes Rep 2014;3:206–22.

61. Adams A, Cronin KA. HCSF Community Research Group. Healthy children, strong families: obesity prevention for preschool American Indian children and their families. In: Brennan VM, Kumanyika SK, Zambrana RE, editors. Obesity interventions in underserved communities: evidence and directions. Baltimore (MD): Johns Hopkins University Press; 2014. p. 344–52.

62. Kaholokula JK, Kekauoha P, Dillard A, et al. The PILI 'Ohana Project: a community-academic partnership to achieve metabolic health equity in Hawai'i. Hawaii J Med Public Health 2014;73(12 Suppl 3):29–33.

63. Branch RA, Chester AL, Hanks S, et al. Obesity management organized by adolescents in rural Appalachia. In: Brennan VM, Kumanyika SK, Zambrana RE,

editors. Obesity interventions in underserved communities: evidence and directions. Baltimore (MD): Johns Hopkins University Press; 2014. p. 205–13.

64. Popkin BM. The world is fat. Sci Am 2007;297(3):88–95.
65. Ng M, Fleming T, Robinson M, et al. Global, regional, and national prevalence of overweight and obesity in children and adults during 1980-2013: a systematic analysis for the Global Burden of Disease Study 2013. Lancet 2014;384(9945): 766–81.
66. Committee on Accelerating Progress in Obesity Prevention and Institute of Medicine. Accelerating progress in obesity prevention: solving the weight of the nation. Baltimore (MD): National Academies Press; 2012.
67. Post RE, Mainous AG 3rd, Gregorie SH, et al. The influence of physician acknowledgment of patients' weight status on patient perceptions of overweight and obesity in the United States. Arch Intern Med 2011;171(4):316–21.
68. Wadden TA, Volger S, Tsai AG, et al. Managing obesity in primary care practice: an overview with perspective from the POWER-UP study. Int J Obes 2013; 37(Suppl 1):S3–11.
69. Vine M, Hargreaves MB, Briefel RR, et al. Expanding the role of primary care in the prevention and treatment of childhood obesity: a review of clinic- and community-based recommendations and interventions. J Obes 2013;2013: 172035.

The Effects of Exercise on Adolescent Physical Development, Brain Development and Adult Health in Underserved Populations

Vincent Morelli, MD[a],*, Daniel L. Bedney, MD[b],
Arie (Eric) Dadush, MD[b]

KEYWORDS

• Exercise • Underserved • Sports medicine • Socioeconomic status

KEY POINTS

• Primary care providers can make a strong argument for exercise promotion in underserved communities.
• The benefits are vitally important in adolescent physical, cognitive, and psychological development as well as in adult disease prevention and treatment.
• In counseling such patients, we should take into account a patient's readiness for change and the barriers to exercise.

EXERCISE IN UNDERSERVED COMMUNITIES

As discussed in other articles in this issue, the untoward health effects brought on by lower socioeconomic status (SES) and higher allostatic load (AL) can be significant. In this article the authors briefly recap the effects of low SES on adolescent development (both physical and psychological) and on adult burden of disease. The authors then examine how exercise might help to ameliorate these untoward health effects in underserved populations.

This article originally appeared in *Primary Care: Clinics in Office Practice*, Volume 44, Issue 1, March 2017.
Disclosure: The authors of this work report no direct financial interest in the subject matter or any material discussed in this article.
[a] Sports Medicine Fellowship, Department of Family and Community Medicine, Meharry Medical College, 1005 Dr D. B. Todd Boulevard, Nashville, TN 37208, USA; [b] Department of Family and Community Medicine, Meharry Medical College, 1005 Dr D. B. Todd Boulevard, Nashville, TN 37208, USA
* Corresponding author.
E-mail address: vmorelli@mmc.edu

DEMOGRAPHICS

The World Health Organization and the American College of Sports Medicine recommend 150 minutes per week of moderate to vigorous physical activity (MVPA) in adults and 60 minutes per day in children and adolescents.[1,2] (MVPA is any activity whereby one is breathing harder than usual but can still carry on a conversation.) In the United States, only 42% of children and 8% of adolescents meet these modest recommendations,[3,4] with underserved children (black and Hispanics) exhibiting the lowest levels of physical activity. The lowest levels of physical activity are seen in children with poorly educated mothers, those living in high-crime neighborhoods, those from low-income families, those with few adult role models, those in schools lacking sufficient physical education (PE) classes, and those living in communities with low community-based physical activity opportunities.[5,6] In addition, as children age from 9 to 15 years, the time spent in MVPA drops significantly, again with the greatest declines seen in children of low-income families (and girls).[7] Contributing to the problem is the fact that in 2014 only 3.6% of elementary schools, 3.4% of middle schools, and 4.0% of high schools nationwide required daily PE for all students (US DHHS, Centers for Disease Control and Prevention. Results from the School Health Policy and Practices Study 2014. Available at: www.cdc.gov/healthyyouth/data/shpps/pdf/shpps-508-final_101315.pdf. Accessed November 8, 2016.), thus, disregarding the recommendations of the nation's Healthy People 2020 goals.[8]

Among adults, less than 50% of US adults meet current exercise recommendations (less than 15% in some studies); those of low SES have even lower levels of compliance.[9] African American women have the lowest exercise rates (only 34% exercise) of any race/sex demographic group.[10–12]

PHYSICAL DEVELOPMENT IN UNDERSERVED POPULATIONS
Normal Adolescent Physical Development, the Effects of Low Socioeconomic Status and the Role of Exercise

Adolescence, the developmental stage leading to physical, sexual, and psychosocial maturation, is mediated by hormonal, genetic, and environmental factors. Whether or not socioeconomic factors affect physical development and maturation is the topic of this section of inquiry.

The normal child to adolescent transition is mediated by neuroendocrine changes. Gonadotropin-releasing hormone (GnRH), essentially dormant since birth, is activated (by largely unknown triggers) leading to an increased secretion of gonadotrophs: follicle-stimulating hormone and luteinizing hormone from the pituitary. Increased secretion, in turn, promotes the production of androgens and estrogens from the ovaries and testes. Concomitantly, the same triggers that stimulate GnRH secretion also incite corticotrophin-releasing hormone secretion from the hypothalamus, which then stimulates the anterior pituitary to secrete adrenocorticotropic hormone, acting on the adrenal glands to increase the secretion of the *adrenal* androgens dehydroepiandrosterone and androstenedione. The elevated levels of estrogens and gonadal and adrenal androgens begin to initiate sexual development and simultaneously stimulate an increase in the release of growth hormone from the pituitary. Together these well-orchestrated changes lead to an increase in physical stature, the development of secondary sexual characteristics, and the ultimate transition into adulthood.[13–16]

The questions before us are as follows: (1) Are there any untoward effects if this normal developmental cascade is altered? (2) Can SES or AL affect this cascade and contribute to these untoward effects? (3) If so, can exercise favorably influence or mitigate such alterations? In answer to the first question, if normal development is altered, there *are* possible untoward effects. Early menarche has been associated with an increased risk of breast cancer,[17] heart disease,[18–20] asthma,[21,22] insulin resistance,[23] metabolic syndrome,[23] coping strategies,[24] and all-cause mortality.[25] No similar data regarding future health risks in boys could be found.

The second question, positing if SES can increase the likelihood of early menarche and its untoward effects, can be answered by reviewing epidemiologic data. Generally, the age of the onset of puberty in the United States has been decreasing since the 1950s (menarche 12.9 years in 1948 and 12.4 years in 1994); although African American girls reach menarche 8 months earlier than Caucasian girls,[26] most studies attribute this to race *not* SES.[27] In fact, some studies specifically examining the role of SES on menarche found earlier menarche in girls of *high* SES.[28] Overall, however, although there is fear of low SES facilitating early menarche, as of 2015 the literature has not definitively documented this.[29] Except in cases of significant malnutrition, the authors found no studies unequivocally demonstrating any adverse effects of AL or low SES on age of menarche (with its increased burden of disease), the development of secondary sexual characteristics, or physical development in adolescence.[30]

In light of the answers to the first two questions, the answer to the third question seems moot. However, let us make a few points with respect to exercise, physical development, and disease prevention in this population. It is well established that adolescent and adult health issues occur disproportionately in underserved communities (eg, heart disease, diabetes, adolescent and adult obesity, asthma, cancers) and that AL is a known contributor to this burden of disease. It is also established that physical activity can decrease AL and ameliorate many of these adult health issues. Therefore, because those with lower SES have lower levels of physical activity,[31] and because childhood habits are proven to carry strongly forward into adulthood,[32–34] instilling a habit of exercise during adolescence is perhaps the primary care provider's best way of enhancing mental health and school performance in adolescents and fostering long-term economic success and health in adults who have carried forward a habit of activity from childhood.[35,36]

BRAIN DEVELOPMENT IN UNDERSERVED POPULATIONS

In order to look at brain development in underserved populations, normal brain development must be briefly reviewed first. The cognitive and structural deficits that occur in underserved or impoverished populations can then be discussed. Finally, it is then possible to examine the effects that exercise has on brain structure and function and to examine how these effects may ameliorate some of the deficits caused by stressful or underserved conditions.

Normal Adolescent Brain Development

As a child grows from adolescence to adulthood, the amount of gray matter (neurons) decreases as selective elimination of redundant pathways (pruning) takes place. Conversely, the amount of cortical white matter (myelin coated axons) increases as more and more cell-to-cell connections are formalized.[37] These connections continue to form through early adulthood and are important in learning, imagination, memory, and physical memory. Any arrest in white matter growth during this time could lead to potential interconnectivity deficits and impaired learning.

One specific area of importance when looking at white matter development is the prefrontal cortex. The white matter connections formed in this area (the seat of impulse control, decision making, delayed gratification, goal-directed behavior) are not complete until a person reaches their mid 20s.[38–40] In addition to this delayed white matter development, the adolescent brain has also been found to have a relative lack of mood modulating and behavioral control neurotransmitters (eg, serotonin) and an excess excitatory neurotransmitters (eg, glutamate, dopamine). It is important for parents, teachers, and policy makers to keep in mind that the end result of all this is that the normal adolescent brain is relatively more excitable and is lacking in impulse control and executive function. Any factors that further delay or impede maturation in these areas could be expected to compound these deficits and lead to further learning and behavioral problems and risky behaviors.[41]

THE EFFECT OF BEING UNDERSERVED ON ADOLESCENT BRAIN DEVELOPMENT

It has been shown that children in socioeconomically stressed conditions (eg, less than 150% of US federal poverty levels) have lower brain electrical activity, altered verbal centers,[42,43] up to 10% less gray matter, and smaller brain volumes in areas critical to learning, such as memory (eg, hippocampus), executive functioning, and impulse control (eg, frontal lobes).[44–48]

In addition, these children form fewer network connections between emotional and control centers (eg, the prefrontal cortex)[49] and have slower overall brain growth. These structural difference have been associated with lower test scores,[48,50] shorter attention spans,[51,52] lower reading comprehension, more disruptive behavior, rule breaking, aggression, and hyperactive behavior. Not only do these structural deficits affect the developing child but these disparities in brain structure have also been proven to persist into adulthood with resultant heightened threat response activity, lower responses to positive social stimuli, lower college enrollment and graduation rates,[53] lower wages and income, and more physical and psychological maladies.[54]

One interesting study examining the cognitive effects of socioeconomic stress followed more than 5000 adopted children and showed that those adopted into low-income homes scored 13 IQ points lower than their counterparts adopted into higher-income families,[55] effects postulated to be due to higher levels of stress, lack of parenteral interaction, limited mental stimulation, and poor nutrition.[56,57]

The Effects of Physical Activity and the Developing Brain

The question we face is as follows: Can exercise ameliorate any of the earlier noted stress-induced metabolic, structural, and behavioral changes?

The authors could find no prospective studies examining the effects of exercise on the *structure* of the "low socioeconomic brain," but several prospective studies looked at the effects of exercise on *academic and cognitive performance* in low-income adolescents. One study examining attention span and reading comprehension in low-income adolescents[52] found that aerobic exercise improved both attention span and reading comprehension to a greater degree in low-income students than their higher-income counterparts. The study recommended that "schools serving low-income adolescents should consider implementing brief sessions of aerobic exercise during the school day."[52]

Another study[58] examining fitness and cognitive performance in 83,000 children in the New York City Public School found that, although all children improved academic performance with increased fitness, the effect was most pronounced in impoverished youths, especially boys.

As mentioned earlier, although the authors could find no prospective studies evaluating exercise's effect on allostatic load or brain structure, relevant observations can be made from existing studies examining the differences between fit and unfit *nonimpoverished* children.

Structurally, regular physical activity has been shown to enhance neurogenesis via increased levels of brain-derived neurotropic factor[59,60] and serotonin.[61] This enhanced neurogenesis may account for the structural advantages seen in the brains of fit children. In other words, physically fit children have been shown to have larger hippocampal volumes (memory storage and association area)[62] and larger basal ganglia volumes (areas important in task completion).

Cognitively, again in nonimpoverished children, exercise has been shown to improve attention span[63] and mental processing speed.[64] It has been shown to enhance learning, especially with challenging subjects,[65] and to strengthen multitasking ability[66] resulting in higher test scores.[67–69] Fit children also have superior relational or associative memory (able to associate dissimilar bits of information), an area important in learning and imagination. In summary, physically fit children have an increased ability to focus, learn, process, and shut out distractions and conflicting impulses,[70,71] all qualities that would be especially desirable in impoverished populations.

THE IMPORTANCE OF EXERCISE IN UNDERSERVED POPULATIONS

Although, as mentioned earlier, the authors could find no prospective trials specifically evaluating the impact of exercise on AL in *underserved communities*, the literature does make a strong case for promoting exercise in these communities for disease prevention and neurologic, academic, and psychological development.

Various reviews note that our stress response has evolved as a means to enhance survival in the face of physical threat, readying ourselves for action (ie, fight or flight) that could save us. Today, however, when physical threat is less imminent and stress is more often caused by prolonged exposure to emotional or social factors, an action outlet is often unavailable to dissipate our pent-up hormonal readiness. It is thought that the energy meant to be mobilized for *fight or flight* is today, instead, stored in visceral fat. It is thought that the prolonged hormonal changes that occur during chronic stress can lead to central obesity, hypertension, dyslipidemia, metabolic syndrome, cardiovascular maladaptation, and neurologic changes resulting in cognitive and mood disturbances.[72] Physical inactivity likely fuels this fire, whereas exercise has been shown to mitigate the effects of such chronic stress and individual markers of AL.[73–76] It is, therefore, vital in our underserved communities, where chronic psychosocial stress is prevalent, that primary care providers educate patients about the heightened risks of inactivity and energetically promote AL-reducing exercise.

In summation, lack of exercise in underserved communities most certainly contributes to developmental delay, increased behavioral problems, and poor academic performance in our children. This finding is vitally important for policy makers to keep in mind because often PE classes are the first to be eliminated when school budgets come under scrutiny. Such curriculum shrinkage will disproportionately affect our underserved populations because 51% of US public school children come from low-income families (2013 data)[48] and because alternative recreation sites/access to safe playgrounds may be limited. It is the authors' opinion that the ameliorating effects of exercise are a critical unguent in our underserved communities and that thoughtful policy must focus on exercise promotion, the elimination of AL, and the abolition of poverty. This point is critical if a nation's children, and, thus, a nation, are to reach their full intellectual potential.

THE MAJOR HEALTH PROBLEMS IN UNDERSERVED *ADULT* POPULATIONS

Most of the significant health issues faced in underserved communities have been addressed in detail in other articles in this issue. The authors' intent here is not to rehash these issues but instead to briefly mention them, then to discuss the role that exercise might play in treatment and prevention. Hypertension, diabetes, asthma, hyperlipidemia, and depression are 5 of the most common medical problems disproportionately encountered in underserved communities.[77] In addition, as explained in Oluwadamilola O. Olaku and Emmanuel A. Taylor's article, "Cancer in the Medically Underserved Population," in this issue, colorectal and breast cancer are the two most common presenting cancers, with increased mortality in these communities.[78,79]

EXERCISE *AS TREATMENT* IN ADULT UNDERSERVED POPULATIONS

Although exercise has been documented to have beneficial effects in a multitude of medical conditions, including the 5 common maladies mentioned earlier,[80] the authors could find no studies documenting the benefits of exercise *selectively* in these conditions in medically underserved populations (MUPs). Therefore, the benefits of exercise discussed later are discussed in reference to normal or nonunderserved communities, which may or may not accurately project onto underserved populations.

Hypertension

Hypertension is the most common medical problem at underserved clinics[77]; studies have shown that aerobic exercise, strength training, and isometric exercise will all reduce blood pressure.[80] The decrease in pressure brought on by exercise (15 mm Hg systolic and 4 mm Hg diastolic) has been shown to persist for 4 to 10 hours and up to 22 hours after exercise.[81] This exercise-induced reduction is of eye-opening importance because a reduction in systolic blood pressure of only 2 mm Hg has been shown to reduce risk of cardiovascular mortality by 7%.[82] The potential impact of exercise is significant.

Diabetes Type II

Physical activity along with diet and medication are the mainstays for the treatment of type II diabetes.[83–85] Exercise results in increased insulin sensitivity and enhanced uptake of glucose by muscle.[80] It has been shown to reduce glycosylated hemoglobin (HbA1c) by 0.4% to 0.6%, a reduction comparable with metformin,[80] and to reduce fasting glucose. Combining aerobic and resistance training produces the greatest reduction of HbA1c.[86] Recent data also suggest that postprandial glucose (rather than fasting glucose or HbA1c) may better correlate with diabetes mortality. Unlike most medications, physical activity has been shown to significantly reduce this postprandial parameter as well.[87,88] Again, whether the effects of exercise seen here can be extrapolated equally to underserved communities is unknown.

Asthma

Physical training has been shown to improve asthmatic symptoms and asthmatic quality of life.[89] Asthmatic patients can enjoy 6 to 9 more symptom-free days per month with aerobic training than those who do not participate in aerobic training.[90–92] Exercise, of course, can trigger bronchoconstriction[93] in patients with exercise-induced asthma; but despite this, exercise has been proven to be safe and beneficial, even in high-intensity workouts if symptoms are controlled.[94] As discussed earlier, studies are needed to specifically address the effects of exercise on asthmatic patients in underserved communities.

Hyperlipidemia

Elevations of cholesterol and triglycerides are known risk factors for atherosclerosis and heart disease. Physical activity[95,96] has been shown to improve these lipid profiles[97,98] by selectively improving skeletal muscles utilization of lipids.[99] Both low-density lipoprotein and triglycerides are lowered with intense exercise,[100] whereas cardioprotective high-density lipoprotein (HDL) is increased with prolonged aerobic exercise (a minimum of 120 minutes weekly). Every HDL increase of 0.025 mmol/L decreases cardiovascular risk by 2% in men and 3% in women.[101,102] Although specific studies addressing physical activity's benefit in cardiovascular disease selectively in underserved communities are lacking, potential benefits are significant.

Depression

Common in underserved communities, one of the main symptoms of major depressive disorder is fatigue.[103] It has been theorized that inactivity can exacerbate this problem[80] and that, conversely, physical activity can help reduce these symptoms and enhance feelings of well-being.[104] There is evidence that aerobic exercise is as effective as pharmacotherapy in the short-term and that patients who exercise (with or without pharmacotherapy) have less depressive symptoms over the long-term as well.[105,106] These benefits of exercise are thought to be due to multiple factors, including hormonal changes,[107] distraction from sad thoughts,[80] and actually inducing neurologic structural changes (eg, increasing hippocampal volume: there is a noted decrease in hippocampal volume in depression).[108,109]

EXERCISE AS *DISEASE PREVENTION* IN ADULT UNDERSERVED POPULATIONS

Primary care physicians not only treat acute and chronic disease but also endeavor to screen and prevent such disease. The topic of screening inadequacies in underserved communities is beyond the scope of this article; however, they are well addressed in the literature.[77] For the authors' purposes in this article, it is important to recognize the preventative effects of exercise on 2 cancers that are commonly screened for: the two most common cancers presenting in underserved conditions.

Colorectal Cancer

In the United States, a higher incidence of colorectal cancer (CRC) is found in underserved communities. (In Europe such an association is not found.)[79,110–112] This finding is due both to inadequate screening and greater exposure to risk factors (see Oluwadamilola O. Olaku and Emmanuel A. Taylor's article, "Cancer in the Medically Underserved Population," in this issue). One of these risk factors, inactivity, is notably more prevalent in underserved communities and can clearly be addressed by exercise promotion. In the general population, physical activity has been demonstrated to prevent CRC in men and women,[113] with moderate or vigorous exercise shown to reduce colon cancer risk by 40%.[114] In addition, exercise *after* diagnosis has been shown to decrease total CRC-specific mortality (by 39%) in patients who increase in their physical activity to as little 5 hours of normal-pace walking per week.[115]

Breast Cancer

Although the incidence of breast cancer is greater in white women and women of high SES,[116] most studies have found that black women and those of lower SES have higher mortality.[117] This finding is likely linked to late stage of presentation, obesity, lower levels of physical activity, lower levels of education,[118,119] and differing treatment regimes.[120]

Physical activity offers a dose-dependent risk reduction in breast cancer.[121] The average risk reduction with moderate to vigorous physical activity is 25% to 30%, although the exact frequency and duration of exercise to achieve this benefit is unclear.[122] With higher cancer mortality among underserved women, one would assume that studies examining the effects of exercise on this mortality would have been done. However, once again, the authors could find no literature specifically addressing the effects of exercise on breast cancer incidence or mortality *specifically* on women of low SES.[121]

BARRIERS TO EXERCISE IN UNDERSERVED POPULATIONS

With all the known benefits of exercise, why do not more underserved patients exercise? The top reasons for not exercising in MUPs are as follows: not having access to exercise equipment, not having time to exercise, excessive cost, general health concerns (not healthy enough to exercise), lack of exercise companionship, feeling uncomfortable or embarrassed exercising, child care responsibilities, lack of motivation, concerns of safety in neighborhood, and low personal functioning.[72,123–125]

SUMMARY

In conclusion, primary care providers can make a strong argument for exercise promotion in underserved communities. The benefits are vitally important in adolescent physical, cognitive, and psychological development as well as in adult disease prevention and treatment. In counseling such patients, we should take into account a patient's readiness for change and the barriers to exercise as discussed earlier.

REFERENCES

1. Fact Sheet Physical Activity. Global recommendations on physical activity for health. Available at: http://www.euro.who.int/__data/assets/pdf_file/0005/288041/WHO-Fact-Sheet-PA-2015.pdf. Accessed February 29, 2016.
2. ACSM, AHA Support federal physical activity guidelines. Available at: https://www.acsm.org/about-acsm/media-room/acsm-in-the-news/2011/08/01/acsm-aha-support-federal-physical-activity-guidelines. Accessed February 29, 2016.
3. Whitt-Glover MC, Taylor WC, Floyd MF, et al. Disparities in physical activity and sedentary behaviors among US children and adolescents: prevalence, correlates, and intervention implications. J Public Health Policy 2009;30:S309–34.
4. Troiano RP, Berrigan D, Dodd KW, et al. Physical activity in the United States measured by accelerometer. Med Sci Sports Exerc 2008;40:181.
5. Gordon-Larsen P, McMurray RG, Popkin BM. Adolescent physical activity and inactivity vary by ethnicity: the National Longitudinal Study of Adolescent Health. J Pediatr 1999;135:301–6.
6. Gordon-Larsen P, McMurray RG, Popkin BM. Determinants of adolescent physical activity and inactivity patterns. Pediatrics 2000;105:e83.
7. Nader PR, Bradley RH, Houts RM, et al. Moderate-to-vigorous physical activity from ages 9 to 15 years. JAMA 2008;300(3):295–305.
8. Centers for Disease Control and Prevention. Healthy People 2020. Available at: http://www.cdc.gov/nchs/healthy_people/hp2020.htm. Accessed February 29, 2016.
9. Taylor WC, Baranowski T, Young DR. Physical activity interventions in low-income, ethnic minority, and populations with disability. Am J Prev Med 1998; 15:334–43.
10. Schrop SL, Pendleton BF, McCord G, et al. The medically underserved: who is likely to exercise and why? J Health Care Poor Underserved 2006;17:276–89.
11. Parks SE, Housemann RA, Brownson RC. Differential correlates of physical activity in urban and rural adults of various socioeconomic backgrounds in the United States. J Epidemiol Community Health 2003;57:29–35.

12. Healthy People 2020. Physical activity. Available at: http://www.healthypeople. gov/2020/topics-objectives/topic/physical-activity. Accessed February 29, 2016.

13. Chulani VL, Gordon LP. Adolescent growth and development. Prim Care 2014; 41:465–87.

14. Colvin CW, Abdullatif H. Anatomy of female puberty: the clinical relevance of developmental changes in the reproductive system. Clin Anat 2013;26:115–29.

15. Tena-Sempere M. Ghrelin, the gonadal axis and the onset of puberty. Endocr Dev 2013;25:69–82.

16. Lee Y, Styne D. Influences on the onset and tempo of puberty in human beings and implications for adolescent psychological development. Horm Behav 2013; 64:250–61.

17. Kotsopoulos J, Lubinski J, Lynch HT. Age at menarche and the risk of breast cancer in BRCA1 and BRCA2 mutation carriers. Cancer Causes Control 2005; 16(6):667–74.

18. Ong KK, Ahmed ML, Dunger DB. Lessons from large population studies on timing and tempo of puberty (secular trends and relation to body size): the European trend. Mol Cell Endocrinol 2006;254-255:8–12.

19. Allison CM, Hyde JS. Early menarche: confluence of biological and contextual factors. Sex Roles 2013;68:55–64.

20. Canoy D, Beral V, Balkwill A, et al, Million Women Study Collaborators*. Age at menarche and risks of coronary heart and other vascular diseases in a large UK cohort. Circulation 2015;131(3):237–44.

21. Castro-Rodriguez JA. A new childhood asthma phenotype: obese with early menarche. Paediatr Respir Rev 2016;18:85–9.

22. Lieberoth S, Gade E. Early menarche is associated with increased risk of asthma: prospective population-based study of twins. Respir Med 2015;109:565–71.

23. Lim SW, Ahn JH, Lee JA, et al. Early menarche is associated with metabolic syndrome and insulin resistance in premenopausal Korean women. Eur J Pediatr 2016;175:97–104.

24. Alcalá-Herrera V, Marván ML. Early menarche, depressive symptoms, and coping strategies. J Adolesc 2014;37:905–13.

25. Tamakoshi K, Yatsuya H, Tamakoshi A, et al. Early age at menarche associated with increased all-cause mortality. Eur J Epidemiol 2011;26:771–8.

26. Ramnitz MS, Lodish MB. Racial disparities in pubertal development. Semin Reprod Med 2013;31:333–9.

27. Wu T, Mendola P, Buck GM. Ethnic differences in the presence of secondary sex characteristics and menarche among US girls: the Third National Health and Nutrition Examination Survey, 1988-1994. Pediatrics 2002;110:752–7.

28. Krzyżanowska M, Mascie-Taylor CG, Thalabard JC. Biosocial correlates of age at menarche in a British cohort. Ann Hum Biol 2015;31:1–6.

29. Krieger N, Kiang MV, Kosheleva A. Age at menarche: 50-year socioeconomic trends among US-born black and white women. Am J Public Health 2015; 105:388–97.

30. McIntyre MH. Adult stature, body proportions and age at menarche in the United States National Health and Nutrition Survey (NHANES) III. Ann Hum Biol 2011;38:716–20.

31. Sallis JF, Zakarian JM, Hovell MF, et al. Ethnic, socioeconomic, and sex differences in physical activity among adolescents. J Clin Epidemiol 1996;49:125–34.

32. Tripodi A, Severi S, Midili S, et al. "Community projects" in Modena (Italy): promote regular physical activity and healthy nutrition habits since childhood. Int J Pediatr Obes 2011;6(Suppl 2):54–6.

33. te Velde SJ, Twisk JW, Brug J. Tracking of fruit and vegetable consumption from adolescence into adulthood and its longitudinal association with overweight. Br J Nutr 2007;98:431–8.

34. Cleland V, Dwyer T, Venn A. Which domains of childhood physical activity predict physical activity in adulthood? A 20-year prospective tracking study. Br J Sports Med 2012;46:595–602.

35. Koivusilta LK, Nupponen H, Rimpelä AH. Adolescent physical activity predicts high education and socio-economic position in adulthood. Eur J Public Health 2012;22:203–9.

36. Aarnio M, Winter T, Kujala U, et al. Associations of health related behaviour, social relationships, and health status with persistent physical activity and inactivity: a study of Finnish adolescent twins. Br J Sports Med 2002;36:360–4.

37. Gogtay N, Giedd JN, Lusk L, et al. Dynamic mapping of human cortical development during childhood through early adulthood. Proc Natl Acad Sci U S A 2004;101:8174–9.

38. Casey BJ, Thomas KM, Welsh TF, et al. Dissociation of response conflict, attentional selection, and expectancy with functional magnetic resonance imaging. Proc Natl Acad Sci 2000;97:8728–33.

39. Casey BJ, Tottenham N, Fossella J. Clinical, imaging, lesion and genetic approaches toward a model of cognitive control. Dev Psychobiol 2002;40:237–54.

40. Casey BJ, Tottenham N, Liston C, et al. Imaging the developing brain: what have we learned about cognitive development? Trends Cogn Sci 2005;9:104–10.

41. Hare TA, Tottenham N, Galvan A, et al. Biological substrates of emotional reactivity and regulation in adolescence during an emotional go-nogo task. Biol Psychiatry 2008;63:927–34.

42. Hackman DA, Farah MJ, Meaney MJ. Socioeconomic status and the brain: mechanistic insights from human and animal research. Nat Rev Neurosci 2010;11:651–9.

43. Noble KG, Wolmetz ME, Ochs LG, et al. Brain-behavior relationships in reading acquisition are modulated by socioeconomic factors. Dev Sci 2006;9:642–54.

44. Kishiyama MM, Boyce WT, Jimenez AM, et al. Socioeconomic disparities affect prefrontal function in children. J Cogn Neurosci 2009;21:1106–15.

45. Noble KG, Engelhardt LE, Brito NH, et al. Socioeconomic disparities in neurocognitive development in the first two years of life. Dev Psychobiol 2015;57:535–51.

46. Noble KG, Houston SM, Brito NH, et al. Family income, parental education and brain structure in children and adolescents. Nat Neurosci 2015;18:773–8.

47. Hanson JL, Hair N, Shen DG, et al. Family poverty affects the rate of human infant brain growth. PLoS One 2013;8:e80954.

48. Hair NL, Hanson JL, Wolfe BL, et al. Association of child poverty, brain development, and academic achievement. JAMA Pediatr 2015;169:822–9.

49. Javanbakht A, King AP, Evans GW, et al. Childhood poverty predicts adult amygdala and frontal activity and connectivity in response to emotional faces. Front Behav Neurosci 2015;9:154.

50. Haveman R, Wolfe B. The determinants of children's attainments: a review of methods and findings. J Econ Lit 1995;33:1829–78.

51. Mezzacappa E. Alerting, orienting, and executive attention: developmental properties and socio demographic correlates epidemiological sample of young, urban children. Child Dev 2004;75:1373–86.

52. Tine M. Acute aerobic exercise: an intervention for the selective visual attention and reading comprehension of low-income adolescents. Front Psychol 2014;5:575.

53. Institute of Education Sciences. National Center for Education Statistics. Assessment of educational progress. Nations Report Card. 2015. Available at: http://nces.ed.gov/nationsreportcard/. Accessed February 29, 2016.
54. Restuccia D, Urrutia C. Intergenerational persistence of earnings: the role of early and college education. Am Econ Rev 2004;94:1354–78.
55. Duyme M, Dumaret AC, Tomkiewicz S. How can we boost IQs of "dull children"? A late adoption study. Proc Natl Acad Sci U S A 1999;96:8790–4.
56. Luby JL, Barch DM, Belden A, et al. Maternal support in early childhood predicts larger hippocampal volumes at school age. Proc Natl Acad Sci U S A 2012;109:2854–9.
57. Luby JL, Belden A, Botteron K, et al. The effects of poverty on childhood brain development: the mediating effect of caregiving and stressful life events. JAMA Pediatr 2013;167:1135–42.
58. Bezold CP, Konty KJ, Day SE, et al. The effects of changes in physical fitness on academic performance among New York City youth. J Adolesc Health 2014;55:774–81.
59. Cotman CW, Berchtold NC, Christie L. Exercise builds brain health: key roles of growth factor cascades and inflammation. Trends Neurosci 2007;30:464–72.
60. Phillips C, Baktir MA, Srivatsan M, et al. Neuroprotective effects of physical activity on the brain: a closer look at trophic factor signaling. Front Cell Neurosci 2014;20(8):170.
61. Klempin F, Beis D, Mosienko V, et al. Serotonin is required for exercise-induced adult hippocampal neurogenesis. J Neurosci 2013;33:8270–5.
62. Erickson KI, Prakash RS, Voss MW, et al. Aerobic fitness is associated with hippocampal volume in elderly humans. Hippocampus 2009;19:1030–9.
63. Hillman CH, Buck SM, Themanson JR, et al. Aerobic fitness and cognitive development: event-related brain potential and task performance indices of executive control in preadolescent children. Dev Psychol 2009;45:114–29.
64. Hillman CH, Castelli DM, Buck SM. Aerobic fitness and neurocognitive function in healthy preadolescent children. Med Sci Sports Exerc 2005;37:1967–74.
65. Raine LB, Lee HK, Saliba BJ, et al. The influence of childhood aerobic fitness on learning and memory. PLoS One 2013;8:e72666.
66. Chaddock L, Neider MB, Lutz A, et al. Role of childhood aerobic fitness in successful street crossing. Med Sci Sports Exerc 2012;44:749–53.
67. Castelli DM, Hillman CH, Buck SM, et al. Physical fitness and academic achievement in third-and fifth-grade students. J Sport Exerc Psychol 2007;29:239–52.
68. Donnelly JE, Greene JL, Gibson CA, et al. Physical Activity Across the Curriculum (PAAC): a randomized controlled trial to promote physical activity and diminish overweight and obesity in elementary school children. Prev Med 2009;49:336–41.
69. Etnier JL, Nowell PM, Landers DM, et al. A meta-regression to examine the relationship between aerobic fitness and cognitive performance. Brain Res Rev 2006;52:119–30.
70. Chaddock L, Erickson KI, Prakash RS, et al. Basal ganglia volume is associated with aerobic fitness in preadolescent children. Dev Neurosci 2010;32:249–56.
71. Chaddock L, Erickson KI, Prakash RS, et al. A functional MRI investigation of the association between childhood aerobic fitness and neurocognitive control. Biol Psychol 2012;89:260–8.
72. Tsasoulis A, Fountoulakis S. The protective role of exercise on stress system dysregulation and comorbidities. Ann N Y Acad Sci 2006;1083:196–213.

73. Salmon P. Effects of physical exercise on anxiety, depression, and sensitivity to stress: a unifying theory. Clin Psychol Rev 2001;21:33–61.

74. Crews DJ, Landers DM. A meta-analytic review of aerobic fitness and reactively to psychosocial stressors. Med Sci Sports Exerc 1987;19:S114–20.

75. Traustadóttir T, Bosch PR, Matt KS. The HPA axis response to stress in women: effects of aging and fitness. Psychoneuroendocrinology 2005;30:399–402.

76. Blumenthal JA, Fredrickson M, Kuhn CM, et al. Aerobic exercise reduces levels of cardiovascular and sympathoadrenal response to mental stress in subjects without prior evidence of myocardial ischemia. Am J Cardiol 1990;65:93–8.

77. HRSA Health Center Program. National data. Available at: http://bphc.hrsa.gov/uds/datacenter.aspx?q=tall&year=2014&state. Accessed March 1, 2016.

78. Siegel R, Naishadham D, Jemal A. Cancer statistics, 2012. CA Cancer J Clin 2012;62:10–29.

79. Doubeni CA, Laiyemo AO, Major JM, et al. Socioeconomic status and the risk of colorectal cancer: an analysis of more than a half million adults in the National Institutes of Health-AARP Diet and Health Study. Cancer 2012;118:3636–44.

80. Pedersen BK, Saltin B. Exercise as medicine—evidence for prescribing exercise as therapy in 26 different chronic diseases. Scand J Med Sci Sports 2015;25:1–72.

81. Pescatello LS, Franklin BA, Fagard R, et al. American College of Sports Medicine position stand. Exercise and hypertension. Med Sci Sports Exerc 2004; 36:533–53.

82. Lewington S, Clarke R, Qizilbash N, et al. Age-specific relevance of usual blood pressure to vascular mortality: a meta-analysis of individual data for one million adults in 61 prospective studies. Lancet 2002;360:1903–13.

83. Joslin EP, Root EF, White P. The treatment of diabetes mellitus. Philadelphia: Lea & Febiger; 1959.

84. Albright A, Franz M, Hornsby G, et al. American College of Sports Medicine position stand. Exercise and type 2 diabetes. Med Sci Sports Exerc 2000;32: 1345–60.

85. American Diabetes Association. Clinical practice recommendations. Diabetes Care 2013;36(Suppl 1):S3.

86. Church TS, Blair SN, Cocreham S, et al. Effects of aerobic and resistance training on hemoglobin A1c levels in patients with type 2 diabetes: a randomized controlled trial. JAMA 2010;304:2253.

87. MacLeod SF, Terada T, Chahal BS, et al. Exercise lowers postprandial glucose but not fasting glucose in type 2 diabetes: a meta-analysis of studies using continuous glucose monitoring. Diabetes Metab Res Rev 2013;29:593–603.

88. Kearney ML, Thyfault JP. Exercise and postprandial glycemic control in type 2 diabetes. Curr Diabetes Rev 2016;12(3):199–210.

89. Carson KV, Chandratilleke MG, Picot J, et al. Physical training for asthma. Cochrane Database Syst Rev 2013;(9):CD001116.

90. Mendes FA, Gonçalves RC, Nunes MP, et al. Effects of aerobic training on psychosocial morbidity and symptoms in patients with asthma: a randomized clinical trial. Chest 2010;138:331–7.

91. Mendes FA, Almeida FM, Cukier A, et al. Effects of aerobic training on airway inflammation in asthmatic patients. Med Sci Sports Exerc 2011;43:197–203.

92. Gonçalves RC, Nunes MPT, Cukier A, et al. Efeito de um programa de condicionamento físico aeróbio nos aspectos psicossociais, na qualidade de vida, nos sintomas e no óxido nítrico exalado de portadores de asma persistente moderada ou grave. [Effects of an aerobic physical training program on psychosocial

characteristics, quality of life, symptoms and exhaled nitric oxide in individuals with moderate or severe persistent asthma]. Rev Bras Fisioter 2008;12:127–35 [in Portuguese].

93. Carlsen KH, Carlsen KC. Exercise induced asthma. Paediatr Respir Rev 2002;3: 154.

94. Emtner M, Herala M, Stalenheim G. High-intensity physical training in adults with asthma. A 10-week rehabilitation program. Chest 1996;109:323–30.

95. Thelle DS, Foorde OH, Try K, et al. The Tromsøo heart study. Methods and main results of the cross-sectional study. Acta Med Scand 1976;200:107–18.

96. Forde OH, Thelle DS, Arnesen E, et al. Distribution of high density lipoprotein cholesterol according to relative body weight, cigarette smoking and leisure time physical activity. The Cardiovascular Disease Study in Finnmark 1977. Acta Med Scand 1986;219:167–71.

97. Prong NP. Short term effects of exercise on plasma lipids and lipoproteins in humans. Sports Med 1993;16:431–48.

98. National Institutes of Health Consensus Development Panel. Triglyceride, DLD, and CHD. JAMA 1993;269:505–20.

99. Earnest CP, Artero EG, Sui X, et al. Maximal estimated cardio-respiratory fitness, cardiometabolic risk factors, and metabolic syndrome in the Aerobics Center Longitudinal Study. Mayo Clin Proc 2013;88:259–70.

100. Mann S, Beedie C, Jimenez A. Differential effects of aerobic exercise, resistance training and combined exercise modalities on cholesterol and the lipid profile: review, synthesis and recommendations. Sports Med 2014;44:211–21.

101. Pasternak RC, Grundy SM, Levy D, et al. Spectrum of risk factors for CHD. J Am Coll Cardiol 1990;27:964–1047.

102. Nicklas BJ, Katzel LI, Busby-Whitehead J, et al. Increases in high-density lipoprotein cholesterol with endurance exercise training are blunted in obese compared with lean men. Metabolism 1997;46:556–61.

103. American Psychiatric Association. Diagnostic and statistical manual of mental disorders. 5th edition. Washington, DC: American Psychiatric Association; 2013.

104. Cooney GM, Dwan K, Greig CA, et al. Exercise for depression. Cochrane Database Syst Rev 2013;(9):CD004366.

105. Blumenthal JA, Babyak MA, Moore KA, et al. Effects of exercise training on older patients with major depression. Arch Intern Med 1999;159:2349–56.

106. Babyak M, Blumenthal JA, Herman S, et al. Exercise treatment for major depression: maintenance of therapeutic benefit at 10 months. Psychosom Med 2000; 62:633–8.

107. Mynors-Wallis LM, Gath DH, Day A, et al. Randomised controlled trial of problem solving treatment, antidepressant medication, and combined treatment for major depression in primary care. BMJ 2000;320:26–30.

108. Pajonk FG, Wobrock T, Gruber O, et al. Hippocampal plasticity in response to exercise in schizophrenia. Arch Gen Psychiatry 2010;67:133–43.

109. Manji HK, Moore GJ, Chen G. Clinical and preclinical evidence for the neurotrophic effects of mood stabilizers: implications for the pathophysiology and treatment of manic-depressive illness. Biol Psychiatry 2000;48:740–54.

110. Aarts MJ, Lemmens VE, Louwman MW, et al. Socioeconomic status and changing inequalities in colorectal cancer? A review of the associations with risk, treatment and outcome. Eur J Cancer 2010;46:2681–95.

111. Leufkens AM, Van Duijnhoven FJ, Boshuizen HC, et al. Educational level and risk of colorectal cancer in EPIC with specific reference to tumor location. Int J Cancer 2012;130:622–30.

112. Brooke HL, Talbäck M, Martling A. Socioeconomic position and incidence of colorectal cancer in the Swedish population. Cancer Epidemiol 2016;40:188–95.
113. Samad AK, Taylor RS, Marshall T, et al. A meta-analysis of the association of physical activity with reduced risk of colorectal cancer. Colorectal Dis 2005;7: 204–13.
114. Thune I, Furberg AS. Physical activity and cancer risk: dose-response and cancer, all sites and site-specific. Med Sci Sports Exerc 2001;33(6 Suppl):S530–50.
115. Van Blarigan EL, Meyerhardt JA. Role of physical activity and diet after colorectal cancer diagnosis. J Clin Oncol 2015;33:1825–34.
116. Goldberg M, Calderon-Margalit R. Socioeconomic disparities in breast cancer incidence and survival among parous women: findings from a population-based cohort, 1964-2008. BMC Cancer 2015;15:921.
117. Thomson CS, Hole DJ, Twelves CJ, et al. Prognostic factors in women with breast cancer: distribution by socioeconomic status and effect on differences in survival. J Epidemiol Community Health 2001;55:308–15.
118. Centers for Disease Control and Prevention. Vital signs: racial disparities in breast cancer severity—United States, 2005-2009. MMWR Morb Mortal Wkly Rep 2012;61:922.
119. Parise CA, Caggiano V. Disparities in race/ethnicity and socioeconomic status: risk of mortality of breast cancer patients in the California Cancer Registry, 2000–2010. BMC Cancer 2013;13:449.
120. Bradley CJ, Given CW, Roberts C. Race, socioeconomic status and breast cancer treatment and survival. J Natl Cancer Inst 2002;94:490.
121. Brown JC, Winters-Stone K, Lee A, et al. Cancer, physical activity, and exercise. Compr Physiol 2012;2:2775–809.
122. Friedenreich CM, Cust AE. Physical activity and breast cancer risk: impact of timing, type and dose of activity and population sub-group effects. Br J Sports Med 2008;42:636–47.
123. Brownson RC, Baker EA, Housemann RA, et al. Environmental and policy determinants of physical activity in the United States. Am J Public Health 2001;91: 1995–2003.
124. Burton NW, Turrell G, Oldenburg B. Participation in recreational physical activity; why do socioeconomic groups differ? Health Educ Behav 2003;30:225–44.
125. Seefeldt V, Malina RM, Clark MA. Factors affecting levels of physical activity in adults. Sports Med 2002;32:143–68.

An Overview of Environmental Justice Issues in Primary Care – 2018

Vincent Morelli, MD[a],*, Carol Ziegler, DNP, APRN, NP-C, RD[b],
Omotayo Fawibe, MD[c]

KEYWORDS

• Environmental justice • Toxins • Air pollution • Ingested pollutants

KEY POINTS

• Environmental justice has wide social, economic, and educational implications.
• Air pollution has the highest environmental risk with dangers from gases, organic compounds, and toxic materials.
• Carbon monoxide, nitric oxide, or nitrogen dioxide, sulfur dioxide, and ozone pose higher dangers for the poor.
• Exposure to metals in air pollution (eg, mercury, lead, cadmium, and manganese) can cause cognitive disorders, nervous system diseases, cancers, and mental illness.
• There is currently some controversy about the possible carcinogenic dangers of ingesting pollutants from water, soil, and food (eg, bisphenol A, arsenic).

INTRODUCTION

On February 17, 2017, the US Senate confirmed Scott Pruitt as the 14th Administrator of the US Environmental Protection Agency (EPA). Although this caused consternation among environmentalists and more than 90% of climate scientists, his well-known

This article originally appeared in *Primary Care: Clinics in Office Practice*, Volume 44, Issue 1, March 2017.
Disclosure Statement: The authors of this work report no direct financial interest in the subject matter or any material discussed in this article.
[a] Sports Medicine Fellowship, Department of Family and Community Medicine, Meharry Medical College, 1005 Dr D. B. Todd Boulevard, Nashville, TN 37208, USA; [b] Vanderbilt University School of Nursing, 461 21st Avenue, South, Nashville, TN 37240, USA; [c] Department of Family and Community Medicine, Meharry Medical College, Nashville, TN 37208, USA
* Corresponding author.
E-mail address: vmorelli@mmc.edu

views on the environment* fit well into the Republican agenda of deregulation and less government interference. Pruitt's effectiveness in this regard was clearly illustrated by the CEO of the National Automobile Association, who stated, "Pruitt has spearheaded over 2 dozen regulatory reforms, with over a billion dollars in savings during his first year here at EPA, and all told, issued more deregulatory actions than any other federal agency under the Trump administration."

Although Pruitt's stance on environmental issues flies in the face of the opinions of our best scientists, our goal in this article is not to weigh in on this argument. Instead, our aim is to examine the topic of environmental justice and how administration changes might affect the Office of Environmental Justice (OEJ) and, by extension, the underserved communities in which we serve. Our introduction briefly addresses the effect the current administration might have on underserved communities. Following this, the bulk of the article serves as a broad environmental overview, so that primary care providers might begin to understand the complexity involved and be more aware of the issues they might face in the underserved communities in which they serve.

Shortly after Scott Pruitt's confirmation, a series of memorandums were issued. One memorandum on the EPA's Environmental Justice (EJ) Policies and Priorities (February 23, 2018, MEMORANDUM: EPA's Environmental Justice and Community Revitalization Priorities) stated, "In the spirit of cooperative federalism" the Office of Environmental Justice (OEJ) will strengthen the ability of partner agencies to incorporate EJ into their work through enhanced collaboration with states...and local governments." In other words, putting more oversight power into the hands of state and local officials rather than the federal government. No surprise. This is in accordance with the Republican ideology of strengthening states' rights and lessening what they see as overly restrictive federal oversight.

The memorandum went on to state that the EPA, "will improve EPA science to better understand the needs of underserved communities." This language seemed intent on spinning the EPA as a champion of the underserved, while in actuality opening the door to allow for *less* protection of underserved communities. This wording could be interpreted to mean that unless the science is unequivocally supportive, a condition that is often nearly impossible to achieve, EJ regulations could be rolled back. Despite this rather loose language, after talking with officials at the EPA it seems that the current political will, despite Scott Pruitt, is in favor of preserving current OEJ policies and fairness.

---

* In November of 2017, EPA Director Scott Pruitt said that despite a government report** stating that "the blame for the rise of global temperatures (can be ascribed to) human activity, (this) won't deter him from continuing to roll back the Obama-era Clean Power Plan, a major rule aimed at combating climate change." Pruitt had sued to block the plan years earlier when first implemented, arguing that the Obama Administration and the EPA were never given the authority by Congress to implement such a sweeping regulation.

** The federally mandated report prepared by the nation's top scientists every 4 years for Congress and the public concluded, "based on extensive evidence, that it is extremely likely that human activities, especially emissions of greenhouse gases, are the dominant cause of the observed (global) warming since the mid-20th century." Hundreds of scientists and the National Academy of Sciences reviewed >1500 studies to produce the report. The report also said carbon dioxide concentration has now passed 400 parts per million, a level that last occurred approximately 3 million years ago when the planet was quite different. Changes in rainfall patterns, water supplies, and sea levels can be expected and are already occurring; sea levels are expected to rise 1 to 8 feet by 2100. All of this can be expected to impact underserved communities disproportionately (*USA Today* November 8, 2018).

A final section of the EPA memorandum stated that the OEJ has been "elevated" into the Office of Policy; a move meant to improve the office's effectiveness and better coordinate EJ work with other governmental departments. In theory, this makes good sense. In practice, EPA officials have informed me that the administrative structure makes less difference than the political support an office receives, and that OEJ currently has the political support needed to continue to push its agenda of environmental fairness without fear of being manipulated. However, there is some concern in the EPA over the current administration's use of "authoritative directives" rather than scientific review before enacting rule changes.

ENVIRONMENTAL JUSTICE

The idea of environmental justice (EJ) arose in the 1980s, bringing to light the concept that the burdens of environmental exposure should be fairly distributed without undue costs being placed on those with low socioeconomic status (SES). The concept was formally written into US policy by executive order in 1994, with policy creation, implementation, and enforcement tasked to the Interagency Working Group on Environmental Justice under the US Department of Agriculture.

When EJ issues are studied, the location of waste disposal sites, manufacturing facilities, energy plants, highways, airports, and toxic waste sites, are mapped against SES or minority groupings. Most North American, Asian, and African studies have documented higher concentrations of pollutants in underserved or low SES communities.[1] Such disparities have important health implications. For example, the prevalence of asthma in some underserved communities in the United States is twice that of the national average (9% of US children have asthma vs 22% in some underserved communities).[2]

EJ issues also have wider social implications due to the interrelatedness of crime, education, poverty, and pollution. For example, a recent air toxin per youth crime mapping study found an association between airborne manganese, mercury, and particulate matter (PM) with higher rates of youth involvement with the juvenile justice system.[3] Although the study methodology could not definitively link exposure to EJ concerns, the implications demand further study. Other studies have noted that mononitrogen oxide (NO_x), ozone, heavy metals, and other pollutants are associated with neurologic deficits, behavioral problems, aggressive behavior, slowed learning, and other cognitive deficits, all important from health, human potential, and social policy perspectives.

ENVIRONMENTAL TOXINS

The Centers for Disease Control and Prevention (CDC) Fourth National Report on Human Exposure to Environmental Chemicals (2009, updated in 2015) includes data on 265 toxins. Exposures may be the result of inhalation (eg, motor vehicle emission, industrial air pollution), ingestion (eg, from tainted foods, ground water), or percutaneous absorption. Compounds, such as pesticides, heavy metals, phenols, fungicides, herbicides, parabens, phthalates, polyaromatic hydrocarbons, volatile organic compounds (VOCs), and tobacco smoke, are included in the analysis. For each chemical in the report, the CDC provides mean blood and urine levels, as well as the 75th, 90th, and 95th percentile levels, so that individuals or groups can be compared with population standards. The best method of detection (blood or urine) for each of the chemicals is also noted and 93 of the compounds have more in-depth biomonitoring data.[4]

The report, however, does not establish what levels may be harmful to an individual's health. These must be obtained from other sources. For example, the CDC provides population comparison levels for arsenic; the Environmental Protection Agency (EPA) monitors and sets the safe levels for air, drinking water, and soil; the Food and Drug Administration (FDA) sets safe food and bottled water levels; and the Occupational Safety and Health Administration (OSHA) is tasked with formulating and monitoring harmful workplace levels. (The EPA, FDA, and OSHA are also tasked with enforcement, so that companies found in violation of guidelines may be fined as set out in their respective policies.)

There are many mechanisms by which toxins may cause injury. Exposures may induce an inhalant allergic response, direct toxic effects on cellular mechanics (eg, lead, arsenic, mercury), endocrine disrupting effects (bisphenol A [BPA], phthalates),[5] direct DNA damage, or may create epigenetic changes (see later discussion). In most cases, free radical formation, oxidative stress, and inflammation[6] are thought to contribute to the injury. Other factors, such as whether the particles are solid, liquid, or gas; electrostatic charge; particle size; site of deposition; and lung response must also be taken into consideration.[7]

The concept of epigenetic change is a relatively recent construct that primary care providers (PCPs) working with underserved populations would do well to keep in mind. This is a growing area of research in which changes in gene expression without alterations in DNA sequence have been shown to contribute to untoward health effects.[8] Briefly, the concept is that environmental, social, physical, nutritional, or chemical stressors can lead to modifications (eg, methylation, acetylation) of the proteins surrounding DNA.[9,10] These modifications can lead to changes in gene expression, which can then be passed on to future generations. Environmentally induced epigenetic mechanisms have been proposed for diabetes and obesity,[11] asthma and food allergies,[12,13] autoimmune disease,[14] psychiatric diseases,[15] cardiovascular disease,[16] cancer,[17,18] and others.

In light of the vast number of potentially noxious compounds, the various mechanisms of injury and the complexities involved in monitoring, a detailed discussion of individual toxins is beyond the scope of this article. However, it will serve the PCP working in underserved communities, in which EJ issues are of concern, to have a general understanding of environmental toxins and their health effects. Armed with an appropriate perspective and a heightened index of suspicion, the PCP should then be able to locate helpful resources, to undertake proper methods of screening and detection, and to educate patients in methods of avoidance or amelioration. This article is meant to help guide the PCP in this pursuit.

AIR POLLUTION

In 2013, 87% of the world's population lived in areas that exceeded World Health Organization (WHO) Air Quality Guidelines. WHO data published in 2014 estimate that 7 million deaths per year are attributable to air pollution, making air pollution the world's largest single environmental health risk.[19] As previously stated, many studies have shown that this burden is borne disproportionately by underserved populations, with both outdoor and indoor air pollution contributing to the disparity.[20]

The chemical makeup of air pollution consists of:

1. Gases (carbon monoxide [CO], sulfur oxides, nitrogen oxides, ground-level or bad ozone, and VOCs)
2. Organic compounds (polycyclic aromatic hydrocarbons, VOCs)
3. Toxic metals (chromium, copper, manganese, lead, vanadium, antimony).

It is a complex, cross-reacting, ever-changing mixture, depending on weather patterns and industrial release. Ninety-eight percent of the urban air pollution consists of gases or vapor-phase compounds: CO, nitrogen dioxide (NO2), nitric oxide (NO), ozone, sulfur dioxide (SO2), or volatile hydrocarbons. Each of these components can act independently to produce adverse health effects, or they can chemically interact to form combined or secondary pollutants. The effects of these combined pollutants are less studied (with the exception of ozone) and largely unknown.

Besides grouping air pollution by chemical makeup, pollutants can also be grouped according to particle size. This is relevant because only small particles (<10 microns) are able to enter the lower airways and cause the most significant damage. Particles with a diameter of 2.5 to 10 μm (PM10) are called coarse particles. Those less than 2.5 μm (PM2.5), the most harmful category, are designated as fine particles. Those less than 1 μm are called ultrafine or nanoparticles.

This article briefly reviews the categories of gases, organic compounds, metals, and PM, so that the PCP may have a fundamental knowledge of terminology, properties, health effects, and approach to monitoring and mitigation.

THE GASES

Ninety-eight percent of urban air pollution consists of gases (CO, NO2, NO, ozone, SO2), which vary depending on regional differences in traffic, industry, wind, weather patterns, and so forth. It is a ubiquitous, itinerant, ever-changing, noxious ether, which bleeds across borders and cycles into the earth's very respirations.

Carbon Monoxide

CO, colloquially known as the silent killer, arises from the incomplete combustion of gas, coal or wood, traffic exhaust, furnaces, heaters, and wood or propane stoves. CO is a colorless, odorless gas that binds tightly to hemoglobin, creating carboxyhemoglobin, essentially displacing oxygen and rendering an affected person hypoxic. Because symptoms can be nonspecific (headache, nausea, vomiting, dizziness, depression, memory loss, irritability, fatigue, subjective weakness) and because carboxyhemoglobin's bright red hue may mask tissue hypoxia (making patients appear a healthy pink while being hypoxic at the cellular level), PCPs must maintain a high level of suspicion in effected areas.

Normal carboxyhemoglobin to hemoglobin ratio is less than 5%, while smokers or auto mechanics may have up to 9%. Symptoms usually occur in the 10% to 30% range.[21]

In addition to its direct toxic effects, CO is also a short-lived greenhouse gas. It has an additional indirect greenhouse effect by slowing the breakdown of methane and ozone, both more potent greenhouse gases. Greenhouse gases contribute to increased ozone formation (see later discussion) and all of the climate change effects noted in this article.

Mononitrogen Oxides, Nitric Oxide, and Nitrogen Dioxide

Any combustion in the presence of nitrogen found in coal or oil in power plants, vehicular exhaust (especially biodiesel), or natural sources will create NOx. NOx adds the brownish hue to urban smog and can contribute to acid rain formation (see later discussion).

NOx can react to form nitric acid, which can penetrate lung tissue and cause cardiorespiratory effects, including bronchitis, chronic obstructive pulmonary disease (COPD), and heart disease. It can also react with sunlight to create ozone, which further contributes to cardiorespiratory disease and neurotoxic effects, including impaired executive function and lower learning abilities (see later discussion). The implications of these neurotoxic effects are particularity worrisome in underserved communities where EJ concerns have been documented.[1,22]

Ozone

Good ozone in the upper atmosphere (stratosphere) is protective because it serves to absorb harmful UVB light, which, if unchecked, can cause significant human skin problems and can damage plant and animal DNA. Depletion of this ozone layer is concerning.

Bad ozone in the lower atmosphere (troposphere) is formed when sunlight reacts with partially combusted fossil fuels (NOx and organic compounds) from autos or industrial plants. This ozone has been proven to interfere with plant photosynthesis, stunt plant growth, and decrease crop yields.[23] In humans, it has been linked to increased inflammation, oxidative stress, asthma, bronchitis, overall respiratory morbidity and mortality, heart attacks and cardiovascular mortality,[24,25] and possibly diabetes.[26] The EPA has stated that both short-term and long-term ozone exposure can "harm the respiratory system causing significant symptoms and imposing significant costs on American families." It goes on to say that there is "likely a causal relationship"[27] between ozone and cardiovascular disease.

Finally, and especially important in underserved communities with higher pollution levels, ozone has been linked to neurotoxic effects, including decreased attention and short-term memory.[28]

Allowable air pollution levels of 70 parts per billion (ppb) have been set by the EPA and recent studies[29,30] have validated that these levels are safe, documenting no harmful cardiopulmonary effects from either short or prolonged ozone exposure at levels near or below EPA standards.

It should be noted that besides ozone's direct health effects on plants and animals, bad or low-level ozone is also a harmful greenhouse gas, trapping heat radiating from the earth and contributing to climate change. An increase in ozone would then result in a disastrous cycle, with increased ozone as a greenhouse gas contributing to global warming. Global warming leads to warmer, stagnant air, which, in turn, creates conditions for the formation of more ozone, further contributing to global warming. It is projected that if pollution remains at its current levels, climate change could nearly double the number of unhealthy AQI (air quality index) days (days when ozone levels are hazardous for everyone) by 2050.[31]

Currently, ozone mapping is the only reasonable way to track ozone because there are no clinically useful biomarkers for individual patient ozone detection.[32] In its 2015 updated ozone regulations, the EPA increased ground monitoring in 33 at-risk states.

Because ozone is largely formed by the conversion of traffic toxins by sunlight, it makes sense that ozone should peak in the late morning to early afternoon, after sunlight has had a chance to play its generative role on the fresh inflow of morning vehicle exhaust.[33]

PCPs caring for underserved patients in high ozone areas should advise them to stay indoors during these times and on high pollution days. They may also advise patients to use indoor air filters if possible, limit physical exertion near roads or industrial sources, and to mitigate parenteral and psychosocial stressors (see later discussion).[34]

Sulfur Dioxide

Sources for SO2 include coal burning power plants, other industries, and volcanoes. It is also used as a preservative in wine, dried fruit, and other foods. SO2 exposure can result in respiratory symptoms and asthma exacerbations.[2,35] Exposure has also been linked to preterm birth, which this is especially important in underserved communities where higher rates of exposure and health care access disparities exist. No neurologic or cardiovascular effects have been documented with SO2. SO2 can also react to form sulfuric acid, which contributes to the formation of acid rain, with its well-known detrimental effects on biodiversity, plant, and animal species. The EPA 1-hour exposure limit is 75 ppb.

Organic Compounds in Air Pollution

These compounds arise from vehicle and industrial fuels, soil erosion, or secondary formation (eg, benzene, toluene, xylene, VOCs). VOCs can cause direct harmful effects (suspected carcinogens linked to leukemia) or can be oxidized to join the ranks of particulate air pollution (see later discussion). They can also contribute to the formation of ozone-causing effects as previously noted. VOCs are grouped as either methane or nonmethane VOCs (NMVOCs). Methane is a greenhouse gas contributing to global warming, whereas NMVOCs, as alluded to, may be a direct carcinogen.

METALS IN AIR POLLUTION

Metals, such as chromium, zinc, copper, nickel, manganese, lead, vanadium, antimony, and barium, are known toxins and are monitored by the EPA. Fifty metals have been identified in coal, 35 in crude oil, and 18 in gasoline.[36,37] Because of combustion, these metals enter the atmosphere, usually as constituents of PM (see later discussion).

Although a complete review of air-metal pollutants is beyond the scope of this article, a few of the more common offenders are discussed so that PCPs working in underserved and overburdened communities may get a general idea and become more aware of potential health impacts.

Mercury

Most harmful mercury exposure in the United States comes from methyl mercury after consumption of fish. However, other inorganic sources of mercury are important in underserved communities and include noncompliant coal burning power plants and other industrial sources.

Prenatal exposure to mercury has been associated with lower IQ, delayed cognitive development, and decreased memory, attention, language, and spatial cognition.[38–40] It has been associated with spontaneous abortions, stillbirths, and congenital malformations (eg, cerebral palsy and mental retardation),[39,41] as well as leukemia.[42] Mercury can cause clinical symptoms, including loss of appetite, weight loss, sleeping disorders, personality changes, memory deficits, depression, headache, tremor, and dermatitis. It has also been linked to antisocial behavior and youth involvement with the juvenile justice system.[3] In the United States, it is estimated that industrial mercury emissions could contribute to lower IQ in 300,000 to 600,000 children,[43] and that the cost of lost productivity and lower intelligence caused by mercury is $8.7 billion annually.[44] All of this is especially important in underserved communities with potentially higher exposure and potentially decreased awareness, monitoring, and access to health care.

Lead

Lead exposure may come from house paint used before 1978 when lead-based paint was banned, plumbing installed before 1987 when lead pipe soldering was banned, soil contaminated with lead from urban sources (eg, leaded gasoline, decaying lead-based paint), and industrial facilities making lead-based products.

Lead toxicity is a well-known entity. Toxic levels can cause cardiovascular, renal, skeletal, and neurologic complications. Nonspecific symptoms, such as nausea, vomiting, abdominal pain, irritability, lethargy, headache, and difficulty concentrating and learning, usually develop early and slowly progress as lead builds up in the body. Lead's effects are especially toxic to the developing nervous system and can cause permanent learning deficits and behavior problems in children. It is known to reduce the prefrontal cortical gray matter area, an area involved in impulse control and executive function, and as such has been strongly associated with aggressive and antisocial behavior, delinquency, and violent crimes.[45,46] Again, all of this is of great interest in underserved communities where both lead toxicity and behavioral problems are more likely to exist.

A toxic level for children, as set by the CDC, is above 5 μg/dL of blood. However no safe level of lead has been established.

Cadmium

Exposure to cadmium comes from cigarette smoke, fossil fuel combustion, mining, manufacturing of nickel-cadmium batteries, pigments, and the creation of plastic stabilizers. Cadmium exposure has been associated COPD; renal failure; osteopenia; and prostate, lung, and testicular cancer.[47] Again, this is important in underserved communities where both combustion byproducts and second-hand smoke (SHS) are more prevalent.

Manganese

Toxic manganese exposure is usually related to steel or aluminum production plants and, although it is among the least toxic elements, high manganese exposure can lead to neurologic effects by altering serotonin and dopamine levels, leading to depression, mood swings, compulsive behaviors, psychosis, and Parkinson-like symptoms. It has also been documented to have neurobehavioral effects, including anxiety, aggression, impulsivity, emotional instability, poor planning, and fatigue.[3]

AIR POLLUTION GROUPING BY PARTICLE SIZE

Common sources of PM10 are ground dust, tire wear emissions, soot from wood combustion, construction works, and mining operations. PM2.5, the most injurious category of PM and thus the most studied, commonly originates from diesel exhaust (contributing to more than 40 toxic pollutants), car exhaust, oil refineries, metal processing facilities, power plants (especially coal burning plants in China, India, and unfiltered plants in the United States), ground dust (eg, sands arising from the Arabian and Saharan deserts), and wild fires. Ultrafine particles may originate from automobile exhaust, jet exhaust, printer toner, photocopiers, and natural sources.[48]

Particulate Matter 2.5

Particles are perhaps the most studied air pollutants and are particularly pathogenic because they are able to evade the body's defenses and penetrate deep into the lungs where, in the case of smaller particles, they may enter the bloodstream. The American Heart Association estimates that in the United States, PM2.5 air pollution contributes to 60,000 deaths per year in the United States with global estimates at 3.3 million premature deaths per year.[49]

Although PM2.5 levels have decreased in most developed countries, industrial practices in Southeast Asia and China have contributed to the recent 20% global increase.[50] The makeup of PM2.5 varies depending on local conditions. In Mexico City in 2006, for example, 55% of PM2.5 was made up of from fossil fuel carbons, 16% from mineral dust, 10% from sulfates, 7% from nitrates, 3% from ammonium, and 9% from various other sources. Bundled into these various other sources are the heavy metals produced by traffic and industrial sources as previously discussed.

PM2.5 has been associated with increased morbidity and mortality from cardiovascular disease (eg, hypertension, coronary artery disease, atherosclerosis and carotid artery intimal thickening, congestive heart failure, myocardial infarction),[51–53] pulmonary disease (eg, asthma, bronchitis,[54] respiratory infections including tuberculosis,[55] pulmonary embolism,[56] and lung cancer).[57,58] It has also been shown to decrease lung function (eg, forced vital capacity, forced expiratory volume in 1 second, respiratory flow rate).[59]

Of special note is that the harmful cardiovascular and pulmonary effects are seen even at low levels of long-term PM2.5 exposure (ie, 5–35 µg/m3). As a reference, the US EPA standard is 12 µg/m3 annual average, whereas Beijing's average from 2010 to 2012 was 100 µg/m3.[60] It is estimated that a 10 µg/m3 increase in average 24-hour PM2.5 exposure increases the relative risk for cardiovascular mortality up to 1.0% and will contribute to 1 premature death per day in a region of 5 million people, potentially leading to the early mortality of tens of thousands of individuals per year in the United States alone.[61,62]

In addition to cardiopulmonary disease, long-term exposure to air pollution has also been linked to neurologic and cognitive function deficits. Pollutants can enter the central nervous system (CNS) via the lung-circulation-CNS pathway or can directly access the CNS through the olfactory mucosa. In either case, the pollutants cause either direct toxicity or may induce damage by activating inflammatory cascades and eliciting free radical formation. These changes will eventually lead to impaired neurogenesis, clinical manifestations, and cognitive-behavioral changes (see later discussion).[63–65]

In utero, PM2.5 exposure in specific windows may have different neurologic sequela. PM2.5 exposure at 31 to 38 weeks has been associated with lower IQ, at 32 to 36 weeks with slower reaction times, at 20 to 26 weeks with decreased attention, and at 12 to 20 weeks with decreased general memory in girls.[66] Overall, PM2.5 exposure in utero has been linked to poorer memory, attention, executive function,[66] psychomotor development,[67] learning, and IQ.[68] It has also been associated with increased autism[69,70] and attention deficit hyperactivity disorder (ADHD). The long-lasting learning impairment, self-esteem issues, and behavioral problems of these latter 2 maladies can be devastating to the individual and costly to society.[71] As could be expected, PM2.5 and PM10 exposure has been associated with increased criminality.[3] All of this is especially evident and worrisome in underserved children living less than 500 m from a freeway or major road.[54]

In adults, the strongest neurologic links to air pollution have been noted with stroke, Parkinson disease, and multiple sclerosis. It has also been linked to Alzheimer disease in genetically susceptible individuals. Cognitively, PM2.5 particles have been associated with poor verbal learning, spatial learning, and memory.[72]

Peak carbon and PM2.5 concentrations occur in the mornings with rush hour traffic.[73] Therefore, PCPs should caution patients to avoid strenuous exercise during these times. For interested PCPs, global satellite maps of PM2.5 have been created and are available online.[74] It should be remembered that when considering the effects of air pollutants, both indoor (SHS or indoor fires for cooking) and outdoor air quality must be considered.

A note on second-hand cigarette smoke particulate matter 2.5

Although the composition of cigarette PM2.5 differs from that of air pollution PM2.5, it has been noted to have similar harmful effects.[60] To underscore the highly toxic effect of SHS, it is noted that living for a year in a polluted city such as Beijing, with an average PM2.5 concentration of 100µg/m3, is the equivalent of smoking just 1.2 cigarettes per week; thus one can only imagine the noxious effect of smoking a pack per day or living in a household where SHS exposure is constant. PCPs working in underserved areas with vastly higher rates of smoking and SHS (11 × greater risk of child SHS exposure in low SES households)[75] need to be aware of these dangers so that avoidance and behavior modification can be emphasized.

GENERAL AIR POLLUTION COUNSELING

As previously stated, when counseling patients regarding air pollution in general, PCPs caring for underserved patients in high pollution areas should advise them to stay indoors on high pollution days, clean indoor air with filters if possible, and limit physical exertion near roads or industrial sources, especially in the late morning or early afternoons when pollutant concentrations and ozone conversion may be highest.

INGESTED POLLUTANTS: WATER, SOIL, AND FOOD CONTAMINATION

Ingested water, soil, and food pollutants can all have adverse effects. As with air pollutants, these toxins vary widely in composition (eg, infectious agents, organic contaminants, inorganic heavy metals) and can come from a variety of sources, including industrial contamination, agricultural runoff, and food storage methods (plastic lining of canned goods). BPA and arsenic (see later discussion) are meant to serve as examples of potential harmful ingestible compounds. These 2 examples are meant only to heighten PCP awareness, not to imply that these examples are more prevalent or more toxic than other ingestible pollutants. The EPA monitors 87 microorganisms, disinfectants, organic compounds, inorganic chemicals, and radionuclides in rivers and public water supplies, each of which is potentially offensive. The FDA tests food and food packaging materials for more than 60 infectious agents, 484 pesticide residues, and many other heavy metals and other chemical contaminants.

Bisphenol A

BPA is used in making polycarbonates, which are found in products such as plastic dinnerware, eyeglass lenses, compact discs, toys, epoxy-based paints, water bottles, and home flooring. One of the most ubiquitous uses of BPA are in the protective linings of canned foods and beverages from which it has been found to leach into canned foods, especially acidic foods such as canned tomato products. In a recent study, 75 participants were split into 2 groups. The first group consumed 5 days of canned soup followed by 5 days without canned consumption. The second group did the reverse. Those consuming canned soup were found to have urinary BPA levels 1000% greater than those consuming only fresh foods.[76] BPA's weak estrogenic properties have been the intense focus of studies since the early 2000s when the concept of endocrine-disrupting compounds came to the forefront. BPA has been detected in 41% of US streams surveyed in 30 states[77] and has been found in the urine of 92% of people older than 6 years of age.[78]

Although the FDA and European Food and Safety Authority currently conclude that, "exposure to BPA at current levels is safe,"[79,80] the Chapel Hill Consensus Statement on BPA disagrees, stating that "BPA concentrations found in the human body are similar to those found in laboratory animals that have been associated with organizational changes of prostate, breast, testis, mammary glands, immune systems and brain."[81] A recent 2015 review concluded, "BPA may increase susceptibility to mammary and prostate cancer."[82] In addition links to hypertension, thyroid function obesity, asthma, and other cardiovascular diseases have been noted.[83–85]

The greatest concern of BPA exposure, however, is the potential risk for pregnant women, infants, and children. Several studies have stated that BPA's neurodevelopmental and behavioral effects are of the greatest concern,[83] and have shown early BPA exposure to be associated with aggressive behavior, ADHD, depression, and anxiety, indicating disruption of brain development during critical, formative windows.[86] It has also been classified as a reproductive toxicant and a recent 2014 review highlights the evidence for decreased uterine receptivity, increased implantation failure, adverse birth outcomes, sexual dysfunction, and testicular toxicant effects.[87] Such effects also may be passed on to future generations through genetic and epigenetic mechanisms (see later discussion).[88,89]

Although BPA has been shown to be biodegradable and is thought not to bioaccumulate,[90] it is still possible that untoward human effects might occur. This is because BPA is so prevalent and exposure is ongoing and prolonged. All of this, especially the prolonged exposure and neurobehavioral effects, is important when assessing BPAs effects in underserved communities. All of the recent studies the authors could find explicitly addressing BPA in underserved communities[91,92] found that those with low SES had significantly higher BPA levels.

The EPA reference dose of 50 µg/kg/d is the recommended safe level of exposure to BPA; however, animal studies have shown effects at much lower doses.

Arsenic

Arsenic is used in many industrial processes (ie, making metal alloys) and in the production of pressure-treated woods (scheduled to be phased out beginning in 2003 but still prevalent in many older houses). Once in the soil, it can be absorbed and concentrated in plants, most notably in leafy vegetables and rice. The main source of arsenic exposure, however, is from the natural diffusion of inorganic arsenic into groundwater. Groundwater in the US Southwest, Nevada, New England, Michigan, Wisconsin, Minnesota, and the Dakotas is known to have higher levels. In a Nevada town, for example, naturally elevated groundwater levels accounted for an average urinary arsenic level 4 times that of the average US population level.[93] It is significantly higher in other countries (ie, Bangladesh, Mongolia, Vietnam, Cambodia). In Bangladesh, levels have been noted to be 50 times higher than US standards and for Inner Mongolia the average level may be up to 70 times higher.[94]

Arsenic has been linked to skin and bladder cancer,[95,96] as well as dermal keratosis, vasospasm, and peripheral neuropathy. These effects have been associated with urinary levels as low as 50 to 100 µg/L in chronically exposed populations, a level found in roughly 5% to 10% of the US population in 2009 to 2010. WHO and EPA standards for arsenic safety is 10 ppb for both food and water consumption. China has a food standard of 150 ppb.

Overall, the authors could find relatively few studies assessing public drinking water or soil contamination in underserved communities[97–102] but those found validated EJ concerns and found excessive toxin levels in underserved communities. Much of this discrepancy was found in rural communities with small or underfunded municipal water systems.

SUMMARY

Because underserved communities are likely to have higher pollution levels, PCPs working in these areas should be prepared to investigate potential occurrences, educate patients, and mitigate effects while waiting for or advocating for larger scale policy changes. Again, PCPs should understand that no standard approach to air, water, or food toxin exposure is possible. Instead, because different communities experience different exposure, depending on industrial contributions; agricultural runoff; traffic patterns; and the prevalence of other infectious, organic, or inorganic toxins, a more individualized and site-specific approach in necessary. It is important for the PCP to be aware of her of his particular community and the environmental factors at play.

REFERENCES

1. Hajat A, Hsia C, O'Neill MS. Socioeconomic disparities and air pollution exposure: a global review. Curr Environ Health Rep 2015;2:440–50.
2. Bai Y, Hillemeier MM, Lengerich EJ. Racial/ethnic disparities in symptom severity among children hospitalized with asthma. J Health Care Poor Underserved 2007;18:54–61.
3. Haynes EN, Chen A, Ryan P, et al. Exposure to airborne metals and particulate matter and risk for youth adjudicated for criminal activity. Environ Res 2011;111:1243–8.
4. Centers for Disease Control and Prevention. National Biomonitoring Program. Biomonitoring Summaries. Available at: http://www.cdc.gov/biomonitoring/biomonitoring_summaries.html. Accessed May 28, 2016.
5. Rosenfeld CS. Bisphenol A and phthalate endocrine disruption of parental and social behaviors. Front Neurosci 2015;9:57.
6. Bengalli R, Molteni E, Longhin E, et al. Release of IL-1 β triggered by Milan summer PM10: molecular pathways involved in the cytokine release. Biomed Res Int 2013;2013:158093.
7. Suhaimi NF, Jalaludin J. Biomarker as a research tool in linking exposure to air particles and respiratory health. Biomed Res Int 2015;2015:962853.
8. Olden K, Lin YS, Gruber D, et al. Epigenome: biosensor of cumulative exposure to chemical and nonchemical stressors related to environmental justice. Am J Public Health 2014;104:1816–21.
9. Feil R. Environmental and nutritional effects on the epigenetic regulation of genes. Mutat Res 2006;600:46–57.
10. Vandegehuchte MB, Janssen CR. Epigenetics and its implications for ecotoxicology. Ecotoxicology 2011;20:607–24.
11. Slomko H, Heo HJ, Einstein FH. Minireview: epigenetics of obesity and diabetes in humans. Endocrinology 2012;153(3):1025–30.
12. Bégin P, Nadeau KC. Epigenetic regulation of asthma and allergic disease. Allergy Asthma Clin Immunol 2014;10:27.
13. Hong X, Wang X. Early life precursors, epigenetics, and the development of food allergy. Semin Immunopathol 2012;34:655–69.
14. Javierre BM, Hernando H, Ballestar E. Environmental triggers and epigenetic deregulation in autoimmune disease. Discov Med 2011;12:535–45.
15. Klengel T, Pape J, Binder EB, et al. The role of DNA methylation in stress-related psychiatric disorders. Neuropharmacology 2014;80:115–32.
16. Saban KL, Mathews HL. Epigenetics and social context: implications for disparity in cardiovascular disease. Aging Dis 2014;5:346–55.

17. Herceg Z, Vaissière T. Epigenetic mechanisms and cancer: an interface between the environment and the genome. Epigenetics 2011;6:804–19.
18. Kanwal R, Gupta K, Gupta S. Cancer epigenetics: an introduction. Methods Mol Biol 2015;1238:3–25.
19. World Health Organization. Media Centre. 7 million premature deaths annually linked to air pollution. Available at: http://www.who.int/mediacentre/news/releases/2014/air-pollution/en/. Accessed March 7, 2016.
20. Calderón-Garcidueñas L, Kulesza RJ. Megacities air pollution problems: Mexico City metropolitan area critical issues on the central nervous system pediatric impact. Environ Res 2015;137:157–69.
21. Hampson NB, Piantadosi CA, Thom SR, et al. Practice recommendations in the diagnosis, management, and prevention of carbon monoxide poisoning. Am J Respir Crit Care Med 2012;186:1095–101.
22. Gatto NM, Henderson VW, Hodis HN, et al. Components of air pollution and cognitive function in middle aged and older adults in Los Angeles. Neurotoxicology 2014;40:1–7.
23. Iglesias DJ, Calatayud A, Barreno E, et al. Responses of citrus plants to ozone: leaf biochemistry, antioxidant mechanisms and lipid peroxidation. Plant Physiol Biochem 2006;44:125–31.
24. Jerrett M, Burnett RT, Pope CA, et al. Long-Term ozone exposure and mortality. N Engl J Med 2009;360:1085–95.
25. Weinhold B. Ozone nation: EPA standard panned by the people. Environ Health Perspect 2008;116:A302–5.
26. Kodavanti UP. Air pollution and insulin resistance: do all roads lead to Rome? Diabetes 2015;64:712–4.
27. United States Environmental Protection Agency. The National Ambient Air Quality Standards for Ozone. Ozone and Health. Available at: https://www.epa.gov/sites/production/files/2016-04/documents/20151001healthfs.pdf. Accessed October 26, 2016.
28. Chen JC, Schwartz J. Neurobehavioral effects of ambient air pollution on cognitive performance in US adults. Neurotoxicology 2009;30:231–9.
29. Goodman JE, Prueitt RL, Sax SN. Weight-of-evidence evaluation of short-term ozone exposure and cardiovascular effects. Crit Rev Toxicol 2014;44:725–90.
30. Prueitt RL, Lynch HN. Weight-of-evidence evaluation of long-term ozone exposure and cardiovascular effects. Crit Rev Toxicol 2014;44:791–822.
31. Lei H, Wuebbles DJ, Liang XZ. Projected risk of high ozone episodes in 2050. Atmospheric Environment 2012;59:567–77.
32. Goodman JE, Prueitt RL. Ozone exposure and systemic biomarkers: evaluation of evidence for adverse cardiovascular health impacts. Crit Rev Toxicol 2015;45: 412–52.
33. Molina LT, Kolb CE, deFoy B, et al. Air quality in North America's most populous city – Overview of the MCMA 2003 campaign. Atmos Chem Phys 2007;7: 2447–73.
34. Shankardass K, McConnell R, Jerrett M, et al. Parental stress increases the effect of traffic-related air pollution on childhood asthma incidence. Proc Natl Acad Sci U S A 2009;106:12406–11.
35. American Lung Association. Trends in asthma morbidity and mortality. Chicago (IL): Epidemiology and Statistical Unit, Research and Health Education Division; 2012. Available at: http://www.lung.org/assets/documents/research/asthma-trend-report.pdf. Accessed on January 30, 2016.

36. Jungers RH, Lee RE, von Lehmden DJ. The EPA national fuel surveillance network. Trace constituents in gasoline and commercial gasoline fuel additives. Environ Health Perspect 1975;10:143–50.

37. Cheung KL, Ntziachristos L, Tzamkiozis T, et al. Emissions of particulate trace elements, metals and organic species from gasoline, diesel, and biodiesel passenger vehicles and their relation to oxidative potential. Aerosol Sci Technol 2010;44:500–13.

38. Grandjean P, Weihe P, White RF, et al. Cognitive deficit in 7-year-old children with prenatal exposure to methylmercury. Neurotoxicol Teratol 1997;19:417–28.

39. Harada M. Minamata disease: Methylmercury poisoning in Japan caused by environmental pollution. Crit Rev Toxicol 1995;25:1–24.

40. Davidson PW, Myers GJ, Cox C, et al. Effects of prenatal and postnatal methylmercury exposure from fish consumption on neurodevelopment: outcomes at 66 months of age in the Seychelles Child Development Study. JAMA 1998; 280:701–7.

41. Sikorski R, Juszkiewicz T, Paszkowski T, et al. Women in dental surgeries: reproductive hazards in occupational exposure to metallic mercury. Int Arch Occup Environ Health 1987;59:551–7.

42. Yorifuji T, Tsuda T, Kawakami N. Age standardized cancer mortality ratios in areas heavily exposed to methyl mercury. Int Arch Occup Environ Health 2007;80:679–88.

43. Trasande L, Schechter C, Haynes KA, et al. Applying cost analyses to drive policy that protects children: Mercury as a case study. Ann N Y Acad Sci 2006; 1076:911–23.

44. Trasande L, Landrigan PJ, Schechter C. Public health and economic consequences of methyl mercury toxicity to the developing brain. Environ Health Perspect 2005;113:590–6.

45. Brower MC, Price BH. Neuropsychiatry of frontal lobe dysfunction in violent and criminal behaviour: a critical review. J Neurol Neurosurg Psychiatry 2001;71: 720–6.

46. Braun JM, Froehlich TE, Daniels JL, et al. Association of environmental toxicants and conduct disorder in U.S. children: NHANES 2001–2004. Environ Health Perspect 2008;116:956–62.

47. Bertin G, Averbeck D. Cadmium: cellular effects, modifications of biomolecules, modulation of DNA repair and genotoxic consequences (a review). Biochimie 2006;88:1549–59.

48. United States Environmental Protection Agency, 2002. Health Assessment Document for Diesel Engine Exhaust. Washington, DC: National Center for Environmental Assessment, USEPA; 2002. p. 669.

49. Lelieveld J, Evans JS. The contribution of outdoor air pollution sources to premature mortality on a global scale. Nature 2015;525:367–71.

50. Brauer M, Freedman G, Frostad J, et al. Ambient air pollution exposure estimation for the global burden of disease 2013. Environ Sci Technol 2016;50:79–88.

51. McGuinn LA, Ward-Caviness CK, Neas LM, et al. Association between satellite-based estimates of long-term PM2.5 exposure and coronary artery disease. Environ Res 2016;145:9–17.

52. Giorgini P, Di Giosia P, Grassi D, et al. Air Pollution Exposure and Blood Pressure: An Updated Review of the Literature. Curr Pharm Des 2015;22:28–51.

53. Kunzli N, Jerrett M, Mack WJ, et al. Ambient air pollution and atherosclerosis in Los Angeles. Environ Health Perspect 2005;113:201–6.

54. Chen Z, Salam MT, Eckel SP, et al. Chronic effects of air pollution on respiratory health in Southern California children: findings from the Southern California Children's Health Study. J Thorac Dis 2015;7:46–58.
55. Ghio AJ. Particle exposures and infections. Infection 2014;42:459–67.
56. Spiezia L, Campello E, Bon M, et al. Short-term exposure to high levels of air pollution as a risk factor for acute isolated pulmonary embolism. Thromb Res 2014;134:259–63.
57. Zhou F, Li S, Jia W, et al. Effects of diesel exhaust particles on microRNA-21 in human bronchial epithelial cells and potential carcinogenic mechanisms. Mol Med Rep 2015;12:2329–35.
58. Brunekreef B, Beelen R, Hoek G, et al. Effects of long-term exposure to traffic-related air pollution on respiratory and cardiovascular mortality in the Netherlands: the NLCS-AIR study. Res Rep Health Eff Inst 2009;139:5–71.
59. Wu S, Deng F, Hao Y, et al. Chemical constituents of fine particulate air pollution and pulmonary function in healthy adults: the Healthy Volunteer Natural Relocation study. J Hazard Mater 2013;260:183–91.
60. Pope CA 3rd, Burnett RT, Turner MC, et al. Lung cancer and cardiovascular disease mortality associated with ambient air pollution and cigarette smoke: shape of the exposure–response relationships. Environ Health Perspect 2011;119:1616–21.
61. Pope CA 3rd, Dockery DW. Health effects of fine particulate air pollution: lines that connect. J Air Waste Manag Assoc 2006;56:709–42.
62. Brook RD, Franklin B, Cascio W, et al, Expert panel on population and prevention science of the American Heart Association. Air pollution and cardiovascular disease: a statement for healthcare professionals from the expert panel on population and prevention science. Circulation 2004;109:2655–71.
63. Genc S, Zadeoglulari Z, Fuss SH, et al. The adverse effects of air pollution on the nervous system. J Toxicol 2012;2012:782462.
64. Costa LG, Cole TB, Coburn J, et al. Neurotoxicity of traffic-related air pollution. Neurotoxicology 2015 [pii: S0161-813(15) 30024–30033].
65. Gerlofs-Nijland ME, van Berlo D, Cassee FR, et al. Effect of prolonged exposure to diesel engine exhaust on proinflammatory markers in different regions of the rat brain. Part Fibre Toxicol 2010;7:12.
66. Chiu YM, Hsu HL, Coull BA, et al. Prenatal particulate air pollution and neurodevelopment in urban children: examining sensitive windows and sex-specific associations. Environ Int 2015;87:56–65.
67. Guxens M, Garcia-Esteban R, Giorgis-Allemand L, et al. Air pollution during pregnancy and childhood cognitive and psychomotor development. Epidemiology 2014;25:636–47.
68. Edwards SC, Jedrychowski W, Butscher M, et al. Prenatal exposure to airborne polycyclic aromatic hydrocarbons and children's intelligence at 5 years of age in a prospective cohort study in Poland. Environ. Health Perspect 2010;118:1326–31.
69. Volk HE, Lurmann F, Penfold B, et al. Traffic related air pollution, particulate matter, and autism. JAMA Psychiatry 2013;70:71–7.
70. Suades-González E, Gascon M, Guxens M, et al. Air pollution and neuropsychological development: a review of the latest evidence. Endocrinology 2015;156:3473–82.
71. Siddique S, Banerjee J, Ray MR, et al. Attention deficit hyperactivity disorder in children chronically exposed to high level of vehicular pollution. Eur J Pediatr 2011;170:923–9.

72. Win-Shwe TT, Yamamoto S, Fujitani Y, et al. Spatial learning and memory function-related gene expression in the hippocampus of mouse exposed to nanoparticle-rich diesel exhaust. Neurotoxicology 2008;29:940–7.

73. Eiguren-Fernandez A, Miguel AH, Froines JR, et al. Seasonal and spatial variation of poly cyclic aromatic hydrocarbons in vapor-phase and PM2.5 in southern California and rural communities. Aerosol Sci Technol 2004;38:447–55.

74. van Donkelaar A, Martin RV, Brauer M, et al. Global estimates of ambient fine particulate matter concentrations from satellite-based aerosol optical depth: development and application. Environ Health Perspect 2010;118:847–55.

75. Pisinger C, Hammer-Helmich L, Andreasen AH, et al. Social disparities in children's exposure to second hand smoke at home: a repeated cross-sectional survey. Environ Health 2012;11:65.

76. Carwile JL, Ye X, Zhou X, et al. Canned soup consumption and urinary bisphenol A: a randomized crossover trial. JAMA 2011;306:2218–20.

77. Kolpin DW, Furlong ET, Meyer MT, et al. Pharmaceuticals, hormones, and other organic wastewater contaminants in U.S. streams, 1999-2000: a national reconnaissance. Environ Sci Technol 2002;36:1202–11.

78. Trasande L, Attina TM, Blustein J. Association between urinary bisphenol A concentration and obesity prevalence in children and adolescents. JAMA 2012;308:1113–21.

79. US Food & Drug Administration.Bisphenol A (BPA): Use in Food Contact Application. Available at: http://www.fda.gov/NewsEvents/PublicHealthFocus/ucm064437.htm. Accessed October 26, 2016.

80. EFSA. Bisphenol A. Available at: http://www.efsa.europa.eu/en/topics/topic/bisphenol. Accessed March 9, 2016.

81. vom Saal FS, Akingbemi BT, Belcher SM, et al. Chapel Hill bisphenol A expert panel consensus statement: integration of mechanisms, effects in animals and potential to impact human health at current levels of exposure. Reprod Toxicol 2007;24:131–8.

82. Seachrist DD, Bonk KW, Ho SM, et al. A review of the carcinogenic potential of bisphenol A. Reprod Toxicol 2016;59:167–82.

83. Rochester JR. Bisphenol A and human health: a review of the literature. Reprod Toxicol 2013;42:132–55.

84. Lang IA, Galloway TS, Scarlett A, et al. Association of urinary bisphenol A concentration with medical disorders and laboratory abnormalities in adults. JAMA 2008;300:1303–10.

85. vom Saal FS, Myers JP. Bisphenol A and risk of metabolic disorders. JAMA 2008;300:1353–5.

86. Mustieles V, Pérez-Lobato R, Olea N, et al. Human exposure and neurobehavior. Neurotoxicology 2015;49:174–84.

87. Peretz J, Vrooman L, Ricke WA, et al. Bisphenol A and reproductive health: update of experimental and human evidence, 2007-2013. Environ Health Perspect 2014;122:775–86.

88. Bernal AJ, Jirtle RL. Epigenomic disruption: the effects of early developmental exposures. Birth Defects Res A Clin Mol Teratol 2010;88:938–44.

89. Ryan KK, Haller AM, Sorrell JE, et al. Perinatal exposure to bisphenol-A and the development of metabolic syndrome in CD-1 mice. Endocrinology 2010;151:2603–12.

90. Negri-Cesi P. Bisphenol A interaction with brain development and functions. Dose Response 2015;13. 1559325815590394.

91. Nelson JW, Scammell MK, Hatch EE, et al. Social disparities in exposures to bisphenol A and polyfluoroalkyl chemicals: a cross-sectional study within NHANES 2003-2006. Environ Health 2012;11:10.
92. Tyrrell J, Melzer D, Henley W, et al. Associations between socioeconomic status and environmental toxicant concentrations in adults in the USA: NHANES 2001-2010. Environ Int 2013;59:328–35.
93. Caldwell KL, Jones RL, Verdon CP, et al. Levels of urinary total and speciated arsenic in the U.S. Population: National Health and Nutrition Examination Survey 2003-2004. J Expo Sci Environ Epidemiol 2009;19:59–68.
94. Sun G, Xu Y, Li X, et al. Urinary arsenic metabolites in children and adults exposed to arsenic in drinking water in Inner Mongolia, China. Environ Health Perspect 2007;115:648–52.
95. Ioch LM, Zierold K, Anderson HA. Association of arsenic-contaminated drinking-water with prevalence of skin cancer in Wisconsin's Fox River Valley. J Health Popul Nutr 2006;24:206–13.
96. Chu HD, Crawford-Brown DJ. Inorganic arsenic in drinking water and bladder cancer: a meta-analysis for dose-response assessment. Int J Environ Res Public Health 2006;3:316–22.
97. Heaney C, Wilson S, Wilson O, et al. Use of community-owned and -managed research to assess the vulnerability of water and sewer services in marginalized and underserved environmental justice communities. J Environ Health 2011;74:8–17.
98. Delpla I, Benmarhnia T. Investigating social inequalities in exposure to drinking water contaminants in rural areas. Environ Pollut 2015;207:88–96.
99. Cushing L, Morello-Frosch R, Wander M, et al. The haves, the have-nots, and the health of everyone: the relationship between social inequality and environmental quality. Annu Rev Public Health 2015;36:193–209.
100. Balazs CL, Ray I. The drinking water disparities framework: on the origins and persistence of inequities in exposure. Am J Public Health 2014;104:603–11.
101. Balazs CL, Morello-Frosch R, Hubbard AE, et al. Environmental justice implications of arsenic contamination in California's San Joaquin Valley: a cross-sectional, cluster-design examining exposure and compliance in community drinking water systems. Environ Health 2012;11:84.
102. Diawara MM, Litt JS, Unis D, et al. Arsenic, cadmium, lead, and mercury in surface soils, Pueblo, Colorado: implications for population health risk. Environ Geochem Health 2006;28:297–315.

Climate Change and Underserved Communities

Carol Ziegler, DNP, APRN, NP-C, RD[a,b], Vincent Morelli, MD[c,*], Omotayo Fawibe, MD[b]

KEYWORDS

- Climate change • Global warming • Greenhouse gases • Greenhouse gas emissions
- Patient education

KEY POINTS

- Climate change is a threat to the basic necessities of life, especially for the most vulnerable. These necessities include health, shelter, food, and water.
- Climate change will have direct health impact on populations seen in primary care.
- The effects of climate change must be dampened with adaptation and mitigation strategies.

A GLOBAL PERSPECTIVE ON CLIMATE CHANGE

The Intergovernmental Panel on Climate Change defines climate change as a change in the state of the climate that persists for an extended period, typically decades, and can be identified by the variability of its properties. It is also any change in climate over time, whether due to natural variability or as a result of human activity.[1] Climate change is not currently widely accepted as a health hazard by health care professionals in the United States; yet it is the single greatest global health threat of the twenty-first century.[2] The effects of climate change on global health are so enormous that in the next few decades billions of lives will be affected.[2] The concept of climate change, despite skepticism and political opposition, is valid. Available science concludes with 90% certainty that the earth's climate has warmed over the past few decades as a result of greenhouse gas emissions from human activities.[1,3] Moreover, no credible body of climate scientists have found an alternate explanation for the rising global temperature.

This article originally appeared in Primary Care: Clinics in Office Practice, Volume 44, Issue 1, March 2017.

Disclosure Statement: The authors of this work report no direct financial interest in the subject matter or any material discussed in this article.

[a] Vanderbilt University School of Nursing, Nashville, 461 21st Ave South, Nashville, TN 37240, USA; [b] Department of Family & Community Medicine, Meharry Medical College, 1005 Dr D. B. Todd Boulevard, Nashville, TN 37208, USA; [c] Sports Medicine Fellowship, Department of Family and Community Medicine, Meharry Medical College, 1005 Dr D. B. Todd Boulevard, Nashville, TN 37208, USA
* Corresponding author.
E-mail address: vmorelli@mmc.edu

Physician Assist Clin 4 (2019) 203–216
https://doi.org/10.1016/j.cpha.2018.08.008
2405-7991/19/© 2018 Elsevier Inc. All rights reserved.

Climate change occurs due to an imbalance between incoming and outgoing radiation in the atmosphere.[4] When solar radiation from sunlight enters the atmosphere, some of the radiation is absorbed by the earth's surface and emitted as infrared radiation. Greenhouse gases, such as carbon dioxide (CO_2), methane (CH_4) and nitrous oxide (N_2O), absorb the infrared radiation, heating up the lower atmosphere.[5,6] These greenhouse gases can occur naturally or from human activities. Fluctuations in the temperature of the lower atmosphere have occurred in the past due to variations in concentrations of naturally occurring greenhouse gases. The significant rise in global temperatures now experienced, however, is due to a rise in the concentration of global greenhouse gases in the atmosphere due to various human activities. CO_2 accounts for 76% of greenhouse gas emissions and is a product of petroleum product combustion, natural gas, and coal. CH_4 is a product of landfills, coal mines, and oil and gas operations and accounts for 16% of emissions, whereas N_2O accounts for 5% of emissions and is a product of nitrogen fertilizers, burning biomass, and waste management processes. Finally, fluorinated gases account for 2% of emissions and are a product of industrial processes like refrigeration (**Fig. 1**).[7]

Since the industrial revolution, atmospheric concentration of CO_2 has increased from 280 parts per million to approximately 395 parts per million today.[3,5] This has led to record-high global temperatures. The planet's average temperature has increased by 0.8°C since 1880 and if the current trend of CO_2 emission levels remains stable, it is predicted that the planet's average temperature will increase by an additional 1.8°C to 5.8°C by the end of the twenty-first century.[5] This is expected to have an impact on basic human needs like food, water, shelter, and health. Increased global temperature will disrupt the water cycle because warmer air retains more moisture, causing flooding in some areas and drought in others; this will affect crop yield from farming and even livestock productivity. Increased temperature can also lead to heat waves increasing the incidence of heat-related illnesses. Heat waves can also increase the ambient level of some air pollutants, which can increase morbidity and mortality related to cardiorespiratory conditions. Also, flooding or drought can affect the geographic distribution of vector-borne diseases, such as malaria and dengue fever. Increased global temperature will also increase ocean

■ Carbon dioxide (from fossil fuel burning, forestry, industrial processes)

■ Methane (from landfills, coal mines, oil & gas operations)

▨ Nitrous oxide (from nitrogen fertilizers, burning biomass & waste management processes)

■ Fluorinated gases (from industrial processes like refrigeration)

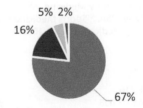

Fig. 1. Global greenhouse gas emissions.

temperatures, potentially disrupting the aquatic ecosystem and affecting industries like fishing. The increased global temperature will also cause sea levels to rise as a result of melting sea ice, forcing migration of coastal dwellers and leading to a host of other challenges (**Fig. 2**).[3,5,7]

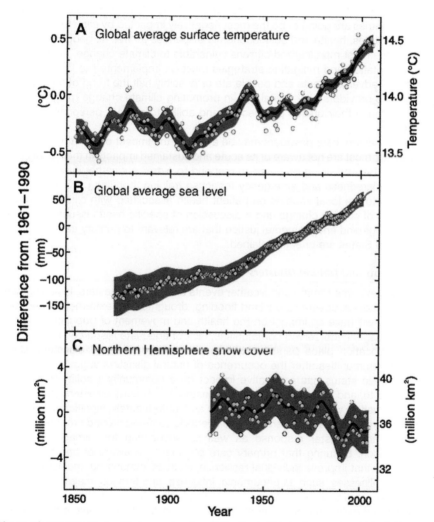

Fig. 2. Changes in temperature, sea level, and Northern Hemisphere snow cover.[1] Observed changes in (a) global average surface temperature, (b) global average sea level from tide gauge (*blue*) and satellite (*red*) data, and (c) Northern Hemisphere snow cover for March–April. All differences are relative to corresponding averages for the period 1961 to 1990. Smoothed curves represent decadal averaged values whereas circles show yearly values. The shaded areas are the uncertainty intervals estimated (a and b) from a comprehensive analysis of known uncertainties and (c) from the time series. (*Figure SPM.1 from* Climate Change 2007: Synthesis Report. Contribution of Working Groups I, II and III to the Fourth Assessment Report of the Intergovernmental Panel on Climate Change. IPCC, Geneva, Switzerland; with permission.)

CLIMATE CHANGE IN THE PRIMARY CARE SETTING

Climate change is a phenomenon that is real but is still approached with skepticism. It is the duty of health care practitioners to learn about the various impacts of climate change and serve as an informant for their patients as well as serving as sentinels for the public health sector when health crises erupt due to climate change. Although the impact of climate change will be seen across the globe, low-income and middle-income countries (LMICs) with minimal resources along with the susceptible groups in wealthy countries are going to be the most negatively impacted by climate change. In the United States, health and socioeconomic disparities as well as geographic location leave the most marginalized citizens vulnerable to climate change. Policies promoting adaptation and mitigation strategies must be implemented to both dampen some of the adverse effects and decelerate or possibly halt the trend of the change. Primary care providers play a vital role in promoting climate change mitigation and activism through their unique perspective and ability to make it personally relevant to health.

Although primary care providers may be aware of the impact of climate change on global health, most are not aware of its acute and sustained impacts in their local practice setting. Beyond being prepared to respond to extreme weather events through disaster preparedness and emergency response training, frontline providers should be attentive to the local impacts on patient health associated with climate change. The process of climate change and a discussion of specific health issues related to climate change and environmental justice that are relevant to primary care providers in the United States are briefly explained.

Climate Events and Natural Disasters

Increases in extreme climate and weather events and natural disasters, including hurricanes, tornadoes, coastal and inland flooding, droughts, and extreme temperature fluctuations, will have an impact on the health and movement of populations in the United States. In underserved communities, lack of adequate resources for evacuation and relocation place persons at increased risk from natural disasters. Case studies of communities after the occurrence of natural disasters suggest that lower socioeconomic status has a negative impact on a community's ability to prepare for, respond to, and recover from natural disasters.[8–11] Natural disasters often result in mass casualties with a spectrum of injuries and, unfortunately, significant mortality. The role of primary care providers in these events is centered around emergency preparedness and disaster response as well as advocating for climate mitigation and adaptation. Ensuring that primary care providers are aware of and promoting interventions that improve individual resilience, such as immunizing against vaccine-preventable illnesses, such as pneumonia, influenza, and tetanus; maintaining infection control in health care settings; and educating patients about nutrition and exercise as well as optimally managing chronic illnesses, is imperative to maximizing patient resilience.[12] Mitigation and adaptation are discussed later; however, emergency preparedness and disaster response are outside of the scope of this article. Primary care providers should avail themselves of training and information related to specific disaster risk and response relevant to their respective regions. Mental health impacts associated with such events are discussed later.

Extreme Temperatures

The American Meteorological Society declared 2014 the hottest year on record.[13] Extreme fluctuations in temperature, both increases in intensity of heat and duration of heat waves, rapid shifts in hot and cold temperatures, and altered patterns of extreme cold are occurring globally and across the United States. Several studies have demonstrated that cold (for normal) and hot (for normal) ambient temperatures are associated with increased risk of mortality in regions across the globe.[14] Although both hot and cold temperatures seem associated with increased risk of mortality across regions, the impact associated with heat, termed *thermal injury*, is observed more rapidly and is typically shorter in duration (the isolated impact of heat on mortality), whereas cold temperatures seem to have a more delayed but longer-lasting impacts.[14]

In addition to impacts from hyperthermia and hypothermia, both of which are emergent conditions not managed in primary care, temperature extremes increase morbidity and mortality with respect to respiratory and cardiovascular systems. Extreme or unseasonably cold temperatures place persons at increased risk of death from cardiovascular disease and respiratory illnesses. Persons with chronic respiratory illnesses, such as asthma and chronic obstructive pulmonary disease (COPD), as well as cardiovascular and cerebrovascular diseases are observed to experience increased mortality in colder temperatures.[15–18] Extreme temperature fluctuations have been observed to increase cardiovascular mortality and morbidity and these impacts disproportionately affect the elderly, small children, people with low socioeconomic status, and those with comorbidities, such as diabetes, hypertension, and kidney disease.[19]

Outside of the direct impact of heat and cold stress on the body's thermoregulatory system, heat waves have been associated with increased exacerbations in cardiovascular disease, asthma, and COPD, and these increases seem related to the temperature itself as well as outdoor and indoor air pollution and humidity.[20] Primary care providers should be aware of the potential impacts of extreme temperature on patients with cardiovascular and respiratory illnesses so that they are able to rapidly optimize management strategies and assist patients in adapting to temperature changes. Educating patients about safety in extreme temperatures, air quality information, and warnings and how to react to them and communicating with local agencies to assist patients in obtaining housing or climate control devices are critical aspects of providing care for those at risk to climate and temperature-related stress.

Vector-Borne Illnesses

Changes in temperature, humidity, and seasonal weather and flooding patterns have broadened the geographic range and seasonal survivability of many vectors of disease. This increase in seasonal and geographic range of common vectors, combined with increased human population density in urban centers and increased human mobility, will broaden the distribution and increase the prevalence of vector-borne and water-borne illnesses. Human mobility and migration patterns due to extreme and insidious changes in climate, as well as conflict, will likely exacerbate this problem.

Warmer winters and changes in seasonal weather patterns will likely broaden the geographic range and encourage expansion of common vectors (in the United States, notably, rodents, ticks, and mosquitoes) to wider latitudes. Globally, malaria, dengue fever, diarrheal diseases, and cholera are on the rise and this increase is directly attributable to climate change.[5] Barriers to vaccinations and other primary care services as well as increased exposures due to inadequate housing and poor vector control in impoverished communities leave persons living in distressed regions of poverty in the United States, such as in communities of color in the Mississippi Delta, impoverished communities in Appalachia, and the urban poor, at increased risk from infections known as neglected infections of poverty.[21]

In the United States, primary care providers must be aware of the signs, symptoms, and most up-to-date transmission patterns and treatment guidelines for illnesses like leptospirosis, Lyme disease, mosquito-borne encephalitis, and hantavirus as the transmission patterns of these illnesses have been noted to increase with respect to the changing climate.[22] Data on the direct impact of climate change on tick and mosquito-related illness in the United States are limited, but modeling suggests that climate change may shift the onset of tick-related illnesses in the United States, expanding the season for tick-borne infections.[23] It is also expected that emerging and re-emerging infections, such as Zika virus, avian flu, malaria, West Nile virus, and others, will likely increase in prevalence and range, appearing in areas where primary care providers may not be familiar with presenting symptoms. In addition, primary care providers must respond rapidly to apparent changes in seasonal patterns of vector-borne illnesses and new cases of vector-borne illnesses by communicating with their local health departments as well as providing patients with education about prevention of these illnesses and the most up-to-date and evidence-based care and management of the illness once a patient is sick. Ensuring that patients are up to date with regular vaccination schedules will prevent the resurgence of vaccine-preventable illnesses.

Impacts on Mental Health

The impact of climate change on mental health is more difficult to assess and more insidious than the direct impact on physical health. The devastating effects of drought, flooding, and other natural disasters coupled with increased migration from conflicts and food shortages will likely have disturbing impacts on populations. Posttraumatic stress disorder, depression, and acculturation stress may result from the devastating impacts that climate change will have on individuals, families, communities, and even entire countries in cases of conflict, drought, or famine.[24] Survivors of floods and hurricanes have increased rates of stress-associated psychiatric disorders.[25–27] In the United states, unusually warm temperatures are associated with increases in mental health disorders, and exacerbations, such as mood and anxiety-related disorders, as well as dementia are increased in heat waves.[28] Heat waves are also associated with higher levels of community violence in low-income neighborhoods.[29] There is a strong association between climate change and collective violence. Increases in social instability and political unrest are associated with elevated temperatures and extreme precipitation.[30,31] It is highly likely that armed conflict will continue to increase with the destabilization of the global climate system.[32]

In addition to effects directly related to extreme weather events and heat, the economic and social consequences of climate change to individuals and entire industries (like agriculture) as well as the impact of increased social conflict have the potential for deleterious effects on the mental health of individuals and populations.[33–35] Climate change will likely have long-term impacts on seasonality, temperatures, and rainfall, thus having an impact on food security and the health of the agricultural industry.[36] The downstream impact of destabilization of broad-based food security systems globally will disproportionately have an impact on the poor and likely lead to malnutrition as well as increases in metabolic diseases from diminished nutrient density of food and food quality.[37] Additionally, economic distress diminishes patient access to primary care services, limiting their ability to manage chronic illnesses and placing them at increased risk for poor health outcomes. Primary care providers practicing in regions experiencing extreme heat and weather events, conflict, and/or community violence or practicing in regions where industries, such as agriculture, are significant sources of employment and income must be cognizant of the pressures felt by the populations they serve. Conducting mental health evaluations and providing trauma-informed counseling for patients experiencing stress from climate-related events and assessing families for food security are critical roles for the primary care provider practicing in the age of climate change.

ADDRESSING HEALTH DISPARITIES RELATED TO CLIMATE CHANGE

The health effects of climate change will not be uniform across the globe. LMICs that already lack the basic infrastructure to meet the essential health care needs of its citizens, are likely to suffer to a greater extent from the impact of climate change than developed countries. These LMICs have little capacity to prevent and/or treat illnesses due to climate change. Ironically, LMICs are the least responsible for climate change, producing less than 10% of global greenhouse gas emissions.[38]

Certain groups in both LMICs and wealthier countries are more susceptible to adverse health effects from climate change. These susceptible groups include the poor, elderly, children, and patients with underlying chronic diseases. The poor have limited access to quality health care, are more likely to be malnourished, and are more likely to live in residences with poor indoor air quality, all factors that contribute to the greater burden of disease experienced by the poor in relation to climate change. The elderly are also at a greater risk of disease from climate change due to frail health and limited mobility, making them less likely to be able to evacuate in the case of a storm or any extreme weather event related to climate change.[39] Children often have developing immune, respiratory, and neurologic systems, making them more sensitive to the adverse health effects of climate change like extreme weather events, heat, and vector-borne diseases.[40,41] In addition to physiologic immaturity, which makes children living in poor countries vulnerable to the health-related consequences of climate change, their poor living conditions often compound health risks.[42] Children accounted for 88% of yearly deaths attributed to climate change in the early 2000s[43] and 99% of the children lived in LMICs.[44,45] In addition, climate change is thought to worsen the top causes of under–5-year-old child mortality, such as acute respiratory infection, diarrhea, malaria, malnutrition, and neonatal deaths.[38] Patients with underlying chronic diseases, such as COPD or asthma, often have impaired lung function that becomes even further impaired by the effects of climate change.[3] It is known that patients with asthma are particularly sensitive to changes in weather, with hot humid days increasing airway resistance of asthmatics.[3] Rapid rises in temperature and humidity have been associated with increased emergency department visits for asthma.[46] Also, exposure to ground-level ozone, production of which is catalyzed by warmer temperatures, has been found associated with increased emergency department visits and hospitalization due to asthma,[47–49] worse asthma control,[50] and reduced lung function.[51,52] Patients with COPD have been found to have more exacerbations, hospitalizations, and even increased all-cause mortality with exposure to heat.[53,54]

Additional Vulnerable Populations in the United States

Vulnerability to climate change may be increased by marginalized mental and/or physical health status, geographic location, or access to adaptation resources (resources that decrease vulnerability to the impacts of climate change). Although climate change will likely have an impact on persons living in low-resource settings globally, in the United States, several populations have been identified who are at increased risk for morbidity and mortality due to climate change and associated stress (in addition to those described previously): older adults (over age 65), children under age 5, pregnant women, persons living with chronic physical and mental illness and/or addiction, the homeless, and people employed in industries requiring exposure to the outdoors. Additionally, specific geographic regions are at increased risk based on proximity to shorelines, coastal and inland waterways, weather patterns, and availability of natural resources, such as water.[55,56] Specific climate-associated risks related to these vulnerable groups are discussed later.

Regional risk depends on availability of resources, proximity to waterways and flood zones, and regional weather patterns. Climate change will have a disproportionate impact on vulnerable populations, but what traits make a community more vulnerable in the United States? Communities of color, indigenous peoples, those who are isolated geographically, and the poor are least able to respond and adapt to climate change. Currently in the Unites States, the southeastern region is at greatest risk from collective impacts of climate change.[57] The southeastern United States is susceptible to climate-related events, such as hurricanes and extreme weather, tornadoes, and also sea level rise along the coastal states. Heat waves and drought also disproportionately have an impact on the southeastern United States[58]; southern cities, such as Atlanta, Miami, New Orleans, and Tampa, reported increased deaths from extreme heat from 1975 to 2004 relative to an increase in days with temperatures at 95°F or greater.[59] Climate change in the southeastern region will have long-term impacts on water availability and associated stresses from water shortages.[60] Additionally, the southern United States has more people living in rural areas and more people working outdoors in agriculture, both at increased risk for health problems from climate change.[61]

Persons employed in industries, such as utilities, transportation, emergency response, health care, environmental remediation, construction or demolition, landscaping and agriculture, forestry and wildlife management, heavy manufacturing, and warehouse work, are at increased risk from extreme weather and temperature events due to the nature of their work and being exposed regularly to the outdoors.[62,63] Workers in these fields may have increased exposure to temperature variations and precipitation, injury due to extreme weather, and exposure to vector-borne illnesses and outdoor pollutants, including from forest fires and industries.

The homeless and the poor will be disproportionately impacted by climate change. Homeless persons typically have increased severity of chronic disease, specifically cardiovascular disease and respiratory illnesses, due to stress, lifestyle factors, and difficulties accessing health care and other resources. Additionally, the homeless disproportionately suffer from substance use and mental health disorders, giving them multiple risk factors for climate change vulnerabilities.[64–67] Homeless persons tend to congregate in urban areas and, due to their lack of shelter, are at increased risk from extreme temperatures and weather events, outdoor air pollution, and vector-borne illnesses, such as West Nile virus.[68]

ADAPTATION STRATEGIES

Considering that LMICs and susceptible groups are more vulnerable to the adverse health effects of climate change, policies promoting adaptation and mitigation strategies should be implemented. Adaptation refers to actions taken by individuals, communities, and governments to lessen or protect against the impacts of climate change. On the other hand, mitigation refers to actions taken by individuals, communities, and governments to reduce or eliminate greenhouse gas emission, thereby limiting the damage from future climate change. Adaptation strategies for adverse health effects of climate change include improving access to quality health care for vulnerable populations, improving disease surveillance, improving weather forecasting, advancing emergency management, ensuring that health facilities are equipped to handle disasters, educating the public about climate change health impacts, development and dissemination of appropriate vaccines, ensuring food and water safety, and having a good vector control program.[38] Mitigation strategies for adverse health effects of climate change include using energy-efficient and renewable energy sources, reducing deforestation, reforestation, and development of greenhouse gas capture and greenhouse gas sequestration technologies.[33,69]

Aside from individual and community adaptation strategies for dealing with the effects of climate change, primary care providers and primary health systems must be prepared to respond to climate-related shifts in both the short term and long term. Great variability exists in the response and adaptation abilities of primary care systems across the globe.[70] Communities in the United States and abroad need functional adaptation assessments prior to climactic events to determine readiness to respond and react to climate change.[70,71] Knowing the significant impact of climate-associated changes on the health of individual patients and the larger impacts on community and population health, frontline care providers have a responsibility to advocate for climate mitigation policies to reduce greenhouse gas emissions and adaptation strategies aimed at preparing for anticipated impacts on the most vulnerable.[72] Several organizations, such as the International Society of Doctors for the Environment (http://www.isde.org/) and the Climate and Health Council (http://www.climateandhealth.org/), are currently engaged in linking primary care providers with climate change policy activism.

Educating Patients About Impact of Climate Change and Ways to Make a Difference

Because patient with underlying chronic diseases like COPD and asthma are more likely to be impacted by climate change, primary care providers have a vital role to

Table 1
Impact of climate change

Type	Effect
Health	1. Increasing burden of disease from malnutrition (as a result of drought and flooding)[41]
	2. Increasing burden of disease from diarrheal diseases (as a result of drought and flooding)[41]
	3. Increase mortality and morbidity from cardiovascular diseases and respiratory diseases (as a result of heat waves, fluctuations in weather, and air pollution)
	4. Increasing burden of disease from vector-borne diseases (as a result of drought, flooding, and increased or decreased precipitation causing change in distribution of some disease vectors)
Shelter	1. Loss of coastal wetlands (as a result of flooding and storms),[41] which means people who live in coastal communities are less protected from adverse events, such as storms
	2. Forced migration (as a result of flooding, drought, and hurricanes)
Food	1. Decline in crop yields and livestock productivity (as a result of drought and flooding)
	2. Reduction in fish supply (as a result of warming of ocean bodies)
Water	1. Increased water stress, especially in arid and semiarid areas (as a result of drought)[44]
	2. Decrease in availability of safe water (as a result of flooding, rise in sea level, and increase in water temperature, which can cause alga blooms and increase bacteria population in water)[44]

play in informing patients about the impact of climate change on their health. **Table 1** lists and discusses the direct health impacts of climate change.

People can make a difference in slowing climate change by adopting environmental-friendly practices. These include improving home energy efficiency by properly insulating homes; using energy-efficient appliances and recycling; using renewable energy sources when feasible, such as photovoltaic solar panels for electricity and compressed natural gas for automobiles; where possible, walking, cycling, using mass transit, or using energy-efficient cars; using a carbon footprint calculator, which is an online tool found on Web sites, such as the Environmental Protection Agency (https://www3.epa.gov/carbon-footprint-calculator/EPA), to estimate household carbon print to identify areas of improvement; and joining an advocacy group, such as Sierra Club, Greenpeace, or Citizens Climate Lobby, to provide opportunity to learn more about the impact of climate change and also be able to advocate for a change.[5,6,38]

SUMMARY

Primary care providers can act as critical advocates for the populations they serve by promoting climate change mitigation and adaptation strategies to optimize the health spans of patients. As frontline providers, primary care providers are critical informants for policymakers, public health researchers, and patients on the emerging health impacts of climate change. In addition to emergency preparedness in the face of increasing climate-related events, primary care providers must be aware of increased risks to marginalized patients related to both extreme weather and vector-borne illnesses and of mental health and environmental impacts on chronic disease management. By educating emerging health care providers as well as patients about this great threat to public health, primary care providers can increase the resilience of the patients they care for in the face of increasing pressure from climate-related changes.

REFERENCES

1. IPCC. Climate change 2007: Synthesis report. Contribution of working groups I, II and III to the fourth assessment report of the intergovernmental panel on climate change. 2007. Available at: http://www.ipcc.ch/publications_and_data/ar4/syr/en/contents.html. Accessed March 6, 2016.
2. Lim V, Stubbs JW, Nahar N, et al. Politicians must heed health effects of climate change. Lancet 2009;374:973.
3. Bernstein AS, Rice MB. Lungs in a warming world climate change and respiratory health. Chest 2013;143:1455–9.
4. Patz JA. Climate change. In: Frumkin H, editor. Environmental health. San Francisco (CA): Josey-Bass; 2005. p. 238–68.
5. Shuman EK. Global climate change and infectious diseases. Int J Occup Environ Med 2011;2:11–20.
6. Holdstock D. Environmental health: threats and their interactions. Environ Health Insights 2008;2:117–22.
7. Environmental Protection Agency. Climate change. 2010. Available at: www.epa.gov/climatechange. Accessed February 9, 2016.
8. Masozera M, Bailey M, Kerchner C. Distribution of impacts of natural disasters across income groups: a case study of New Orleans. Ecol Econ 2007;63:299–306.
9. Bohle HG, Downing TE, Watts MJ. Climate change and social vulnerability: the sociology and geography of food insecurity. Global Environ Change 1994;4:37–48.

10. Fothergill A, Maestas E, Darlington J. Race, ethnicity and disasters in the United States: a review of the literature. Disasters 1999;23:156–73.
11. Fothergill A, Peek L. Poverty and disasters in the United States: a review of the recent sociological findings. Nat Hazards 2004;32:89–110.
12. Keim M. Building human resilience: the role of public health preparedness and response as an adaptation to climate change. Am J Prev Med 2008;35:508–16.
13. NOAA. International report confirms: 2014 was Earth's warmest year on record. Available at: http://www.noaanews.noaa.gov/stories2015/071615-international-report-confirms-2014-was-earths-warmest-year-on-record.html. Accessed March 6, 2016.
14. Guo Y, Gasparrini A, Armstrong B, et al. Global variation in the effects of ambient temperature on mortality: a systematic evaluation. Epidemiology 2014;25:781–9.
15. The Eurowinter Group. Cold exposure and winter mortality from ischemic heart disease, cerebrovascular disease, respiratory disease, and all causes in warm and cold regions of Europe. Lancet 1997;349:1341–6.
16. Lloyd EL. The role of cold in ischaemic heart disease: a review. Public Health 1991;105:205–15.
17. Pozos RS, Danzl DF. Human physiological responses to cold stress and hypothermia. In: Pandolf KB, Burr RE, editors. Medical aspects of harsh environments. Washington, DC: Borden Institute; 2001. p. 351–82.
18. Barnett A, Dobson A, McElduff P, et al. Cold periods and coronary events: an analysis of populations worldwide. J Epidemiol Community Health 2005;59: 551–7.
19. Liu C, Yavar Z, Sun Q. Cardiovascular response to thermoregulatory challenges. Am J Physiol Heart Circ Physiol 2015;309(11):H1793–812.
20. Kravchenko J, Abernethy AP, Fawzy M, et al. Minimization of heatwave morbidity and mortality. Am J Prev Med 2013;44:274–82.
21. Hotez PJ. Neglected diseases and poverty in "The Other America": the greatest health disparity in the United States? PLoS Negl Trop Dis 2007;1:e159.
22. Gubler DJ, Reiter P, Ebi KL, et al. Climate variability and change in the United States: potential impacts on vector- and rodent-borne diseases. Environ Health Perspect 2001;109(Suppl 2):223–33.
23. Monaghan AJ, Moore SM, Sampson KM, et al. Climate change influences on the annual onset of Lyme disease in the United States. Ticks Tick Borne Dis 2015; 6(5):615–22.
24. Padhy SK, Sarkar S, Panigrahi M, et al. Mental health effects of climate change. Indian J Occup Environ Med 2015;19:3–7.
25. DeSalvo KB, Hyre AD, Ompad DC, et al. Symptoms of posttraumatic stress disorder in a New Orleans workforce following Hurricane Katrina. J Urban Health 2007;84:142–52.
26. McMillen C, North C, Mosley M, et al. Untangling the psychiatric comorbidity of posttraumatic stress disorder in a sample of flood survivors. Compr Psychiatry 2002;43:478–85.
27. Norris FH, Murphy AD, Baker CK, et al. Postdisaster PTSD over four waves of a panel study of Mexico's 1999 flood. J Trauma Stress 2004;17:283–92.
28. Berry HL, Bowen K, Kjellstrom T. Climate change and mental health: a causal pathways framework. Int J Public Health 2010;55:123–32.
29. Mares D. Climate change and levels of violence in socially disadvantaged neighborhood groups. J Urban Health 2013;90:768–83.
30. Levy BS, Sidel VW. Collective violence caused by climate change and how it threatens health and human rights. Health Hum Rights 2014;16:32–40.

31. Hsiang SM, Burke M. Climate, conflict, and social stability: what does the evidence say? Climatic Change 2014;123:39–55.
32. Haines A. Redefining security. 1992. Med Confl Surviv 2009;25:282–5.
33. De Silva MJ, McKenzie K, Harpham T, et al. Social capital and mental illness: a systematic review. J Epidemiol Community Health 2005;59:619–27.
34. Whitley R, McKenzie K. Social capital and psychiatry: review of the literature. Harv Rev Psychiatry 2005;13:71–84.
35. Uphoff EP, Pickett KE, Cabieses B, et al. A systematic review of the relationships between social capital and socioeconomic inequalities in health: a contribution to understanding the psychosocial pathway of health inequalities. Int J Equity Health 2013;12:54.
36. Stevenson TJ, Visser ME, Arnold W, et al. Disrupted seasonal biology impacts health, food security and ecosystems. Proc Biol Sci 2015;282:20151453.
37. Bloem MW, Semba RD, Kraemer K. Castel Gandolfo Workshop: an introduction to the impact of climate change, the economic crisis, and the increase in the food prices on malnutrition. J Nutr 2010;140:132.
38. Kiang K, Graham S, Farrant B. Climate change, child health and the role of the paediatric profession in under-resourced settings. Trop Med Int Health 2013; 18:1053–6.
39. Ebi KL, Sussman FG, Wilbanks TJ. In: Gamble JL, editor. CCSP: Effects of Global Change on Human Health, in Analyses of the effects of global change on human health and welfare and human systems. A report by the U.S. climate change science program and the subcommittee on global change research. Washington, DC: US Environmental Protection Agency; 2008. p. 39–87.
40. National Research Council. Advancing the science of climate change. Washington, DC: National Research Council. The National Academies Press; 2010.
41. Wilbanks TJ, Lankao PR, Bao M, et al. Industry, settlement and society. In: Parry ML, Canziani OF, Palutikof JP, et al, editors. Climate Change 2007: impacts, adaptation and vulnerability. contribution of working group II to the fourth assessment report of the intergovernmental panel on climate change. Cambridge (United Kingdom): Cambridge University Press; 2007. p. 357–90.
42. Bunyavanich S, Landrigan CP, McMichael AJ, et al. The impact of climate change on child health. Ambul Pediatr 2003;3:44–52.
43. McMichael AJ, Woodruff RE, Hales S. Climate change and human health: Present and future risks. Lancet 2006;367:859–69.
44. Patz J, Gibbs H, Foley JA, et al. Climate change and global health: Quantifying a growing ethical crisis. EcoHealth 2007;4:397–405.
45. DARA. Climate Vulnerable Forum. Climate vulnerability monitor. A guide to the cold calculus of a hot planet. 2nd edition. Madrid (Spain): Estudis Graficos Europeos, S.A.; 2012.
46. Mireku N, Wang Y, Ager J, et al. Changes in weather and the effects on pediatric asthma exacerbations. Ann Allergy Asthma Immunol 2009;103:220–4.
47. Moore K, Neugebauer R, Lurmann F, et al. Ambient ozone concentrations cause increased hospitalizations for asthma in children: an 18-year study in Southern California. Environ Health Perspect 2008;116:1063–70.
48. Glad JA, Brink LL, Talbott EO, et al. The relationship of ambient ozone and PM(2.5) levels and asthma emergency department visits: Possible influence of gender and ethnicity. Arch Environ Occup Health 2012;67:103–8.
49. Babin S, Burkom H, Holtry R, et al. Medicaid patient asthma-related acute care visits and their associations with ozone and particulates in Washington, DC, from 1994-2005. Int J Environ Health Res 2008;18:209–21.

50. Meng YY, Wilhelm M, Rull RP, et al. Traffic and outdoor air pollution levels near residences and poorly controlled asthma in adults. Ann Allergy Asthma Immunol 2007;98:455–63.
51. Chan CC, Wu TH. Effects of ambient ozone exposure on mail carriers' peak expiratory flow rates. Environ Health Perspect 2005;113:735–8.
52. Chen PC, Lai YM, Chan CC, et al. Short-term effect of ozone on the pulmonary function of children in primary school. Environ Health Perspect 1999;107: 921–5.
53. Lin S, Luo M, Walker RJ, et al. Extreme high temperatures and hospital admissions for respiratory and cardiovascular diseases. Epidemiology 2009;20: 738–46.
54. Zanobetti A, O'Neill MS, Gronlund CJ, et al. Summer temperature variability and long-term survival among elderly people with chronic disease. Proc Natl Acad Sci U S A 2012;109:6608–13.
55. Balbus JM, Malina C. Identifying vulnerable subpopulations for climate change health effects in the United States. J Occup Environ Med 2009;51:33–7.
56. Kim KH, Kabir E, Ara Jahan S. A review of the consequences of global climate change on human health. J Environ Sci Health C Environ Carcinog Ecotoxicol Rev 2014;32:299–318.
57. Gutierrez KS, LePrevost CE. Climate justice in rural Southeastern United States: a review of climate change impacts and effects on human health. Int J Environ Res Public Health 2016;13(2):189.
58. Carter LM, Jones JW, Berry L, et al. In: Melillo JM, Richmond TC, Yohe GW, editors. Southeast and the Caribbean. Climate change impacts in the United States: the third national climate assessment. U.S. Global Change Research Program; 2014. p. 396–417. Ch. 17.
59. Sheridan SC, Kalkstein AJ, Kalkstein LS. Trends in heat-related mortality in the United States, 1975–2004. Nat Hazards 2009;50:145–60.
60. Sun G. Impacts of climate change and variability on water resources in the Southeast USA. In: Ingram KT, Dow K, Carter L, et al, editors. Climate of the Southeast United States. Washington, DC: Springer; 2013. p. 210–36.
61. Portier CJ, Tart KT, Carter SR, et al. A human health perspective on climate change; environmental health perspectives and the national institute of environmental health sciences. Washington, DC: Environmental Health Perspectives and the National Institute of Environmental Health Sciences; 2010.
62. Roelofs C, Wegman DH. Workers: the "climate canaries"?. In: Levy BS, Patz JA, editors. Climate change and public health. New York: Oxford University Press; 2015. p. 18–9.
63. Lundgren K, Kuklane K, Gao C, et al. Effects of heat stress on working populations when facing climate change. Ind Health 2013;51:3–15.
64. Hwang SW. Homelessness and health. Can Med Assoc J 2001;164:229–33.
65. Lee TC, Hanlon JG, Ben-David J, et al. Risk factors for cardiovascular disease in homeless adults. Circulation 2005;111:2629–35.
66. Raoult D, Foucault C, Brouqi P. Infections in the homeless. Lancet Infect Dis 2001; 1:77–84.
67. North CS, Eyrich KM, Pollio D, et al. Are rates of psychiatric disorders in the homeless population changing? Am J Public Health 2004;94:103–8.
68. Ramin B, Svoboda T. Health of the homeless and climate change. J Urban Health 2009;86:654–64.
69. Shea KM. Global climate change and children's health. Pediatrics 2007;120: 1359–67.

70. Van Minh H, Tuan Anh T, Rocklöv J, et al. Primary healthcare system capacities for responding to storm and flood-related health problems: a case study from a rural district in central Vietnam. Glob Health Action 2014;7:23007.
71. Ebi KL, Schmier JK. A stitch in time: improving public health early warning systems for extreme weather events. Epidemiol Rev 2005;27:115–21.
72. Patz JA, Grabow ML, Limaye VS. When it rains, it pours: future climate extremes and health. Ann Glob Health 2014;80:332–44.

Geriatric Care Issues
An American and an International Perspective

Mohamad A. Sidani, MD, MS*, Brian C. Reed, MD,
Jeffrey Steinbauer, MD

KEYWORDS

- Elderly • Geriatric • Underserved • Falls • Elder abuse • Polypharmacy • Caregiver
- Alcohol use

KEY POINTS

- As the global population ages, there is an opportunity to benefit from the increased longevity of a healthy older adult population.
- Healthy older individuals often contribute financially to younger generations by offering financial assistance, paying more in taxes than benefits received, and providing unpaid childcare and voluntary work.
- Governments must work to create policies that sufficiently address the challenges of income insecurity, adequate access to health care, social isolation, and neglect that currently face elderly adults in many countries across the globe.
- A reduction in disparities in these areas can lead to better health outcomes and allow societies to benefit from longer, healthier lives of their citizens.

INTRODUCTION

The global population is aging rapidly in all regions of the world. The number of older adults (65 years of age and older) will double during the next 25 years to about 72 million, and will comprise 20% of the US population in 2030.[1] The proportion of the world's older adults will double from 12% (900 million) in 2015 to 22% (2 billion) in 2050.[2] In 2013, 21.2% of older adults were members of racial or ethnic minority populations (8.6% African American, 3.9% Asian or Pacific Islander, 0.5% Native American, 0.1% Native Hawaiian/Pacific Islander, and 7.5% Hispanic).[3] Globally, 1.3% of the population is more than 80 years old and the rate of growth among this segment is very rapid. People are living longer as a result of improved sanitation, nutrition, advances in health care, and education. Life expectancy at birth exceeds 80 years in 33 countries.[4]

This article originally appeared in Primary Care: Clinics in Office Practice, Volume 44, Issue 1, March 2017.
Disclosure: The authors have nothing to disclose.
Department of Family and Community Medicine, Baylor College of Medicine, Houston, TX, USA
* Corresponding author. Department of Family and Community Medicine, Baylor College of Medicine, 3701 Kirby Drive, Suite 600, Houston, TX 77098.
E-mail address: masidani@bcm.edu

Societal concerns about income security among older adults, access to quality health care, and the provision of physical environments that foster active aging accompany the shifting demographics of the world's population. Most countries lack a comprehensive safety net that can provide for the economic and social well-being of elderly people once they exit the workforce. Accordingly, a significant proportion of the world's population of older adults is vulnerable to poverty, food insecurity, inadequate health care, and other societal challenges.[4]

LIVING AND FINANCIAL SITUATIONS OF OLDER ADULTS

In 2013, the median income of older adults was $29,327 for men and $16,301 for women.[3] The prevalence of poverty (income below the poverty line) in older adults is 9.5%, ranging from 4.7% in married persons to 19.8% in minorities.[5] In 2013, 84% of older adults receive Social Security income; this constituted 90% or more of income for 21% of aged beneficiary couples and 46% of aged nonmarried beneficiaries.[5] Among the geriatric population, approximately 28% of Hispanic and 22% of African American people lived in poverty.[6]

The world's older individuals often live in poverty because of a lack of pension benefits and a reduced capacity to work and earn wages. The United Nations estimates that even higher percentages of older adults live in poverty in sub-Saharan Africa and Latin America. For example, an estimated 40% of the population aged more than 60 years in El Salvador, the Dominican Republic, Guatemala, Honduras, and Paraguay live in poverty. Several European countries have high rates of poverty among individuals more than 65 years of age as well. In Latvia, Cyprus, and Estonia, poverty affects 39% to 51% of the population more than 65 years old.[4]

In poorer countries, major health care expenses become a financial burden for the entire family and can cause a financial setback that requires several years to overcome. These financial hardships create challenges for access to care and have led to health care disparities in the prevalence of disabilities and health outcomes for patients with chronic disease between industrialized countries and developing countries. For example, the prevalence of significant visual impairment among elderly adults living in developing countries is almost 3 times higher compared with older adults who live in the developed world. Similarly, adults living in developing countries with chronic lung disease or who have had a stroke live shorter lives compared with adults with similar health conditions in more developed countries.[4]

Among health care costs for older Americans, 95% are for chronic diseases. The cost of providing health care for 1 person aged 65 years or older is 3 to 5 times higher than the cost for someone younger than 65 years.[7] By 2030, health care spending will increase by 25%[8] largely because the population will be older. Medicare spending is projected to increase from $555 billion in 2011 to $903 billion in 2020.[3] In 2013, older adults spent an average of $5069 (compared with $3631 for all population) out of pocket on health care (66% for insurance, 16% for medical services, 14% for drugs, and 4.0% for medical supplies).[3]

In 2013, only 3.4% of older adults in the United States (1.5 million) lived in institutional settings (1.3 million in nursing homes, with almost half aged 85 years and older). The percentage increases from 1% for persons 65 to 74 years of age, to 3% for persons 75 to 84 years of age, and up to 10% for persons 85 years of age and older.[3] In 2014, 57% of noninstitutionalized older adults lived with their spouses and this percentage decreases with age. Twenty-eight percent lived alone and this percentage increases with age. Eighty-one percent were owners and 19% were renters.[3]

MORTALITY AND MORBIDITY/CHRONIC CONDITIONS IN ELDERLY

Life expectancy at 65 years of age averages 19.3 years for both genders (17.9 years for men and 20.5 years for women). In 2013, the 5 most common causes of death in the elderly were heart disease, cancer, chronic lower respiratory disease, cerebrovascular disease, and Alzheimer disease (AD).[9]

The prevalence of diabetes mellitus among older adults in the United States was estimated to be 26.7% (5.5% undiagnosed and 21.2% diagnosed by a physician) in 2014.[8] Hypertension was estimated at 61.7% among men 65 to 74 years of age; 66.7% among men 75 years of age and older; 75.1% among women 65 to 74 years of age; and 79.3% among women 75 years of age and older. Uncontrolled hypertension was estimated at 36.9% among men 65 to 74 years of age; 45.4% among men 75 years of age and older; 48.9% among women 65 to 74 years of age; and 57.8% among women 75 years of age and older.[9]

Stroke in older adults accounts for nearly three-quarters of all strokes. After the age of 55 years, the risk of stroke more than doubles with each decade of life. Stroke is the number 1 cause of serious disability in the United States; it reduces mobility in more than half of stroke survivors 65 years of age and older.[10] The incidence of stroke has been decreasing in the United States, Europe, New Zealand, Western Australia, and Japan. The decrease in rates varies with age groups, from no significant decrease in younger persons (aged <65 years) to a significant decrease in older adults.[11,12] Statins have been proved to decrease the incidence of stroke in older adults.[13]

Among older adults, the prevalence of doctor-diagnosed arthritis was estimated at 49.7% and of arthritis-attributable activity limitation at 44.45% between the years 2010 to 2012.[14] Osteoarthritis is the most common type of arthritis among older adults.[15] Fifty percent of older adults with arthritis, compared with 23% of those without arthritis, need assistance with activities of daily living (ADLs). Older adults with arthritis are likely to be living in nursing homes. They are more likely to use prescription drugs (94%), social worker service, adult day care, rehabilitation, transportation, and meals on wheels.[16]

Around 36% of community older adults reported some type of disability in 2013 (vision difficulty, 7%; self-care difficulty, 9%; cognitive difficulty, 9%; hearing difficulty, 15%; and ambulatory difficulty, 23%). In 2012, 33% of noninstitutionalized Medicare beneficiaries reported difficulty with ADLs and 12% reported difficulty with instrumental ADLs (IADLs). By contrast, 96% of institutionalized beneficiaries had difficulties with ADLs and 83% had difficulty with IADLs.[3]

QUALITY-OF-LIFE ISSUES IN UNDERSERVED OLDER ADULTS

Health-related quality of life (HRQOL) is the general well-being of individuals and its relationship with health. One of the proposed definitions of HRQOL is the state of well-being, which is a composite of 2 components: the ability to perform everyday activities that reflect physical, psychological, and social well-being; and patient satisfaction with levels of functioning and control of the disease.[17] HRQOL is subjective and is challenging to measure. Household income and educational attainment have positive relationship with HRQOL in the United States, but not in Canada. This difference was attributed in part to the guaranteed comprehensive universal coverage in the nonelderly population in Canada and not in the United States.[18]

Federal Government agencies are improving the quality of life for older adults by implementing programs that address chronic illnesses. Many of these programs target minorities and underserved populations.[19] Most older adults want to remain in their communities as long as possible. However, when they acquire disabilities, often there is not enough support available to help them. States that invest in such services show lower rates of growth in long-term care expenditures (see www.healthypeople.gov). Early prevention and physical activity can help prevent such declines.[19] Exercise can improve body composition, decrease falls, increase strength, reduce depression, reduce arthritis pain, reduce risks for diabetes and coronary artery disease, and improve longevity. However, less than 20% of older adults engage in enough physical activity, and fewer do routine strength training.[20]

EPIDEMIOLOGY OF PROBLEMS FACED DISPROPORTIONATELY BY THE ELDERLY

There are fairly wide variations in the percentage of people more than 60 years of age across the various regions of the world[4] (Table 1).

Financial insecurity, poor health, injuries, neglect, ageism, and abuse are common challenges faced by elderly individuals across the world. Social exclusion compounds the problem of poverty among older adults. Data from the United Nations Human Development Reports reveals that prevalence of social exclusion tends to be higher in Europe and central Asia. The combination of poverty and social exclusion make the geriatric population more vulnerable to abuse, neglect, and declines in overall health.

An estimated 46% of the population aged 60 years or older has disabilities and more than 250 million people in the world have severe disabilities. In addition to osteoarthritis, there is a high prevalence of visual impairment, hearing impairment, and dementia among elderly adults. The prevalence of disability increases with age in both developed and developing countries. These disabilities affect the ability to perform ADLs, reduce independence, and can worsen social isolation among elderly adults[4] (Table 2).

Elder abuse is a global problem as well. The World Health Organization (WHO) estimates that 4% to 6% of older adults in wealthy countries have experienced some form of elder abuse at home. For example, in Europe, an estimated 4 million people aged 60 years and older experience physical abuse, 1 million experience sexual abuse, 29 million experience psychological abuse, and 6 million experience financial abuse. In 2012, a study in India of 5600 elderly adults revealed that approximately 31% had experienced abuse.[21]

ALCOHOL AND DRUG ABUSE

Substance abuse is not common in the geriatric population, but has been increasing over the past 10 years. This increase may have been caused by the lifestyle choices of

Table 1	
Distribution of older adults around the world	
Individuals Aged More Than 60 y (%)	**Region of the World**
6	Africa
10	Latin America and the Caribbean
11	Asia
15	Oceania/South Pacific
19	North America
22	Europe

Data from UNFPA and HelpAge. 2012. Ageing in the twenty-first century: a celebration and a challenge. Available at: http://www.unfpa.org/publications/ageing-twenty-first-century. Accessed March 9, 2016.

Table 2
Number of older adults with chronic conditions in developed and developing countries

Health Condition	Developed Countries (Millions)	Developing Countries (Millions)
Visual impairment	15.0	94.2
Hearing loss	18.5	43.9
Osteoarthritis	8.1	19.4
Ischemic heart disease	2.2	11.9
Dementia	6.2	7.0
Chronic obstructive pulmonary disease	4.8	8.0
Cerebrovascular disease	2.2	4.9
Depression	0.5	4.8
Rheumatoid arthritis	1.7	3.7

Data from UNFPA and HelpAge. (2012) Ageing in the twenty-first century: a celebration and a challenge. Available at: http://www.unfpa.org/publications/ageing-twenty-first-century. Accessed March 9, 2016.

older patients when they were young adults or/and by the greater availability of addictive substances both through illicit access on the street and prescriptions (eg, opioids).[22-24]

Forty-three percent of older adults reported using alcohol during past year and 6.7% of those reported alcohol abuse, dependence, or dependence symptoms.[25] Alcohol and substance abuse are higher among some underserved populations (eg, homeless). However, precise data on the prevalence and incidence of the problem in underserved groups is lacking. The lifetime prevalence of alcohol abuse and dependence in older adults has been stable at about 3% to 4%. Prevalence varies among older patients, with 5% to 10% in those presenting to outpatient clinics, 7% to 22% among medical inpatients, and 10% to 15% among patients presenting to emergency rooms.[26] Adults older than 75 years have a lower incidence, whereas peak incidence in the older age group is the group aged 65 to 75 years. Being divorced or widowed, white, and male had the highest lifetime risk.

The National Institute on Alcohol Abuse and Alcoholism recommends that people more than 65 years of age should have no more than 7 drinks a week and no more than 3 drinks on any 1 day.[27] Studies have shown varying negative effects on ADLs and IADLs in older people who are heavy drinkers.[22] Chronic alcohol use makes hypertension, diabetes, and congestive heart failure (CHF) worse. It increases the likelihood of falling, and precipitates periods of delirium during withdrawal. Stomach ulcers, pancreatitis, cardiomyopathy, and liver failure are all known complications in younger people and older drinkers are susceptible to these complications.

Alcohol abuse in the elderly is often missed in the primary care physician's office. It is hard to recognize alcoholism in the context of an older patient who has many concurrent illnesses. Older alcoholics tend to present with vague geriatric syndromes of self-neglect, contusions, malnutrition, depression, falls, incontinence, diarrhea, and apparent.[24,28] Physicians may have a bias against asking about alcohol and drug use in the elderly, or may not believe that an elderly person might be a drunk. Interactions between alcohol and other medications may make recognition more difficult.[29] One study found that physicians identified only about one-third of the elderly alcoholics, compared with nearly two-thirds of the younger alcoholics.[29]

Most screening tests for alcohol use have been validated and tested on younger patients. Self-report tests may be misleading, especially if the patient has some degree of dementia. Thus, getting information from a family member or someone who lives with the patient may be the best approach. Because of complex, competing needs during brief office visits with older patients, primary care clinicians may struggle with adequately screening older patients for alcohol abuse. There are many screening tools, including the CAGE (http://www.cdc.gov/ncbddd/fasd/documents/alcoholsbiimplementationguide.pdf); the Short Michigan Alcohol Screening Test–Geriatric (SMAST-G; http://sbirt.vermont.gov/wordpress/wp-content/uploads/2014/04/SMAST-G-1.pdf), Alcohol Use Disorders Identification Test (AUDIT and AUDIT C; http://www.cdc.gov/ncbddd/fasd/documents/alcoholsbiimplementationguide.pdf); and the Alcohol-Related Problems Survey (ARPS; http://www.public-health.uiowa.edu/icmha/outreach/documents/AlcoholUseSurveyforOlderAdults.pdf). Physicians may use an elder-specific screening instrument, such as the SMAST-G, to identify problem drinking or dependence and/or the ARPS to identify hazardous or harmful drinking.[30] However, the main component in successful identification remains a high index of suspicion on the part of physicians.

Illicit drug use is more prevalent among older adults in the United States than in any other country in the world. Cannabis is the most commonly reported illicit drug used in older adults. Prescription drug use may also be a problem. Benzodiazepines are the most commonly prescribed psychiatric medication among all adults. Despite contraindications for use with older adults, they are widely prescribed and are disproportionately prescribed to older adults.[31] Benzodiazepines, opiate analgesics, and some skeletal muscle relaxants may result in physical dependence; however, tolerance, withdrawal syndrome, and dose escalation may be less common in older patients. Screening instruments for prescription drug abuse have not been validated in the geriatric population,[32] which increases the possibility of interactions between alcohol/drugs and prescription medications. Individuals on a low fixed income may not have the funds for discretionary or luxury expenses and may spend money at the neglect of more basic needs, such as adequate food or medication.

INJURY PREVENTION (FALLS)

Around 30% to 40% of community-dwelling adults 65 years of age and older fall annually. About half of these falls result in an injury and 10% of injuries are classified as serious (fractures). Falls threaten independence because of injury and fear of falling. Of those who sustain a fall, 35% to 40% develop a fear of falling, which further limits activities. It is estimated that the annual cost of treating fall-related injuries and disability in the United States is in excess of $30 billion.[33] The costs of care increase dramatically when a patient has an injury that requires hospitalization. In addition, mortality is increased among those who fall repeatedly and/or require hospitalization for their injuries.[34] Older adults with lower income face an increased risk of falls.[35] The WHO, in its global report on falls prevention, reports that older adults who live alone or in rural areas are at increased risk of falls.[36]

Intrinsic (causes within the patient) and extrinsic causes are one way to characterize the causes of falls (**Table 3**).Thus, evaluation of falls and fall risk should include assessment of the intrinsic and extrinsic causes.[33] Elderly patients who have recently incurred a fracture after a fall should be considered at high risk for repeated falls and injury. More than 50% of people who have had a fracture with a fall have another fall within 6 months.[37]

Evaluation of falls includes a detailed history about the current fall and previous falls; review of all medications; physical examination to include blood pressure

Table 3 Causes of falls	
Intrinsic causes	Age-related changes in blood pressure; proprioception and muscle strength Cognitive deficits; changes in vision Chronic health conditions (diabetes, CHF) Acute illness
Extrinsic causes	Medications (eg, sedatives, psychotropic, antihypertensive, diuretics) Footwear Assistive devices Home features (throw rugs, furniture clutter) Alcohol and drugs

Data from Phelan EA, Mahoney JE, Voit JC, et al. Assessment and management of fall risk in primary care settings. Med Clin North Am 2015;99(2):281–93.

measurement, visual acuity, heart examination, neurologic examination, joint examination, and check for orthostatic hypotension; and gait evaluation.[33] Medications, especially blood pressure and psychoactive medications, are associated with an increased risk of falling.[33,38]

The American Geriatrics Society (AGS) and British Geriatrics Society guideline recommends to screen older adults for risk of fall annually. Any patient who has fallen 2 or more times in the past year, or required medical care from a fall, or who has fallen 1 time but has gait abnormalities should be further evaluated. Any patient with a history of only 1 fall in the previous year without injury and without gait or balance problems does not warrant further assessment beyond continued annual fall risk screening.[39] The 3 quick gait, strength, and balance tests that are used frequently are the Timed Up-and-Go, the 30-Second Chair Stand test, and the 4-Stage Balance test (http://www.cdc.gov/steadi/materials.html).

For inpatients, the Morse fall scale (http://www.ahrq.gov/professionals/systems/hospital/fallpxtoolkit/fallpxtk-tool3h.html) has a high sensitivity, but the Stratify test (http://www.ahrq.gov/professionals/systems/hospital/fallpxtoolkit/fallpxtk-tool3g.html) has better specificity.[37] An automated system of extracting data from electronic health records showed sensitivity and predictive value at least as good as the standard paper assessment.[40] The Agency for Healthcare Research and Quality has developed a program to assist with evaluation, project planning, intervention, and outcome measurement to prevent falls in hospitalized patients.[41] An ambulatory accelerometer to measure gait variation and axis deviation while walking was found to be effective in identifying patients who were at risk for falls.[42]

Clinical assessment by a health care provider combined with individualized treatment of identified risk factors, referral if needed, and follow-up have been found to reduce the rate of falls by 24%. Vitamin D supplementation was not found to reduce falls but may be effective in people who have low vitamin D levels before treatment.[43] The US Preventive Services Task Force recommends that vitamin D supplementation is effective in preventing falls in community-dwelling adults aged 65 years or older who are at increased risk for falls.[44] Higher monthly doses of vitamin D supplementation (>24,000 units per month) were found to be more effective in increasing the 25-hydroxyvitamin D level to 30 ng/mL, but had no benefit on lower extremity function and were associated with increased risk of falls.[45] A Cochrane Review found that exercise for patients who have fallen reduces the fear of falling.[46] Exercise programs that include exercises that challenge balance, use a higher dose of exercise (>50 hours, which equates to 2 hours weekly for 25 weeks), and do not include walking were found to be more effective than others.[47] Cognitive impairment increases the risk of falling and thus all patients with dementia should still be evaluated for balance and safe gait. Exercise has been found to reduce fall risk in those with cognitive impairment.[48]

The risk of falls and resultant injuries in the hospital setting can be reduced by using the Acute Care for Elders (ACE) model of care. Using ACE principles resulted in injury reduction, shorter stays, lower costs, less delirium, and more home discharges.[49,50]

COGNITIVE IMPAIRMENT

Lower socioeconomic status (SES) is associated with lower cognitive functioning in older adults.[51–55] Each year, 7.7 million new cases of dementia are diagnosed worldwide. It is estimated that 47.5 million people have dementia worldwide, and 58% of them live in low-income and middle-income countries. The total number of people with dementia is projected to be 75.6 million in 2030 and 135.5 million in 2050. Much of this increase is attributable to the increasing numbers of people with dementia living in low-income and middle-income countries.[56] The incidence of dementia doubles every 10 years after age 60 years.[57] There is very little sex difference in incidence and prevalence of dementia, although by absolute numbers there are more women than men with the disease, particularly in patients more than 85 years of age, because of differences in life expectancy.[2] Low educational achievement is associated with a higher incidence of AD irrespective of the SES.[58]

In 2013, the American Psychiatric Association renamed dementia as a major neurocognitive disorder.[59] Many physicians use standardized mental status scales to document the presence and progression of dementia. The Montreal Cognitive Assessment (MoCA) and the Mini-Mental State Examination (MMSE) are the two most commonly used scales.[60] The MoCA is freely accessible online and in several languages at www.mocatest.org.

AD is a neurodegenerative disorder of uncertain cause and pathogenesis that primarily affects older adults and is the most common cause of dementia in the elderly, accounting for 60% to 80% of cases.[61] There were 5.2 million older adults with AD in 2012. This number is expected to reach 6.7 million by the year 2025.[62,63] Criteria for the diagnosis of probable AD dementia have been established by the National Institute on Aging and the Alzheimer's Association and most recently updated in 2011. One of the core criteria to differentiate from other dementias is the insidious onset.[64]

A detailed clinical assessment (detailed cognitive and neurologic examination) provides reasonable diagnostic accuracy for AD in most patients.[64] Brain imaging, preferably with MRI, is indicated in the evaluation of patients with suspected AD.[65] AD continues to progress as long as the patient is living. Several studies have found that patients decline 3 to 3.5 points on average on the MMSE each year.[66] Around 10% have a rapid decline of 5 to 6 points annually on MMSE.[67] The reported mean survival after diagnosis of AD ranges from 3 to 20 years, with an average life expectancy of 8 to 10 years, depending in part on how impaired the person is at the time of diagnosis.[68,69] Patients generally succumb to terminal-stage complications that relate to advanced debilitation, such as dehydration, malnutrition, and infection.

Vascular dementia is the second most common form of dementia, making up 10% to 20% of cases in North America and Europe.[70] However, it is the most frequent cause of dementia in certain countries, such as Japan and China, with AD being the second most common.[71] Dementia with Lewy bodies (DLB) accounts for 4% to 30% of dementia cases.[72] It is associated with higher rates of morbidity, mortality, caregiver stress, and a poorer quality of life than AD. Pathologically, DLB is characterized by the abnormal presence of protein aggregates (inclusion bodies/Lewy bodies) inside nerve cells.[73] Patients have early visuospatial problems, executive dysfunction with prominent attentional impairment, and less impaired episodic memory than in AD. Core clinical features include recurrent detailed visual hallucinations, cognitive fluctuation, parkinsonism, rapid eye movement sleep behavior disorder, autonomic dysfunction, and recurrent falls.[74]

Individuals with dementia living in rural areas of China had a 3 times greater risk of mortality.[75] Low-income countries accounted for slightly less than 1% of total worldwide costs (but 14% of the prevalence), and high income countries for 89% of the costs (but 46% of the prevalence). About 70% of the global costs occurred in just 2 regions: western Europe and North America. Informal care costs account for 58% of all costs in low-income countries and 40% in high-income countries. Social care (including costs for residential and nursing home care) accounts for 50% of all costs in high-income countries and 10% in low-income countries.[76]

MEDICATION MANAGEMENT/POLYPHARMACY/HIGH-RISK MEDICATIONS

Beers and colleagues[77] first published criteria for inappropriate medication use in nursing home residents in 1991 and then the list was expanded in 1997 to involve all elderly.[78] In 2003, Fick and colleagues[79] published the first update. In 2011, the AGS assumed the responsibility of updating and maintaining the Beers Criteria and published the most recent updates in 2012 and 2015.[80] In 2015, Hanoln and colleagues[81] published a list of alternative medications for high-risk medications in the elderly. Mattison and colleagues[82] found that a computerized provider order entry with clinical decision support system decreased the number of potentially inappropriate medications as defined by a subset of Beers list medications in hospitalized older adults (11.56 before to 9.94 orders per day after; $P<.001$). It has been found that 28% of adverse drug events (ADEs) are preventable and that educational intervention can reduce the occurrence of ADEs.[83]

No consensus definition for polypharmacy is found. The most commonly cited definition is medication that does not match the diagnosis. Other definitions include the term inappropriate, many medications, 6 or more medications, duplication of medications, drug/drug interactions, and excessive duration.[84] Inappropriate medication use was present in more than 40% of older adults taking 5 or more medications.[85] Older adults with lower SES were more likely to receive a greater number of drugs, be exposed to major polypharmacy, receive potentially harmful drugs, and receive potentially interacting agents, and less likely to receive secondary prevention therapies.[86] It has been found that treatment selection by physicians varies depending on patient income.[87]

Underprescription of potentially useful drugs is widespread among older people and may herald several adverse outcomes. Underprescription was observed in 64% of outpatient older adults who were using 5 or more medications[85] and in 62.0% of patients discharged from 11 US veterans' hospitals.[88] Main factors contributing to underprescription include comorbidity, polypharmacy, fear of ADEs by physicians, and economic factors.[89] Hospitalization rates were higher among middle-aged and older adults with cardiovascular disease who reported cutting back on medication use because of cost.[90] Reducing out-of-pocket cost to patients after acute myocardial infarction was found to both improve health and save money from the societal perspective.[91]

PAIN MANAGEMENT IN THE ELDERLY

Pain lasting greater than 3 months among patients 65 years of age or older satisfies the definition of chronic geriatric pain. The prevalence of chronic geriatric pain increases with age. The cause of this condition is often increased joint pains and neu-ralgia. Chronic pain can lead to decreased ambulation, dependence in ADLs, decon-ditioning, falls, worsening of depression, and cognitive decline.

Most geriatric patients experience significant pain and it is often undertreated. Underreporting of pain is fairly common because of an incorrect assumption that pain is a routine part of aging. In some scenarios, like cancer-related pain, the pain is underreported because of fear of progression of the disease. In addition, diagnosis and treatment of chronic geriatric pain in patients with dementia can be particularly difficult.

The treatment of chronic geriatric pain begins with a thorough assessment. Because of the complexity of pain in geriatric patients, the assessment usually requires a multi-disciplinary approach in which physicians collaborate with physical therapists and behavioral therapists in their evaluation. Initial assessment of chronic geriatric pain should include a complete history and physical examination; review of location of pain, intensity (using a visual analog scale, verbal descriptor scale, or numerical rating scale), ameliorating factors, aggravating factors, impact on mood and sleep; screening for cognitive impairment; screening for depression; review of ADLs and IADLs; assessment of gait and balance; and assessment of visual and auditory acuity.

Before initiation of medical management with pharmaceutical agents, the medical personnel must consider physiologic changes such as decline in renal function, reduced hepatic clearance of medications, decreased muscle mass, increase in fat mass, and changes in the central nervous system that can affect drug distribution.[92] The American Geriatric Society considers acetaminophen as the initial treatment of chronic pain because of its effectiveness and safety profile. Nonselective nonsteroidal antiinflammatory drugs should be considered with caution because of the risk of gastrointestinal bleeding in the elderly, chance of further harm to kidney function, and possible worsening of heart failure. Most skeletal muscle relaxants, such as car-isoprodol and cyclobenzaprine, should be avoided because of excessive sedation and potential risk of falls. Tertiary tricyclic antidepressants such as amitriptyline and imip-ramine should be avoided because of the high risk of anticholinergic effects and cognitive impairment. Management of chronic geriatric pain with opioids should be considered for patients with moderate to severe pain, impaired function because of pain, and lower quality of life because of pain. Adjuvant medications, such as antide-pressants, anticonvulsants, corticosteroids, and topical agents, are also used in the management of chronic geriatric pain.

In addition to medications, psychological support and physical rehabilitation should be incorporated into the care plans of patients with chronic geriatric pain. Pain coping strategies such as relaxation and attention diversion techniques may help to reduce the amount of pain experienced by patients. Depression and anxiety should be addressed. Physical rehabilitation can help to adapt to loss of physical skills and help patients to live more independently. Interventional modalities such as nerve blocks and neuroaugmentation can help to reduce pain without the need for medica-tions and unwanted side effects.[93]

HOSPICE AND PALLIATIVE CARE

Hospice care focuses on the provision of expert medical care, pain management, emotional support, and spiritual support within the context of life-limiting illness. In 2011, there were approximately 2,513,000 deaths in the United States with 1,059,000 (46%) deaths occurring under the care of hospices. The number of patients who received hospice care in the United States increased to an estimated 1,600,000 in

2014. A review of Medicare beneficiaries reveals that there have been increases in hospice use over the last 5 years among patients with cancer and dementia. The most common diagnoses for hospice admissions are cancer (less than half of all hospice admissions), dementia, heart disease, lung disease, stroke, and end-stage renal disease.

Most hospice care is delivered at home. In 2014, most hospice patients in the United States were 65 years of age and older, with 41.1% of all hospice recipients in the United States being more than 85 years old.[94] Patients of minority race account for approximately 25% of patients who received hospice care in 2014. Studies have shown that some of the racial and ethnic disparities in hospice use may be related to health beliefs and preferences regarding aggressive end-of-life care. Hispanic people, African Americans, and other minorities tend to pursue more aggressive care at the end of life and may opt out of hospice care more often.[95]

The National Quality Forum defines palliative care as patient-centered and family-centered care that optimizes the quality of life by anticipating, preventing, and treating suffering. Ideally, palliative care is initiated at the onset of a serious life-threatening illness or chronic progressive disease. During the continuum of illness, high-quality palliative care should address the physical, emotional, social, and spiritual needs of the patient.

In the United States, most large hospitals (defined as having >300 hospital beds) have a palliative care team. Inpatient palliative consultation has been associated with higher rates of completion of advance directives and do-not-resuscitate orders among ethnic minorities in safety net hospitals.[96] However, many public safety net hospitals do not have a palliative care team. Furthermore, several studies have shown reduced availability of prescription opioids among pharmacies in predominantly ethnic minority neighborhoods.[97,98]

Lack of access to palliative care is a global problem. Many countries have limited access to pain relief and any form of palliative care. For example, older adults who live in the poorest countries have less access to opioids for the management of severe pain at the end of life.

ELDER ABUSE

Although there is no universally accepted definition of elder abuse, existing definitions are consistent with the (1985) Elder Abuse Prevention, Identification and Treatment Act, which defines abuse as "the willful infliction of injury, unreasonable confinement, intimidation or cruel punishment with resulting physical harm or pain or mental anguish or the willful deprivation by a caretaker of goods or services which are necessary to avoid physical harm, mental anguish or mental illness."

The WHO further describes elder abuse as an act of violence and a human rights violation.[99] The US National Center on Elder Abuse identifies 7 unique types of elder abuse and provides definitions for each: physical abuse, sexual abuse, financial exploitation, caregiver neglect, psychological and emotional abuse, abandonment, and self-neglect.[100,101]

The incidence of abuse in the elderly is expected to increase because of the increasing number of vulnerable adults alone. Some investigators have found that the incidence may be higher in 24-hour care facilities than at home.[102] Considering all these facts, it is estimated that 1 in 10 older adults may be a victim of abuse.[101] The prevalences of the 7 types of abuse are 1.6% for physical abuse, 0.6% for sexual abuse, 3.2% for psychological/emotional abuse, 5.2% for financial exploitation, and 5.1% for neglect.[99] It is suggested that there is a higher incidence of elder abuse among minorities and in poor countries.[101] Wolf and colleagues[103] found that areas with low-income families in Massachusetts have higher rates of elder abuse reporting than affluent areas. This difference was attributed to these families being in more frequent and direct contact with mandated reporters. The WHO reported that some cultural and socioeconomic factors may increase the risk of elder abuse: systems of inheritance that affect the distribution of power and material goods within families; migration of young couples leaving their elderly alone, in societies in which older people are cared for by their offspring; and, in cultures in which women have inferior social status, elderly women are at special risk of being abandoned and having their property seized when they are widowed.[104] Dong and colleagues[105] found that rates of hospitalization were about 2 times higher among abused seniors than for those who were not abused.

Screening tests are available, but they are lengthy and require special training.[99] Elder abuse is a complex problem that is under-recognized and underreported. Some risk factors of abuse have been identified[99] (**Table 4**). The first and most important step is to have a high index of suspicion based on the patient situation, the caregiver's situation, and the medical conditions for which the patient presents for care. **Table 5** lists common patterns of injury related to specific types.

Once suspected, it should be reported to the local health department. Elder abuse is underreported by professionals for a variety of reasons: lack of knowledge, lack of experience, fear of offense, fear of being wrong, fear of cutting a therapeutic relationship, or belief that the procedures to deal with the offense are too punitive.

CAREGIVER ISSUES IN UNDERSERVED OLDER ADULTS

Caregiver burden is a concept that describes the stress on a person who is caring for another aged, sick, and/or disabled person. Caregiver burden is divided into objective burden and subjective burden. Objective burden is the physical effort required to help the dependent person throughout the day in direct self-care, supervision, or IADLs. Subjective burden is divided into personal strain and role strain. Personal strain is

Table 4 Risk factors for abuse	
Characteristics of the victim	Female Advanced age Cognitive impairment Cohabitation with other family members Social isolation and poor social support networks Mental health problems Substance abuse Frailty Dependency on perpetrator for care
Characteristics of the perpetrator	Cognitive impairment Family history of abusive behavior Male Mental illness or mentally challenged >40 y of age Financial dependency Substance abuse Adult child of victim

Data from Burnett J, Achenbaum WA, Murphy KP. Prevention and early identification of elder abuse. Clin Geriatr Med 2014;30(4):743–59.

Table 5
Common patterns of injury related to specific types of abuse

Physical abuse	Bruises (bruises associated with elder abuse are commonly large [>5 cm], and are present on the face, lateral right arm, and posterior torso) burns, fractures, welts, lacerations, bite marks, untreated injuries, internal injuries, repeated history of falls, repeated emergency department visits, traumatic alopecia
Sexual abuse	Difficulty walking or sitting; pain or itching in the genital area; unexplained sexually transmitted diseases; vaginal or anal bleeding; torn, stained, or bloody underclothing; bruising around genital or breast regions
Psychological/ emotional abuse	Emotional upset; agitation; depression; suicidal ideation; hypervigilance toward abuser; withdrawn; unusual behavior such as sucking, biting, rocking, crying, self-mutilation
Financial exploitation	Sudden changes in bank accounts, inability to afford medications, unexplained disappearance of possessions, unexplained asset transfers, and unexplained loss of pension or Social Security checks
Caregiver neglect	Dehydration, malnutrition, ulcers, unexplained deterioration in health, failure to thrive, lack of routine medical care or medications, urine burns, multiple hospital and emergency department admissions, repeated falls, poor hygiene, unexplained weight loss
Abandonment	Cognitively impaired older adult left in emergency department, older adult placed on public transportation with a 1-way ticket, older adult is left alone unsafely for periods of time
Self-neglect	Unkempt appearance, withdrawn, depressed, isolated, hazardous or unsafe living conditions, unexpected to unexplained deterioration in health, untreated health conditions, weight loss, dehydration, poor hygiene

Data from Burnett J, Achenbaum WA, Murphy KP. Prevention and early identification of elder abuse. Clin Geriatr Med 2014;30(4):743–59.

the psychological burden of keeping lists of things in mind for the dependent person; monitoring their schedule and the burden of responsibility. Role strain refers to the time and attention required of caregivers, who often have other people in their lives who also are dependent.[106]

Measuring caregiver burden is important because it directly correlates with a higher incidence of depression in the caregiver, and poor outcomes for the patient, including earlier nursing home placement.[106] A common method of measurement is the Zarit Burden Scale, which is a 22-item test with high internal consistency and good test-test reliability.[106] It has also become available in a short, 12-item version. Each question has a 5-point Likert response from "Never" to "Always." The form can be accessed online at http://www.uconn-aging.uchc.edu/patientcare/memory/pdfs/zarit_burden_interview.pdf.

The Caregiver Self-assessment Questionnaire is a self-assessment tool available free at http://www.healthinaging.org/resources/resource:caregiver-self-assessment/ (also available in Spanish).

Epstein-Lubow and colleagues[107] found that this tool is a valid instrument for assessing caregiver depression. The Neuropsychiatric Inventory for Caregiver Distress is a reliable and valid measure of neuropsychiatric symptoms in patients with AD to caregiver distress.[108]

Taking care of patients with greater degrees of functional dependence (low ADL and IADL scores) results in greater burden on caregivers. Depressed dependents cause greater caregiver burden that those who are not depressed. These findings have been seen across cultures.[109] Different behavioral disturbances have varying effects on caregiver stress. Delusion has been found to cause greatest stress on the caregiver followed by agitation/aggression, anxiety, and then irritability and dysphoria.[110,111] Caring for patients with AD with increasing AD severity was associated with increased subjective caregiver burden and overall caregiving time.[112] There is a higher burden of care in patients who have frontotemporal dementia than in AD. This finding is likely a reflection of increased problems with behavior in the patient causing increased stress for the caregiver.[113–117] Adult-child caregivers experienced a higher burden than spousal caregivers despite spending less time caring.[118,119] Financial challenges are greater in underserved populations and caregiver burden is expected to be higher. Clinicians should always assess both the support the patient needs and who is providing that support. In essence, clinicians taking care of geriatric patients have 2 patients: the index patient and the caregiver. Caregivers are in danger of being the "invisible" patient.

The stressors and opportunities to help caregivers have been studied across cultures and are strikingly similar.[120] It may be assumed that the opportunities for helping caregivers in underserved populations are similar as well. However, the need for social programs to help with increased costs when caregivers are unable to work, or must work part-time, may demand more philanthropic or governmental programs to maintain these caregivers in the best possible health.

ISSUES IN PREVENTIVE HEALTH CARE AND SCREENING IN OLDER UNDERSERVED ADULTS

Despite guidelines from the Centers for Disease Control and Prevention (CDC) and initiatives such as Healthy People 2020, adult immunization rates among individuals more than 65 years of age have failed to reach the desired targets. Furthermore, data from the National Health Interview Survey reveal that racial and ethnic disparities persist for routinely recommended immunizations. Individuals with private insurance typically received recommended immunizations at a higher rate than older individuals with public insurance or no health care insurance. Barriers to higher immunization rates include variations in insurance coverage of vaccines, and the financial cost to providers of vaccination to uninsured older adults. Greater public awareness of recommended vaccines, provider reminders regarding immunizations, and standing order protocols can potentially increase immunization rates among older adults[121] (**Table 6**).

Table 6 Rates of immunization in older adults				
	Pneumococcal Vaccine	Influenza Vaccine	Tetanus Vaccine Within Last 10 y	Herpes Zoster Vaccine
Healthy People 2020 Goal (%)	90.0	90	No target	30
Total Aged >65 y (%)	61.3	71.5	57.7	31.1
White (%)	64.7	73.4	60.6	35.0
African American (%)	49.8	60.5	43.1	13.5
Hispanic/Latin American (%)	45.2	64.0	49.1	16.3
Asian (%)	47.7	72.5	46.6	20.7
Other (%)	69.4	63.6	63.1	19.6

Data from Williams WW, Lu PJ, O'Halloran A, et al. Surveillance of vaccination coverage among adult populations - United States, 2014. MMWR Surveill Summ 2016;65(1):1–36.

Table 7
Common cancers in different populations

Gender	Economically Developed Countries	Economically Developing Countries
Male	Most commonly diagnosed cancers: • Prostate • Lung • Colorectal	Most commonly diagnosed cancers: • Lung • Liver • Stomach
Female	Most commonly diagnosed cancers: • Breast • Colorectal • Lung	Most commonly diagnosed cancers: • Breast • Cervix • Lung

Data from American Cancer Society. Global cancer facts & figures. Available at: http://www.cancer.org/acs/groups/content/@research/documents/document/acspc-044738.pdf/. Accessed February 15, 2016.

In 2012, there were approximately 14.1 million new cases of cancer worldwide according to estimates from the International Agency for Research on Cancer. Approximately 8 million, or 82%, of the new cases of cancer occurred in economically developed countries. The most prevalent types of cancer differ between the economically developing and the developed countries. Higher rates of preventable infections in the economically developing countries, such as human papillomavirus, human immunodeficiency virus, hepatitis B virus, hepatitis C virus, and *Helicobacter pylori* contribute to these differences[122] **(Table 7)**.

Early screening for cancer and infection among high-risk patient populations can potentially lead to earlier detection of cancer and better outcomes. The estimated rates of colorectal cancer screening have increased in the United States from 54% in 2002 to 65% in 2012 among adults aged 50 to 75 years of age. The Healthy People 2020 goal is to achieve a screening rate of 70.5% among adults 50 to 75 years of age. An estimated 27.7% of adults aged 50 to 75 years had never been screened. Reasons for not being screened were a lack of health care insurance (55.0%) and a lack of a usual health care provider (61.0%). A higher percentage of this group was of Hispanic or Native American descent who lived in nonmetropolitan areas. There are proportional increases in screening rates as the educational level and household income increase.[121] Greater public awareness and health promotion may help to improve rates of colon cancer screening.

In the United States, the estimated rate of women receiving screening mammograms has been fairly steady at approximately 75% (The goal is 81.1% for Healthy People 2020) during the last decade. However, there was not a great deal of variation among the racial and ethnic groups.[121]

SUMMARY

As the global population ages, there is an opportunity to benefit from the increased longevity of a healthy older adult population. Healthy older individuals often contribute financially to younger generations by offering financial assistance, paying more in taxes than benefits received, and providing unpaid childcare and voluntary work. Governments must work to create policies that sufficiently address the challenges of income insecurity, adequate access to health care, social isolation, and neglect that currently face elderly adults in many countries across the globe. A reduction in disparities in these areas can lead to better health outcomes and allow societies to benefit from longer, healthier lives of their citizens.[4]

REFERENCES

1. Centers for Disease Control and Prevention. The state of aging and health in America 2013. Atlanta (GA): Centers for Disease Control and Prevention; US Dept of Health and Human Services; 2013 [Online]. Available at: http://www.cdc.gov/aging/pdf/state-aging-health-in-america-2013.pdf. Accessed December 23, 2015.

2. Available at: http://www.who.int/mediacentre/factsheets/fs381/en/. Accessed February 2, 2016.

3. Available at: http://www.aoa.acl.gov/aging_statistics/profile/2014/6.aspx/. Accessed February 1, 2016.

4. UNFPA and HelpAge. 2012. Ageing in the twenty-first century: a celebration and a challenge. Available at: http://www.unfpa.org/publications/ageing-twenty-first-century. Accessed March 9, 2016.

5. Available at: https://www.ssa.gov/policy/docs/chartbooks/fast_facts/2015/fast_facts15.html#page5. Accessed January 12, 2016.

6. Cubanski J, Casillas G, Damico A. Poverty among seniors: an updated analysis of national and state level poverty rates under the official and supplemental poverty measures. Menlo Park (CA): Kaiser Family Foundation; 2015. Available at: http://kff.org/report-section/poverty-among-seniors-issue-brief/.

7. Glass TA, Balfour JL. Neighborhoods, aging, and functional limitations. In: Kawachi I, Berkman LF, editors. Neighborhoods and health. New York: Oxford University Press; 2003. p. 303–34.

8. Hunter RH, Sykes K, Lowman SG, et al. Environmental and policy change to support healthy aging. J Aging Soc Policy 2011;23(4):354–71.

9. National Center for Health Statistics. Health, United States, 2014: with special feature on adults aged 55–64. Washington, DC: US Government Printing Office; 2015.

10. Available at: http://www.cdc.gov/dhdsp/data_statistics/fact_sheets/fs_stroke.htm. Accessed December 23, 2015.

11. Koton S, Schneider AL, Rosamond WD, et al. Stroke incidence and mortality trends in US communities, 1987 to 2011. JAMA 2014;312(3):259–68.

12. Rosengren A, Giang KW, Lappas G, et al. Twenty-four-year trends in the incidence of ischemic stroke in Sweden from 1987 to 2010. Stroke 2013;44(9):2388–93.

13. Afilalo J, Duque G, Steele R, et al. Statins for secondary prevention in elderly patients: a hierarchical bayesian meta-analysis. J Am Coll Cardiol 2008;51(1):37–45.

14. Available at: http://www.cdc.gov/mmwr/PDF/wk/mm6244.pdf/. Accessed January 24, 2016.

15. Available at: https://www.nia.nih.gov/health/publication/arthritis-advice/. Accessed February 25, 2016.

16. Available at: http://www.agingsociety.org/agingsociety/pdf/arthritis.pdf/. Accessed February 25, 2016.

17. Gotay CC, Korn EL, McCabe MS, et al. Quality-of-life assessment in cancer treatment protocols: research issues in protocol development. J Natl Cancer Inst 1992;84:575–9.

18. Huguet N, Kaplan MS, Feeny D. Socioeconomic status and health-related quality of life among elderly people: results from the Joint Canada/United States Survey of Health. Soc Sci Med 2008;66(4):803–10.

19. Available at: https://www.healthypeople.gov/2020/topics-objectives/topic/older-adults#five/. Accessed January 6, 2016.

20. Christmas C, Andersen RA. Exercise and older patients: guidelines for the clinician. J Am Geriatr Soc 2000;48(3):318–24, 6 Minority populations often have lower rates of physical activity.

21. HelpAge India. Elder abuse in India, a help age India report 2012. New Delhi. 2012.

22. Culberson JW. Alcohol use in the elderly: beyond the CAGE. Part 1 of 2: prevalence and patterns of problem drinking. Geriatrics 2006;61(10):23–7.

23. Kalapatapu RK, Sullivan MA. Prescription use disorders in older adults. Am J Addict 2010;19(6):515–22.

24. Bommersbach TJ, Lapid MI, Rummans TA, et al. Geriatric alcohol use disorder: a review for primary care physicians. Mayo Clin Proc 2015;90(5):659–66.

25. Blazer DG, Wu LT. The epidemiology of alcohol use disorders and subthreshold dependence in a middle-aged and elderly community sample. Am J Geriatr Psychiatry 2011;19(8):685–94.

26. Conigliaro J, Kraemer K, McNeil M. Screening and identification of older adults with alcohol problems in primary care. J Geriatr Psychiatry Neurol 2000;13(3): 106–14.

27. Available at: https://www.nia.nih.gov/health/publication/alcohol-use-older-people/. Accessed March 18, 2016.

28. Egbert AM. The older alcoholic: recognizing the subtle clinical clues. Geriatrics 1993;48(7):63–6, 69.

29. Crome IB, Rao R, Crome P. Substance misuse and older people: better information, better care. Age Ageing 2015;44(5):729–31.

30. Culberson JW. Alcohol use in the elderly: beyond the CAGE. Part 2: screening instruments and treatment strategies. Geriatrics 2006;61(11):20–6.

31. Kuerbis A, Sacco P, Blazer DG, et al. Substance abuse among older adults. Clin Geriatr Med 2014;30(3):629–54.

32. Culberson JW, Zicka M. Prescription drug misuse/abuse in the elderly. Geriatrics 2008;63(9):22–31.

33. Phelan EA, Mahoney JE, Voit JC, et al. Assessment and management of fall risk in primary care settings. Med Clin North Am 2015;99(2):281–93.

34. Bohl AA, Fishman PA, Ciol MA, et al. A longitudinal analysis of total 3-year healthcare costs for older adults who experience a fall requiring medical care. J Am Geriatr Soc 2010;58(5):853–60.

35. Reyes-Ortiz CA, Al Snih S, Loera J, et al. Risk factors for falling in older Mexican Americans. Ethn Dis 2004;14(3):417–22.

36. Available at: www.who.int/ageing/publications/falls_prevention7march.pdf. Accessed#April 29, 2016.

37. Demontiero O, Gunawardene P, Duque G. Postoperative prevention of falls in older adults with fragility fractures. Clin Geriatr Med 2014;30(2):333–47.

38. Moncada LV. Management of falls in older persons: a prescription for prevention. Am Fam Physician 2011;84(11):1267–76.

39. Panel on Prevention of Falls in Older Persons, American Geriatrics Society, British Geriatrics Society. Summary of the updated American Geriatrics Society/British Geriatrics Society clinical practice guideline for prevention of falls in older persons. J Am Geriatr Soc 2011;59(1):148–57.

40. Lee JY, Jin Y, Piao J, et al. Development and evaluation of an automated fall risk assessment system. Int J Qual Health Care 2016;28(2):175–82.

41. Available at: http://www.ahrq.gov/professionals/systems/hospital/fallpxtoolkit/index.html/. Accessed March 9, 2016.

42. Weiss A, Brozgol M, Dorfman M, et al. Does the evaluation of gait quality during daily life provide insight into fall risk? A novel approach using 3-day accelerometer recordings. Neurorehabil Neural Repair 2013;27(8):742–52.

43. Gillespie LD, Robertson MC, Gillespie WJ, et al. Interventions for preventing falls in older people living in the community. Cochrane Database Syst Rev 2012;(9):CD007146.

44. Available at: http://www.uspreventiveservicestaskforce.org/Page/Document/UpdateSummaryFinal/vitamin-d-and-calcium-to-prevent-fractures-preventive-medication?ds=1&s=vitamin%20D/. Accessed January 6, 2016.

45. Bischoff-Ferrari HA, Dawson-Hughes B, Orav EJ, et al. Monthly high-dose vitamin D treatment for the prevention of functional decline: a randomized clinical trial. JAMA Intern Med 2016;176(2):175–83.

46. Kendrick D, Kumar A, Carpenter H, et al. Exercise for reducing fear of falling in older people living in the community. Cochrane Database Syst Rev 2014;(11):CD009848.

47. Sherrington C, Whitney JC, Lord SR, et al. Effective exercise for the prevention of falls: a systematic review and meta-analysis. J Am Geriatr Soc 2008;56(12):2234–43.

48. Chan WC, Yeung JW, Wong CS, et al. Efficacy of physical exercise in preventing falls in older adults with cognitive impairment: a systematic review and meta-analysis. J Am Med Dir Assoc 2015;16(2):149–54.

49. Fox MT, Persaud M, Maimets I, et al. Effectiveness of acute geriatric unit care using acute care for elders components: a systematic review and meta-analysis. J Am Geriatr Soc 2012;60(12):2237–45.

50. Tinetti M. ACP Journal Club. Review: acute geriatric unit care reduces falls, delirium, and functional decline. Ann Intern Med 2013;158(12):JC11.

51. Marengoni A, Fratiglioni L, Bandinelli S, et al. Socioeconomic status during lifetime and cognitive impairment no-dementia in late life: the population-based aging in the Chianti area (InCHIANTI) study. J Alzheimers Dis 2011;24(3):559–68.

52. Wee LE, Yeo WX, Yang GR, et al. Individual and area level socioeconomic status and its association with cognitive function and cognitive impairment (low MMSE) among community-dwelling elderly in Singapore. Dement Geriatr Cogn Dis Extra 2012;2(1):529–42.

53. Shih RA, Ghosh-Dastidar B, Margolis KL, et al. Neighborhood socioeconomic status and cognitive function in women. Am J Public Health 2011;101(9):1721–8.

54. Lang IA, Llewellyn DJ, Langa KM, et al. Neighborhood deprivation, individual socioeconomic status, and cognitive function in older people: analyses from the English Longitudinal Study of Ageing. J Am Geriatr Soc 2008;56(2):191–8.

55. Wight RG, Aneshensel CS, Miller-Martinez D, et al. Urban neighborhood context, educational attainment, and cognitive function among older adults. Am J Epidemiol 2006;163:1071–8.

56. Available at: http://www.who.int/mediacentre/factsheets/fs362/en/. Accessed March 1, 2016.

57. Prince M, Bryce R, Albanese E, et al. The global prevalence of dementia: a systematic review and metaanalysis. Alzheimers Dement 2013;9(1):63–75.

58. Karp A, Kåreholt I, Qiu C, et al. Relation of education and occupation-based socioeconomic status to incident Alzheimer's disease. Am J Epidemiol 2004;159(2):175–83.

59. American Psychiatric Association. Diagnostic and statistical manual of mental disorders. 5th edition. Arlington (VA): American Psychiatric Association; 2013 (DSM-5).

60. Rossetti HC, Lacritz LH, Cullum CM, et al. Normative data for the Montreal Cognitive Assessment (MoCA) in a population-based sample. Neurology 2011;77(13):1272–5.

61. Ballard C, Gauthier S, Corbett A, et al. Alzheimer's disease. Lancet 2011; 377(9770):1019–31.

62. Hebert LE, Scherr PA, Bienias JL, et al. Alzheimer disease in the US population: prevalence estimates using the 2000 census. Arch Neurol 2003;60(8):1119–22.

63. Available at: http://www.alz.org/downloads/facts_figures_2012.pdf/. Accessed February 15, 2016.

64. McKhann GM, Knopman DS, Chertkow H, et al. The diagnosis of dementia due to Alzheimer's disease: recommendations from the National Institute on Aging-Alzheimer's Association workgroups on diagnostic guidelines for Alzheimer's disease. Alzheimers Dement 2011;7(3):263–9.

65. Knopman DS, DeKosky ST, Cummings JL, et al. Practice parameter: diagnosis of dementia (an evidence-based review). Report of the Quality Standards Sub-committee of the American Academy of Neurology. Neurology 2001;56(9): 1143–53.

66. Han L, Cole M, Bellavance F, et al. Tracking cognitive decline in Alzheimer's disease using the mini-mental state examination: a meta-analysis. Int Psychogeriatr 2000;12(2):231–47.

67. Schmidt C, Wolff M, Weitz M, et al. Rapidly progressive Alzheimer disease. Arch Neurol 2011;68(9):1124–30.

68. Helzner EP, Scarmeas N, Cosentino S, et al. Survival in Alzheimer disease: a multiethnic, population-based study of incident cases. Neurology 2008;71(19): 1489–95.

69. Larson EB, Shadlen MF, Wang L, et al. Survival after initial diagnosis of Alzheimer disease. Ann Intern Med 2004;140(7):501–9.

70. Lobo A, Launer LJ, Fratiglioni L, et al. Prevalence of dementia and major subtypes in Europe: a collaborative study of population-based cohorts. Neurologic diseases in the elderly research Group. Neurology 2000;54(11 Suppl 5):S4–9.

71. Ikejima C, Yasuno F, Mizukami K, et al. Prevalence and causes of early-onset dementia in Japan: a population-based study. Stroke 2009;40(8):2709–14.

72. Vann Jones SA, O'Brien JT. The prevalence and incidence of dementia with Lewy bodies: a systematic review of population and clinical studies. Psychol Med 2014;44(4):673–83.

73. McKeith IG, Dickson DW, Lowe J, et al. Diagnosis and management of dementia with Lewy bodies: third report of the DLB Consortium. Neurology 2005;65(12): 1863–72.

74. LoGiudice D, Watson R. Dementia in older people: an update. Intern Med J 2014;44(11):1066–73.

75. Chen R, Hu Z, Wei L, et al. Socioeconomic status and survival among older adults with dementia and depression. Br J Psychiatry 2014;204(6):436–40.

76. Available at: http://www.alz.co.uk/research/files/WorldAlzheimerReport2010. pdf/. Accessed May 1, 2016.

77. Beers MH, Ouslander JG, Rollingher I, et al. Explicit criteria for determining inappropriate medication use in nursing home residents. UCLA Division of Geriatric Medicine. Arch Intern Med 1991;151:1825–32.

78. Beers MH. Explicit criteria for determining potentially inappropriate medication use by the elderly. An update. Arch Intern Med 1997;157:1531–6.

79. Fick DM, Cooper JW, Wade WE, et al. Updating the Beers criteria for potentially inappropriate medication use in older adults: results of a U.S. consensus panel of experts. Arch Intern Med 2003;163:2716–24.

80. The American Geriatrics Society. 2015 Beers criteria update expert panel. American Geriatrics Society 2015 updated Beers criteria for potentially inappropriate medication use in older adults. J Am Geriatr Soc 2015;63(11):2227–46.

81. Hanlon JT, Semla TP, Schmader KE. Alternative medications for medications in the use of high-risk medications in the elderly and potentially harmful drug-disease interactions in the elderly quality measures. J Am Geriatr Soc 2015; 63(12):e8–18.

82. Mattison ML, Afonso KA, Ngo LH, et al. Preventing potentially inappropriate medication use in hospitalized older patients with a computerized provider order entry warning system. Arch Intern Med 2010;170:1331–6.

83. Trivalle C, Cartier T, Verny C, et al, for the IMEPAG GROUP. Identifying and preventing adverse drug events in elderly hospitalised patients: a randomised trial of a program to reduce adverse drug effects. J Nutr Health Aging 2010;14:57–61.

84. Bushardt RL, Massey EB, Simpson TW, et al. Polypharmacy: misleading, but manageable. Clin Interv Aging 2008;3(2):383–9.

85. Steinman MA, Landefeld CS, Rosenthal GE, et al. Polypharmacy and prescribing quality in older people. J Am Geriatr Soc 2006;54(10):1516–23.

86. Odubanjo E, Bennett K, Feely J. Influence of socioeconomic status on the quality of prescribing in the elderly – a population based study. Br J Clin Pharmacol 2004;58(5):496–502.

87. Mamdani MM, Tu K, Austin PC, et al. Influence of socioeconomic status on drug selection for the elderly in Canada. Ann Pharmacother 2002;36(5):804–8.

88. Wright RM, Sloane R, Pieper CF, et al. Underuse of indicated medications among physically frail older US veterans at the time of hospital discharge; results of a cross-sectional analysis of data from the Geriatric Evaluation and Management Drug Study. Am J Geriatr Pharmacother 2009;7(5):271–80.

89. Cherubini A, Corsonello A, Lattanzio F. Underprescription of beneficial medicines in older people: causes, consequences and prevention. Drugs Aging 2012;29(6):463–75.

90. Heisler M, Choi H, Rosen AB, et al. Hospitalizations and deaths among adults with cardiovascular disease who underuse medications because of cost: a longitudinal analysis. Med Care 2010;48(2):87–94.

91. Choudhry NK, Patrick AR, Amman EM, et al. Cost-effectiveness of providing full drug coverage to increase medication adherence in post-myocardial infarction Medicare beneficiaries. Circulation 2008;117(10):1261–8.

92. Kaye AD, Baluch A, Scott JT. Pain management in the elderly population: a review. Ochsner J 2010;10(3):179–87.

93. American Geriatrics Society Panel on Pharmacological Management of Persistent Pain in Older Persons. Pharmacological management of persistent pain in older persons. J Am Geriatr Soc 2009;57(8):1331–46.

94. National Hospice and Palliative Care Organization. NHPCO's facts and figures hospice care in America 2015 edition [Online]. Available at: http://www.nhpco.org/sites/default/files/public/Statistics_Research/2015_Facts_Figures.pdf. Accessed January 5, 2016.

95. O' Reilly K. Minority patients less interested in hospice care. Amednews.com, July 9, 2012. Available at: http://www.amednews.com/article/20120709/profession/307099943/4/. Accessed January 5, 2016.

96. Sacco J, Deravin Carr D, Viola D. The effects of palliative medicine consultation on the DNR status of African Americans in a safety-net hospital. Am J Hosp Palliat Care 2013;30(4):363–9.

97. Green CR, Ndao-Brumblay SK, West B, et al. Differences in prescription opioid analgesic availability: comparing minority and white pharmacies across Michigan. J Pain 2005;6(10):689–99.

98. Morrison RS, Wallenstein S, Natale DK, et al. "We don't carry that"–failure of pharmacies in predominantly nonwhite neighborhoods to stock opioid analgesics. N Engl J Med 2000;342(14):1023–6.

99. Burnett J, Achenbaum WA, Murphy KP. Prevention and early identification of elder abuse. Clin Geriatr Med 2014;30(4):743–59.

100. Johannesen M, LoGiudice D. Elder abuse: a systematic review of risk factors in community-dwelling elders. Age Ageing 2013;42(3):292–8.

101. Dong XQ. Elder abuse: systematic review and implications for practice. J Am Geriatr Soc 2015;63(6):1214–38.

102. Cooper C, Livingston G. Mental health/psychiatric issues in elder abuse and neglect. Clin Geriatr Med 2014;30(4):839–50.

103. Wolf RS, Li D. Factors affecting the rate of elder abuse reporting to a state protective services program. Gerontologist 1999;39(2):222–8.

104. Available at: http://www.who.int/violence_injury_prevention/violence/world_report/factsheets/en/elderabusefacts.pdf/. Accessed May 1, 2016.

105. Dong X, Simon MA. Elder abuse as a risk factor for hospitalization in older persons. JAMA Intern Med 2013;173(10):911–7.

106. Brodaty H, Woodward M, Boundy K, et al. Prevalence and predictors of burden in caregivers of people with dementia. Am J Geriatr Psychiatry 2014;22(8):756–65.

107. Epstein-Lubow G, Gaudiano BA, Hinckley M, et al. Evidence for the validity of the American Medical Association's caregiver self-assessment questionnaire as a screening measure for depression. J Am Geriatr Soc 2010;58(2):387–8.

108. Kaufer DI, Cummings JL, Christine D, et al. Assessing the impact of neuropsychiatric symptoms in Alzheimer's disease: the neuropsychiatric inventory caregiver distress scale. J Am Geriatr Soc 1998;46(2):210–5.

109. Kang HS, Myung W, Na DL, et al. Factors associated with caregiver burden in patients with Alzheimer's disease. Psychiatry Investig 2014;11(2):152–9.

110. Huang MF, Huang WH, Su YC, et al. Coping strategy and caregiver burden among caregivers of patients with dementia. Am J Alzheimers Dis Other Demen 2015;30(7):694–8.

111. Miyamoto Y, Tachimori H, Ito H. Formal caregiver burden in dementia: impact of behavioral and psychological symptoms of dementia and activities of daily living. Geriatr Nurs 2010;31(4):246–53.

112. Haro JM, Kahle-Wrobleski K, Bruno G, et al. Analysis of burden in caregivers of people with Alzheimer's disease using self-report and supervision hours. J Nutr Health Aging 2014;18(7):677–84.

113. Lillo P, Mioshi E, Hodges JR. Caregiver burden in amyotrophic lateral sclerosis is more dependent on patients' behavioral changes than physical disability: a comparative study. BMC Neurol 2012;12:156.

114. Mioshi E, Foxe D, Leslie F, et al. The impact of dementia severity on caregiver burden in frontotemporal dementia and Alzheimer disease. Alzheimer Dis Assoc Disord 2013;27(1):68–73.
115. Hsieh S, Leyton CE, Caga J, et al. The evolution of caregiver burden in frontotemporal dementia with and without amyotrophic lateral sclerosis. J Alzheimers Dis 2015;49(3):875–85.
116. Shim SH, Kang HS, Kim JH, et al. Factors associated with caregiver burden in dementia: 1-year follow-up study. Psychiatry Investig 2016;13(1):43–9.
117. Uflacker A, Edmondson MC, Onyike CU, et al. Caregiver burden in atypical dementias: comparing frontotemporal dementia, Creutzfeldt-Jakob disease, and Alzheimer's disease. Int Psychogeriatr 2016;28(2):269–73.
118. Rosdinom R, Zarina MZ, Zanariah MS, et al. Behavioural and psychological symptoms of dementia, cognitive impairment and caregiver burden in patients with dementia. Prev Med 2013;57(Suppl):S67–9.
119. Reed C, Belger M, Dell'agnello G, et al. Caregiver burden in Alzheimer's disease: differential associations in adult-child and spousal caregivers in the GERAS observational study. Dement Geriatr Cogn Dis Extra 2014;4(1):51–64.
120. Torti FM Jr, Gwyther LP, Reed SD, et al. A multinational review of recent trends and reports in dementia caregiver burden. Alzheimer Dis Assoc Disord 2004; 18(2):99–109.
121. Williams WW, Lu PJ, O'Halloran A, et al. Surveillance of vaccination coverage among adult populations - United States, 2014. MMWR Surveill Summ 2016; 65(1):1–36.
122. American Cancer Society. Global cancer facts & figures. Available at: http://www.cancer.org/acs/groups/content/@research/documents/document/acspc-044738.pdf/. Accessed February 15, 2016.

Cardiovascular Health Disparities in Underserved Populations

Charles P. Mouton, MD, MS[a],*, Michael Hayden, MD[b],
Janet H. Southerland, DDS, PhD, MPH[c]

KEYWORDS

- Cardiovascular disease • African Americans • Health disparities
- Primary care management

KEY POINTS

- African Americans have a greater of burden of cardiovascular disease that require targeted primary care management.
- Aggressive management of cardiovascular risk factors, especially blood pressure control and cholesterol levels, are essential.
- Using community resources can be an adjunct to clinical management of key risk factors.
- Future opportunities to target genetic polymorphism may provide additional benefit.

INTRODUCTION

Cardiovascular disease (CVD) is a leading cause of morbidity and mortality in the United States for both men and women. Approximately 610,000 people die from heart disease in the United States annually, estimated at 1 in every 4 deaths attributed to CVD, with the greatest mortality risk in racial and ethnic minority groups. In 2009, CVD caused the deaths of 46,334 African American (AA) males and 48,070 AA females.[1] Annual death rates for AAs were 387.0 per 100, 000 population for males and 267.9 per 100,000 for females, whereas the overall death rate from CVD was 236.1 per 100,000.[1,2]

CVD is the leading cause of death among Hispanics, which mirrors that of the United States as a whole. Estimates show that the overall prevalence of CVD is 33.4% for

This article originally appeared in Primary Care: Clinics in Office Practice, Volume 44, Issue 1, March 2017.
[a] Department of Family and Community Medicine, School of Medicine, Meharry Medical College, 1005 Dr. DB Todd, Jr. Boulevard, Nashville, TN 37208, USA; [b] Department of Internal Medicine, School of Medicine, Meharry Medical College, 1005 Dr. DB Todd, Jr. Boulevard, Nashville, TN 37208, USA; [c] Department of Oral and Maxillofacial Surgery, School of Dentistry, Meharry Medical College, 1005 Dr. DB Todd, Jr. Boulevard, Nashville, TN 37208, USA
* Corresponding author.
E-mail address: cmouton@mmc.edu

Mexican American males and 30.7% for Mexican American females, which is lower than the overall prevalence in non-Hispanics whites and non-Hispanic AAs.[3] Despite having higher rates of many CVD risk factors, the lower prevalence of overall CVD and overall mortality has been described as the Hispanic paradox. Although there are some data available for CVD risks and morbidity and mortality in Hispanic subgroups, most of the cohort data are limited to inclusion of predominantly Mexicans Americans. Given that 10 Hispanic subgroups represent 92% of the total US Hispanic population (eg, Mexican, Puerto Rican, Cuban, Dominican, Columbian, Honduran, Ecuadorian, Guatemalan, Peruvian, and Salvadoran), these data may underestimate the CVD rates in Hispanics.[4] In addition, Hispanics are significantly less aware of CVD as the leading cause of death and their personal risk factors for CVD than are non-Hispanic whites (NHWs).[5]

The Hispanic paradox, if it really exists, may not apply to every Hispanic subgroup equally.[6] Studies that have disaggregated the Hispanic population by national subgroup have reported varying degrees of support for the Hispanic paradox. For example, using the National Longitudinal Mortality Study, Abraído-Lanza and colleagues[7] found lower mortality hazard ratios (HRs) for each of the Hispanic subgroups relative to NHWs after they accounted for age, education, and family income. Hummer[8] compared all-cause mortality outcomes for 5 major Hispanic subgroups and found that only Mexicans and Central/South Americans had significantly lower mortality than NHWs. These data highlight the significant heterogeneity within the Hispanic population and demonstrate that the unique sociocultural characteristics of the diverse Hispanic subgroups may contribute to these differential outcomes. As a result, health research that lumps all individuals Hispanic of origin into a single category potentially masks substantial differences among the diverse Hispanic subgroups, particularly with regard to the notion of the Hispanic paradox.[9]

There are approximately 6.2 million people classified as American Indian/Alaska Native (AI/AN) Profile as of 2011, comprising approximately 2.0% of the US population in 2013 living on 569 federally recognized tribes.[10] According to 2000 data, 43% live in the West, 31% live in the South, 17% live in the Midwest, and 9% live in the Northeast.[2] While 34% of AI/AN reside on reservations or in rural areas, another 55% live in urban communities.[11] In AI/AN, CVD remains a significant cause of morbidity with an incidence of 15 to 28 per 1000 population for men and 9 to 15 per 1000 population for women.

Disproportionate mortality rates in the AA community are owing to a particularly high disease burden of CVD. Nearly one-half of all AA adults, 48% of women and 46% of men, have some form of CVD.[12] In addition, CVD is a major contributor to the overall problem of disparities in AA mortality. Older AAs in the United States have shorter overall life expectancy (74.3 years for NHW males compared with 67.2 AA males) owing higher rates of CVD. AAs have 1.5 times the rate of cardiovascular deaths compared with their NHW counterparts. AA mortality rates are especially elevated for heart disease and cerebrovascular disease while exceeding those for NHW for any age group beyond 44 years old.[2]

Given the impact of CVD in these populations, we will focus this article on specific disease categories (eg, coronary heart disease [CHD], congestive heart failure, cerebrovascular disease [CVD], and peripheral vascular disease [PVD]) that influence CVD mortality in underserved populations (UPs). We pay particular attention to the primary care management of these diseases, especially its primary risk factor, namely, hypertension (HTN). We also discuss some of the behavioral and socioenvironmental factors that place AAs at risk for CVD and strategies for primary care providers to manage these as well.

CORONARY HEART DISEASE

Coronary heart disease (CHD) is a major contributor to CVD in UPs. Angina (chest pain or discomfort caused by reduced blood supply to the heart muscle) is a sign of CHD and is more common in women than in men. Among non-Hispanic AAs age 20 and older, 2.4% of men and 5.4% of women report angina. In Hispanics, 3.5% report angina. These rates are important because angina may be a sign of CHD.

AAs in the United States have the highest rates of CHD mortality, 186.8 versus 182.8 per 100,000 for NHWs and 124.2 for Hispanic Whites. Among AAs age 20 and older, 6.8% of men and 7.1% of women have CHD. Among AAs age 20 and older, 3.9% of men and 2.3% of women have had a myocardial infarction.[2] For Hispanics, 4% of men and 2% of women have had a myocardial infarction. These high rates of CHD reflect the increased risk from the high rates of HTN in the population, which accounts for one-half of the CVD mortality disparity, and is discussed elsewhere in this article. Also, AA and Hispanics have a higher prevalence of dyslipidemia and lower adherence rates to lipid-lowering medication, also discussed elsewhere in this article.[13]

Genetics also play a role with polymorphisms in the lipid-coding region APOL1, which are associated with kidney function, subclinical atherosclerosis, and incident CVD and death. In AA, the high-risk genotype was also associated with increased risk for incident myocardial infarction (adjusted HR, 1.8; 95% confidence interval [CI], 1.1–3.0) and mortality (adjusted HR, 1.3; 95% CI, 1.0–1.7).[14] Other risks for CHD and CVD in general include (1) tobacco abuse, (2) physical inactivity, (3) obesity, (4) diabetes, and (5) socioenvironmental stressors. Because of the importance of these factors for primary care, each of these general CVD risk factors are discussed in the section on risk factors.

In addition, low serum vitamin D levels (more prevalent in AAs) have been associated with increased CHD risk. National Health and Nutrition Examination Survey (NHANES) data showed that severe vitamin D deficiency (<10 ng/mL) was present in 3% of whites, 7% of Hispanics, and 30% of AAs.[12] The Health Professions Follow-up study showed a 2.4-fold increased risk of myocardial infarction for men[15] with vitamin D levels of less than 15 ng/mL. Also, vitamin D supplementation has been shown to improve coronary artery function with supplementation of 60,000 IU monthly oral vitamin D (approximately 2000 IU/d) improving vascular endothelial function in AA adults.[16] However, clinical trials (most having few AA participants) of vitamin D supplementation have not shown a decrease in CVD outcomes or mortality.[17,18]

More than one-half of the Hispanic men and one-third of the women from the Multi-Ethnic Study of Atherosclerosis (MESA) were found to have some coronary calcification (Agatston score >0), although the prevalence was significantly lower than in NHWs (56.5% and 34.9% for Hispanic men and women vs 70.4% and 44.6% for NHW men and women).[19] With adjustment for age, education, and CVD risk factors, Hispanics had a 15% lower risk of coronary artery calcium (CAC) than NHWs, and the amount of CAC among Hispanic participants with any CAC was 74% that of NHWs.[19] There were 335 similar findings reported in a physician-referred population, that is, relative risk (RR) for any CAC among Hispanics was 0.88 (95% confidence interval CI, 0.67–1.15) compared with NHWs.[19]

Data from MESA suggest that the prevalence of any CAC may be greater among Mexicans than Dominicans, Puerto Ricans, or other Hispanic subgroups.[20] Moreover, foreign-born Hispanics have lower CAC scores than US-born Hispanics[21] and this difference was independent of socioeconomic status and standard CVD risk factors (eg, smoking, body mass index [BMI] >30 kg/m^2, elevated serum lipids, HTN, and diabetes mellitus). Among the least acculturated people, these data found an inverse association of higher incomes with lower CAC scores, but this was reversed to a positive association (higher socioeconomic status with higher CAC scores) among the more highly acculturated individuals.[22] Finally, CAC scores have been found to be independent predictors of incident CHD, with magnitudes of association that are similar for NHW (HR for a major coronary event, 1.15; 95% CI, 1.02–1.29) and Hispanic (HR, 1.17; 95% CI, 1.06–1.30) participants.[23]

Treatment

Primary care management for CHD in UPs is consistent with the guidelines for the general population. For primary prevention, clinicians should consider the coronary risk status using risk calculators such as: the Framingham risk score, the Systematic Coronary Risk Evaluation (SCORE), ASCVD risk calculation, and the MESA. Both the Framingham risk score and the SCORE have been criticized for possibly underestimating the cardiac risk in AAs The MESA risk score, which has been validated in AAs and Hispanics and is available online on the MESA web site for easy use, can be used to aid clinicians when communicating risk to patients and when determining risk-based treatment strategies.[24] A more accurate estimate of 10-year CHD risk can be obtained using these risk factor scores in conjunction with an estimate of CAC obtained from a specialized computed tomography scan, yet outcomes data have been conflicting to date. Also of note, patients with a history of atherosclerotic stroke should be included among those deemed to be at high risk ($\geq$20% over 10 years).[25] There is also a strong consensus that men with erectile dysfunction should be considered at high risk for CVD.[26]

Management of UPs with CHD focuses on risk factor reduction. For those without clinical CHD or other major CHD risk factors (low risk), a heart healthy lifestyle (appropriate diet and exercise), statin use based on the 2013 American College of Cardiology/American Heart Association (ACC/AHA) cholesterol guidelines,[27] treatment of HTN and diabetes, weight loss, and smoking cessation should be considered. For those postmyocardial infarction or clinical CHD (high risk), clinicians should consider heart healthy lifestyle, cholesterol control to targets as per ACC/AHA cholesterol guidelines, and antiplatelet agents, in addition to aggressive management of HTN, diabetes, smoking cessation, weight loss, and cardiac rehabilitation.

For some underserved CHD patients, more intense interventions are necessary to limit CVD morbidity and mortality. Guidelines recommend the use of coronary artery bypass grafting (CABG) as the treatment of choice for patients with asymptomatic ischemia, stable angina, or unstable angina/non-ST elevation myocardial infarction who have left main CHD.[28] However, drug-eluting stents seem to be safe in AAs and may improve survival in certain subgroups such as patients with acute coronary syndromes. In a study of AA patients, the mortality rate in the bare metal stents group was 12.8% compared with 7.1% in the drug-eluting stents group (adjusted P = .19); HR for bare metal stents group compared with drug-eluting stents group for death of 1.4 (95% CI, 0.8–2.4).[29] In a subgroup analysis, patients presenting with acute coronary syndrome had a higher mortality when treated with bare metal stents compared with drug-eluting stents (17.1 vs 6.3%; P = .022; HR, 2.2; 95% CI, 1.1–4.4).[29]

Although CABG has been suggested as the treatment of choice, several studies cite the disparities in AA associated with bypass surgery.[30,31] AA experience high morbidity and mortality after CABG.[32,33] AAs had a significantly longer hospitalization postoperatively (odds ratio [OR], 0.79; 95% CI, 0.66–0.96).[33] Even after multiple adjustments, AAs undergoing CABG surgery had significantly greater morbidity compared with Caucasian patients.[34] Also, lack of preoperative inotropic support was an independent preoperative risk factor for long-term mortality among AAs undergoing CABG. This outcome provides information that may be useful for surgeons, primary care providers, and their patients.[35]

With regard to antiplatelet agents, the American College of Chest Physicians (ACCP) recommends for primary prevention of CVD low-dose aspirin (75–100 mg/d) in patients aged greater than or equal to 50 years over no aspirin therapy. For patients with established CHD, with prior revascularization, coronary stenoses greater than 50% by coronary angiogram, and/or evidence for cardiac ischemia on diagnostic testing, the ACCP recommends long-term low-dose aspirin or clopidogrel (75 mg/d). Individuals with acute coronary syndromes who undergo percutaneous coronary intervention with stent placement, the ACCP recommends for the first year dual antiplatelet therapy with low-dose aspirin in combination with ticagrelor 90 mg bid, clopidogrel 75 mg/d, or prasugrel 10 mg/d over single antiplatelet therapy. For patients undergoing elective percutaneous coronary intervention with stent placement, the ACCP recommends aspirin (75–325 mg/d) and clopidogrel for a minimum duration of at least 1 month (with bare metal stents) or 3 to 6 months (with drug-eluting stents). The ACCP also suggests continuing low-dose aspirin plus clopidogrel for 12 months for all stents.

Other guidelines recommend clopidogrel use for 6 to 12 months after the placement of a drug-eluting stent and 1 to 12 months after placement of a bare metal stent. After initial treatment, the ACCP recommends single antiplatelet therapy over continuation of dual antiplatelet therapy.[36] However, others recommend for patients with or undergoing elective percutaneous coronary intervention with stent placement that dual antiplatelet therapy for up to 1 year is warranted. Cruden and colleagues[37] showed longer (>12 months) clopidogrel use was associated with a reduction in death and hospitalization for myocardial infarction in patients with drug-eluding stents.

Once CHD patients have received their initial intervention and treatment for myocardial infarction/acute coronary syndrome, and major CVD risks (eg, blood pressure [BP], lipids, smoking, weight, diabetes) have been addressed, additional benefit can be gained by attention to improving the functional limitations that cardiovascular heart disease places on patients. In post myocardial infarction patients, cardiac rehabilitation improves CHD risk factors and mortality. AAs derive a significant benefit from cardiac rehabilitation, but not to the same degree as whites. Based on changes in risk factors and in exercise capacity, AA women had the least improvement.[38] Other strategies have proven useful in AA patients. A selected mind–body intervention such as the transcendental meditation program significantly reduced the risk for mortality, myocardial infarction, and stroke in AA CHD patients. These changes were also associated with a 4.9 mm Hg lower BP and reduction in psychosocial stress factors.[39]

CONGESTIVE HEART FAILURE

Heart failure (HF) affects over 5.7 million people in the United States with an annual incidence rate of 2.4 per 1000 person-years for NHWs and 9.1 per 1000 person-years for AAs and 3.5 per 1000 person years in Hispanics.[3,40] AAs have a 50% higher frequency of HF compared with NHWs.[41] And AAs are at significantly higher risk of developing HF compared with Whites (HR, 1.81, CI 1.07–3.07).[42] Importantly, the onset of HF occurs at an earlier age and its severity is worse at the time of diagnosis for AAs.[41] In the ADHERE study, AAs were a mean >10 younger at onset of HF and more likely to have non-ischemic cardiomyopathy.[43]

Several factors have been suggested for these differences including the greater prevalence of HTN in AAs (3–7 fold higher), the greater incidence of left ventricular hypertrophy (3 fold higher) and greater salt sensitivity.[43,44] Also, recent studies suggest possible cellular mechanisms for the difference in HF in AAs. Procollagen type III N-terminal peptide (PIIINP) is a biomarker of cardiac fibrosis is associated with poor outcomes in AAs with chronic heart failure (HF).[45] PIIINP levels greater than 4.88 ng/mL was associated with all-cause mortality on univariate (HR, 4.9, 95% CI, 2.2–11.0; $P < .001$) and multivariate (HR 5.8; 95% CI 1.9–17.3; $P = .002$) analyses. Also observed was an increased risk of all-cause mortality or hospitalization for HF with PIIINP level greater than 4.88 ng/mL on univariate (HR 2.6; 95% CI, 1.6–5.0; $P < .001$) and multivariate (HR 2.4; 95% CI, 1.2–4.7; $P = .016$) analyses.[45] In addition to PIIINP, single nucleotide polymorphisms have been suggested as mechanisms for HF in AAs. Candidate genes for SNPs in AAs with HF include transforming growth factor (TGF)-β, endothelin, β-adrenergic receptors, aldosterone synthase, nitric oxide (NO) synthase, and the 825T allele of the GNB-3 protein subunit.[40]

Treatment

HF is a common disease with morbidity and mortality, especially in UPs. Therefore, primary care management is paramount for longitudinal care, with specific regard to preventing hospital admission and readmission. Management of fluid balance is a mainstay of HF treatment. Diuretics have favorable symptomatic benefits in both AA and white patients with HF with evidence of fluid retention. Loop diuretics and thiazide diuretics have benefit in patients with HF. No studies have shown a differential effect in AAs. There is good evidence for the use of spironolactone in all patients with heart failure, but no evidence for a different effect in AA patients. In some studies of HF, angiotensin-converting enzyme (ACE) inhibitors (ACEI) seem to be less effective in the treatment of AA patients with HF. This may be owing to low preexisting activity of the renin–angiotensin system in AAs. The most recent data show that, in adjusted models, ACE/angiotensin receptor blocker exposure was associated with lower risk of death or hospitalization in both groups (AAs HR, 0.47 [$P < .001$]; whites HR, 0.55 [$P < .001$]).[46] Also, certain β-adrenoceptor antagonists (eg, carvedilol) are effective in both AA and white patients with HF. However, a recent analysis showed that the benefit of β-blockers for whites was a decrease in mortality of 31%, whereas AAs had a 3% reduction.[46]

In addition to single drug therapy, the combination of hydralazine and nitrates seem to be particularly effective in AA patients with HF.[47] The ACC and AHA recommend combined isosorbide dinitrate and hydralazine to reduce mortality and morbidity for AAs with symptomatic HF and a reduced ejection fraction, currently receiving optimal medical therapy (class I, level A).[47] Nitrates can alleviate HF symptoms, but continuous use is limited by tolerance. Isosorbide dinitrate–hydralazine improved survival and exercise tolerance in men with dilated cardiomyopathy or HF with reduced left ventricular ejection fraction, most notably in self-identified AA participants. In the AA population treatment with isosorbide dinitrate–hydralazine was associated with a substantial reduction in the first and recurrent HF hospitalizations, and in total all-cause hospitalizations.[47,48] Consequently, it was found that adding a fixed-dose combination isosorbide dinitrate–hydralazine to modern guideline-based care improved outcomes versus placebo, including all-cause mortality. HF morbidity and mortality as well as hospitalizations potentially affect burgeoning HF health care costs.[48] It is important to accept that racial categorization acts as only a surrogate marker for genetic or other factors responsible for individual responses to drug therapy and that any identified differences will not apply to all members of each stratified group. Nonetheless, in managing a complex, common, and often fatal condition such as HF, recognizing potential individual differences in drug responses should enable the responsible clinician to provide a tailored and evidence-based approach to patient treatment.[49]

In addition to medical therapy, clinical trials have demonstrated benefit for cardiac resynchronization therapy (CRT) and implantable cardioverter-defibrillator therapies in patients with heart failure with reduced ejection fraction. There was clinical benefit associated with implantable cardioverter-defibrillator/cardiac resynchronization therapy (adjusted OR, 0.64; 95% CI, 0.52–0.79; P = .0002 for 24-month mortality), which was of similar proportion in white, AA, and other minorities (device–race/ethnicity interaction P = .7861).[50] For cardiac resynchronization therapy with pacemaker function/cardiac resynchronization therapy with defibrillator, there were also associated mortality benefits (adjusted OR, 0.55; 95% CI, 0.33–0.91; P = .0222); however, the device–race/ethnicity interaction was not significant (P = .5413).[50]

The community prevalence of HF among Mexicans was 1.9% for males and 1.1% for females.[51] Using the large database of hospitalized patients from the AHA's Get with the Guidelines–Heart Failure 1 study noted 46% of Hispanic inpatients had heart failure with preserved ejection fraction, whereas 54% had heart failure with reduced ejection fraction, compared with 55% and 45% of NHWs, respectively. Relative to NHWs, Hispanics with heart failure were more likely to be younger, to have diabetes mellitus or HTN, and to be overweight/obese. In a multivariate analysis, a 45% lower mortality risk was observed among Hispanics with heart failure with preserved ejection fraction, but not among Hispanics with heart failure with reduced ejection fraction, compared with NHWs (P = .63).[52] A report from MESA estimated 67 of 257 elderly Hispanics (26%) developed congestive heart failure at the 43-month follow-up.[53]

CEREBROVASCULAR DISEASE

Cerebrovascular disease is a major cause of morbidity and mortality in UPs. AAs have a 1.3 times greater rate of nonfatal stroke and a 1.8 times greater rate of fatal stroke.[1,2] Among non-Hispanic AAs age 20 and older, 4.3% of men and 4.7% of women have had a stroke. AAs have a risk of first-ever stroke that is almost twice that of whites.[1,2] Moreover, between the 1990s and 2005, the incidence rates of stroke decreased for whites, but not for AAs. The age-adjusted death rates from stroke is 35% higher in AA than in whites and the intracerebral hemorrhage rates were 1.7-fold higher.[1,2]

As with other CVDs, risk factors that have an impact on the higher prevalence of stroke in AAs include higher prevalence of HTN and diabetes. The NHANES Epidemiologic Follow-up Study showed that the risk factors of age, gender, education, BP treatment group (eg, normotensive, controlled hypertensive, hypertensives receiving medication, and hypertensives not receiving medication), systolic BP, diabetes mellitus, history of heart disease, Quetelet index (eg, BMI), hemoglobin, and magnesium explained approximately one-third of the excess stroke risk among AAs aged 35 to 74 years at baseline.[42] Also, interindividual variation in leukocyte telomere length has been previously associated with susceptibility to CVD with genetic polymorphisms nominally associated with incident CHD (hazards rate ratio, 1.20; P = .02; 95% CI, 1.03–1.40) and stroke (hazards rate ratio, 1.17; P = .05; 95% CI, 1.00–1.38), in AAs.[54]

The Consortium of Minority Population Genome-Wide Association Studies of Stroke (COMPASS) showed that the 15q21.3 locus linked with lipid levels and HTN was associated with total stroke (rs4471613; P = 3.9×10^{-8}) in AAs. Also associations for total or ischemic stroke were observed for 18 variants in or near genes implicated in cell cycle/messenger RNA presplicing (PTPRG, CDC5L), platelet function (HPS4), blood–brain barrier permeability (CLDN17), immune response (ELTD1, WDFY4, and

IL1F10-IL1RN), and histone modification (HDAC9).[55] Four of 7 previously reported ischemic stroke loci (PITX2, HDAC9, CDKN2A/CDKN2B, and ZFHX3) were nominally associated (P<.05) with stroke in COMPASS.[55] Sickle Cell Trait was associated with an ischemic stroke HR of 1.4 (95% CI, 1.0–2.0) and an incidence rate difference amounting to 1.9 (95% CI, 0.4–3.8) extra strokes per 1000 person-years.[56] In addition to genetic and disease comorbidity, other factors may contribute to stroke disparities, poor stroke awareness, higher vascular risk factor burden, limited access to care, mistrust of the medical system, and inequities in diagnostic testing and treatment usage may account for some of the disparity.[57]

The BASIC (Brain Attack Surveillance in Corpus Christi) project showed an increased incidence of stroke among Mexicans compared with NHWs in this southeast Texas community. The crude 2-year cumulative incidence (2000–2002) was 168 per 10,000 in Mexicans and 136 per 10,000 in NHWs. Specifically, Mexicans had a higher cumulative incidence of ischemic stroke at younger ages (45–59 years of age, crude rate 76 per 10,000 [RR, 2.10; 95% CI, 1.64–2.69]; 60 to 74 years of age, crude rate 224 per 10,000 [RR, 1.59; 95% CI, 1.34–1.90]). However, no difference was observed at older ages (>75 years of age, crude rate 468 per 10,000 [RR, 1.15; 95% CI, 0.98–1.34]). Mexicans also had a higher incidence of intracerebral hemorrhage (25/10,000 vs 19/10,000; RR, 1.37; 95% CI, 1.04–1.80) than NHWs, but not significantly different rates of subarachnoid hemorrhage (5/10,000 vs 4/10,000), adjusted for age.[58] The total cost of stroke from 2005 to 2050 (in 2005 dollars) is projected to be $313 billion for Hispanics and $379 billion for non-Hispanic blacks.[58–60]

Intracranial atherosclerosis (atherothrombotic subtype) and lacunar (small vessel subtype) stroke mechanisms were more common among Hispanics than cardioembolic stroke.[60,61] In NOMAS (Northern Manhattan Study), which included Hispanics of primarily Dominican, Cuban, and Puerto Rican origin, the relative rate of intracranial atherosclerotic stroke was 5.00 (95% CI, 1.69–14.76) and the relative rate of lacunar stroke was 2.32 (95% CI, 1.48–3.63) compared with NHWs.[59,60]

Death certificates for AI/AN were evaluated for rates of stroke and/or CVD based on race/ethnicity looked at death certificates from the National Center for Health Statistics to see if there were differences in stroke types based on gender and race/ethnicity between 1995 and 1998. The instigators found that age-standardized stroke death rate was lower for ischemic stroke in AI/AN women (49.2 vs 79.3 per 100,000) and in AI/AN men (47.6 vs 65.3 per 100,000) as well as for intracranial hemorrhage in AI/AN women (10.7 vs 12.8 per 100,000) and in AI/AN men (9.9 vs 13.6 per 100,000).[62] Rates of subarachnoid hemorrhage were higher in AI/AN women (6.0 vs 4.5 per 100,000) but similar in AI/AN men (2.3 vs 2.9 per 100,000).[38] Although these results suggest that rates of stroke might be similar or even decreased, the reality is that death certificates are known to underreport race. The National Center for Health Statistics reported that death rates might be underreported by as much as 21% for AI/AN populations.[62] Another study looked at mortality from heart disease and stroke and attempted to correct for the underreporting of AI/AN race.[63]

The Strong Heart Study participants without a stroke at the time of recruitment (between 1989 and 1992) and through the end of 2004 to determine the incidence rate of stroke as well as 1-year poststroke mortality. The author found that the incident rate of stroke in this cohort was 384 per 100,000 person-years for 45 to 54 year-olds, 727 per 100,000 person-years for 55 to 64 years, and 1002 per 100,000 person-years for the 65 to 74 year-old.[64] Hispanic white population in Minnesota collected in 1985 and 1989. Competed with the Framingham Heart Cohort, the Strong Heart cohort had a much higher incidence of stroke.[65] Furthermore, the 1-year mortality rate was 33.1% for women and 31% for men, compared with 24%

and 21%, respectively, based on pooled data from the Framingham Heart Study, the Atherosclerosis Risk in Communities Study, and the Cardiovascular Health Study. The author concluded that poststroke mortality among AI was 1.5 times that of other US populations.[65] Similarly, the authors of the Strong Heart follow-up study compared the incidence rates of stroke with a mostly white population and found that the rate for stroke was lower for AI men and similar for AI women, although the average follow-up for comparison cohort was 3.3 years compared with 4.2 years for the Strong Heart Study.[64]

ATRIAL FIBRILLATION

Atrial fibrillation (AF) is associated with an increased risk of stroke owing in part to the pathophysiology of AF with an increase in left atrial size. In AAs, increased left atrial size is significantly related to stroke[66] along with other factors including female sex, obesity, HTN, and diabetes. In patients with AF, the use of anticoagulants to prevent thrombotic stroke could lead to stroke owing to intracranial hemorrhage. Nonwhites are at greater risk for intracranial hemorrhage than whites.[66] In a multiethnic study of nonrheumatic AF, the magnitude of increased risk for intracranial hemorrhage associated with warfarin use was greater for nonwhites than for whites.[66] Possible explanations for this disparity included polymorphisms of the P450 cytochrome CYP2C9, the enzyme responsible for metabolizing warfarin or for variants in the gene for vitamin K epoxide reductase complex 1, the target enzyme for warfarin.[67] Differences in these haplotypes have been seen in AAs. Although the use of warfarin to prevent left atrial thrombi in AF is recommended, approximately one-third of strokes in AF are nonthromboembolic.[67]

Treatment

Primary prevention of stroke is critical for patients with risk factors for atherosclerosis, including HTN, diabetes, smoking, and hypercholesterolemia. As with CHD, antiplatelet agents are often considered as part of the management of patients at risk for stroke. However, studies have found no difference between ticlopidine and aspirin in the prevention of recurrent stroke, myocardial infarction, or vascular death. Based on these data and the risk of serious adverse events with ticlopidine, there is a suggestion that aspirin is a better treatment for aspirin-tolerant AA patients with noncardioembolic ischemic stroke.[68]

Controversy persists regarding the best antiplatelet agent for stroke treatment and prevention. A blinded study of ticlopidine was halted after about 6.5 years when futility analyses revealed a less than 1% probability of ticlopidine being shown superior to aspirin in reducing recurrent stroke, myocardial infarction, or vascular death.

PERIPHERAL VASCULAR DISEASE

Peripheral artery disease (PAD) is clinically defined as a disorder in which stenosis or occlusion in the aorta or arteries of the extremities (especially lower extremities) is present. The condition most often affects patients greater than 40 years of age and the leading cause is atherosclerosis. The highest prevalence occurs during the sixth and seventh decades of life. In addition, other risk factors (common to CAD) that increase the risk of developing PAD include tobacco smoking in diabetic patients, advanced age (>65 years), HTN, or hypercholesterolemia.[69] Complications of longstanding PAD include a gradual decline in walking ability (ie, distance, speed, and/or stair climbing). The reduction in activity thus leads to loss of mobility with the eventual loss in the ability to perform activities of daily living.

Unfortunately, like many of the aforementioned chronic illness and diseases, PAD disproportionately affects AAs compared with NHWs.[69,70] As noted, AAs suffer more from chronic diseases than their counterparts for a variety of reasons although there is no specific causal relationship for these findings. Furthermore, AAs seemingly experience more complications from PAD than NHWs including limb loss attributable to PAD.[70] Because atherosclerosis is the known primary risk factor for PAD, management revolves around controlling those risk factors leading to reduction in ischemic events in patients with PAD. Smoking can increase disease severity up to 4-fold and diabetes mellitus can increase it by 2-fold.[71] Diabetes causes endothelial damage leading to PAD. Uncontrolled HTN, another risk factor, increases symptomatic PAD (eg, intermittent claudication). Finally, dyslipidemia is a known risk factor where elevated low-density lipoprotein cholesterol (LDL-C), triglycerides, and low high-density lipoprotein cholesterol may predispose to PAD. In the Cardiovascular Health Study that genotyped APOL1 polymorphisms, the high-risk genotype with 2 risk alleles was associated with 2-fold higher levels of albuminuria and lower ankle-brachial indices but similar carotid intima media thickness among AAs.[72] Median survival among high-risk AAs was 9.9 years (95% CI, 8.7–11.9), compared with 13.3 years (95% CI, 13.0–13.6) among whites ($P = .03$). As such, current guidelines in the management of PAD include smoking cessation, optimal BP control with a goal of less than 130/80 mm Hg, glycosylated hemoglobin A1c of less than 7%, and LDL-C of less than 100 (or <70 mg/dL in very high-risk patients).[72]

The rate of peripheral vascular revascularization procedures is lower in Hispanics than in NHWs (4 vs 6 per 10,000 person-years).[73] Of course, this could be more reflective of disparities in use of health care than of true differences in incident disease. Conversely, the rate of admission for lower limb amputations is higher in Hispanics than in NHWs (3 vs 2 per 10,000 person-years).[73] Only 1 study to date has examined a relation of lower limb amputations and diabetes mellitus prevalence among a select group of Hispanics.[74] This is an area that requires further study. In the community-based MESA cohort, the prevalence of an ankle-brachial index of less than 0.9 (to define PVD) was substantially higher in non-Hispanic blacks (7.2%) than in NHWs (3.6%), Hispanics (2.4%), or Chinese (2.0%), with Hispanics having 51% lower odds of having PVD than NHWs after adjustment for multiple risk factors, including diabetes mellitus, smoking, and socioeconomic status. Among primary care clinic patients, the prevalence of PVD was reported to be as high as 13.7% among Mexicans, similar to NHWs (13.5%) and less than non-Hispanic blacks (22.8%).[75] PVD prevalence was 16% among older Hispanics in an academic hospital-based geriatric practice.[76] The AHA practice guidelines for PVD do not report prevalence by ethnicity.[77] A higher percentage of Native American ancestry among Hispanics was associated with lower odds of PVD compared with European ancestry.[78]

Treatment

Treatment options primarily involve increasing physical activity; however, many patients with PAD may be asymptomatic (eg, no exertional leg symptoms) or may have exertional symptoms including leg pain, fatigue, weakness, or numbness with walking. Symptomatic disease is categorized as atypical leg pain, classic intermittent claudication, or critical limb ischemia. AAs have an higher prevalence of asymptomatic PAD (eg, objective evidence of disease but without leg symptoms), which may ultimately lead to a delay in care and continuation of high-risk behaviors, including a sedentary lifestyle.[69] In an article by Aronow,[79] greater walking impairment in AAs as compared with NHWs was largely explained by a higher prevalence of asymptomatic disease in AAs. For persons with PAD and leg symptoms, pharmacotherapy such as cilostazol is proven to improve leg symptoms, walking distance, and quality of life in persons with PAD. In addition, statins have been shown to improve claudication symptoms, ambulatory ability, total walking distance, and leg functioning. In a secondary analysis of data from 1 study, ACEIs improved symptomatic PAD.[80]

Walking therapy reduces impairment[81] by increasing lower limb blood flow and walking economy (eg, gait stability without compromising walking velocity). Participants in a study of home-based walking improved their stair climbing ability at 12 weeks.[70] However, few AAs were involved in the studies. Because AAs are more prone to sedentary lifestyles than their NHW counterparts, work is needed to identify the benefits of home-based walking in AAs with PAD.

RISK FACTORS FOR CARDIOVASCULAR DISEASE
Hypertension

HTN is inarguably the leading risk factor for CVD in UPs and likely explains the disparities in CVD epidemiology and outcomes. BP levels vary by race and ethnicity[1] and the prevalence of HTN in US AAs is among the highest in the world. Compared with NHWs, AAs develop HTN at an earlier age and their average BPs are much higher.[1]

Overall, mortality owing to HTN and its consequences is 4 to 5 times more likely in AAs than in whites.[82] And AAs have 5 times as many hospitalizations for HTN compared with whites.[13] The increased risk of HTN is apparent even in childhood. The Bogalusa Heart Study demonstrated elevations in BP in AA children under the age of 10 years.[83] Left ventricular hypertrophy is more common in AAs and an independent predictor of cardiovascular morbidity and mortality, is directly associated with risk factors, HTN in particular. A community-based sample of 467 young adults (29% AA and 71% white) were examined from childhood to adulthood demonstrating that AAs had greater left ventricular mass (index to height; $P<.05$).[84]

This racial/ethnic variation in BP is predominately owing to socioevironmental factors, but genetic factors do contribute to the variation. The Genetics of Hypertension Associated Treatment Study examined 35 candidate gene variants that might modulate BP response to 4 different antihypertensive medications.[85] Several suggestive gene-by-treatment interactions were identified. For example, among participants with 2 minor alleles of renin r, diastolic BP response was much improved on doxazosin compared with chlorthalidone (on average -9.49 mm Hg vs -1.70 mm Hg; $P = .007$). Although several suggestive loci were identified, none of the findings passed significance criteria after correction for multiple testing.[85]

Factors associated with the stress hypothesis, "John Henryism," salt sensitivity, and socioenvironmental factors also have been suggested as contributors to development of HTN in AA. Each of these factors contribute to the disparity in HTN prevalence in AAs and may also contribute independently to CVD disparities.

John Henryism describes a coping mechanism by AAs in response to prolonged exposure to stressors. It describes a process where AAs expend a high levels of effort to overcome the stressor, which in turn results in greater psychological costs. These stressors lead to activation of the hypothalamic–pituitary–adrenal axis, causing release of vasoactive hormones and neurotransmitters (including vasopressin, serotonin, and norepinephrine), which have deleterious effects on the vascular system. Chronic exposure to these factors leads to increased vascular resistance and HTN. Also, activation of the hypothalamic–pituitary–adrenal axis releases high levels of cortisol, having deleterious effects on the endovasculature and metabolic control.[86]

There is a remarkable lack of consistent information regarding the prevalence of HTN among US Hispanics. Studies suggest that the prevalence of HTN is highest in non-Hispanic blacks and lowest in Mexican Americans.[87,88] The prevalence of HTN among Mexicans (30.1% in males, 28.8% in females) is lower than the prevalence of HTN in the general American population (33.0%).[89] Comparison between NHANES examinations[90] conducted in 1988 to 1992 and 1999 to 2000 revealed that among Mexicans, age-adjusted rates of pre-HTN increased from 33.2% to 35.1%, rates of stage 1 HTN increased from 12.4% to 14.8%, and rates of stage 2 HTN increased from 4.2% to 5.3%. Similarly, the age-adjusted prevalence of HTN among Mexicans increased from 17.2% in 1988 to 1991 to 20.7% in 1999 to 2000 and to 27.8% in 2003 to 2004.[87,91] Over a 10-year time span, Hispanic individuals remained more likely to have undiagnosed, untreated, or uncontrolled HTN than other ethnic groups.[92–94]

Three national studies using National Health Interview Survey (NHIS) and Behavioral Risk Factor Surveillance System (BRFSS) data evaluated rates of self-reported HTN and hyperlipidemia with mixed results. One study based on 2003 BRFSS data showed higher rates of self-reported HTN in AI/AN compared with NHWs (26.8% vs 21.9%).[95] Among AI/AN reporting HTN, 61.3% reported taking antihypertensive medications compared with 60.9% of NHW respondents.[95] Of the AI/AN hypertensive respondents, 38.4% reported meeting physical activity recommendations compared with 42.9% of NHWs.[95] Using NHIS data between 2004 and 2008, the Centers for Disease Control and Prevention reported increased rates of HTN among AI/AN compared with NHWs (34.5% vs 25.7%).[10] Data comparing rates of HTN and hyperlipidemia among women were also equivocal. A study using BRFSS data from 2005 to 2007 found that significantly more AI/AN women (ages 18–44) reported having HTN compared with NHW women (12.0% vs 8.2%; $P = .007$). No differences were found for those reporting a diagnosis of hyperlipidemia (19.7% of both groups reported this).[96] In terms of regional data, Harwell and colleagues[97] analyzed 1999 BRFSS data on Indians versus non-Indians in Montana, stratified by age. They found that both younger (<45 years old) and older (>45 years old) groups had higher rates of HTN, yet lower rates of hyperlipidemia. The OR for the younger group was 1.75 (95% CI, 1.16–2.65) for HTN and 1.42 (95% CI, 1.08–1.87) for the older age group.[97]

In the Hispanic Community Health Study/Study of Latinos (HCHS/SOL) study, the overall age-adjusted prevalence of HTN was 25.5% (26.1% for men and 25.3% for women)[98,99]; HTN was defined as average measured BP of 140 mm Hg or greater systolic or 90 mm Hg or greater diastolic or self-reported use of medications for HTN in the last 4 weeks. When compared with national estimates, prevalence rates of HTN reported by HCHS/SOL were comparable with those found in NHANES 2009 to 2010 for Hispanic participants (26.1%) and slightly lower than those reported for NHW participants (27.4%).[66] The prevalence of HTN varied significantly across Hispanic background, with South American women having the lowest rates at 17.2% and Dominican men having the highest at 34.3%.[64]

Exposure to racism also has a role in rates of HTN. Overall, perceived racial discrimination was associated with hypertensive status. Racism's effect on HTN is strengthened by gender (male), race (black), age (older), education (lower). Perceived discrimination was most strongly associated with nighttime ambulatory BP, especially among AAs.[86]

Prevalence estimates of perceived discrimination (those who experienced some form of unfair treatment attributed to race or ethnicity) among the US Hispanic population is approximately 30% to 40%, but may vary by Hispanic subgroup and Hispanic race.[100–103] In 1 study, perceived everyday discrimination was detrimental to the physical health of Puerto Ricans and Mexicans, but the stress-buffering effects of marriage attenuated the associations among Mexicans only.[104] Another study found that there were no variations between non-Hispanic blacks, NHWs, and Hispanics in the inverse associations of perceived discrimination and self-reported general health.[105] Coping mechanisms in response to perceived discrimination among the total Hispanic population or certain subpopulations may have similarities to or differences from those of non-Hispanic blacks, but this has not been studied. Validation of existing perceived discrimination instruments (mostly developed for non-Hispanic blacks) in Hispanics is also needed.

Salt Sensitivity

Salt sensitivity has been long postulated to contribute to the burden of HTN in some UPs. In non-Hispanic AAs, there is evidence that endothelial dysfunction, reduced potassium intake, decreased urinary kallikrein excretion, upregulation of sodium channel activity, dysfunction in atrial natriuretic peptide production, and *APOL1* gene nephropathy risk variants may cause or contribute to salt sensitivity. The low renin hypertensive phenotype commonly seen in AAs has also been linked to salt sensitivity. Increased morbidity and mortality associated with salt sensitivity suggests the potential efficacy of tailored dietary and pharmacologic treatment in AAs.[106]

There are few data estimating the prevalence of salt sensitivity in this large ethnic group (Hispanic). As for determining etiology, unfortunately, in many cases circumstantial evidence is all there is to draw conclusions from. Although speculative, it may be that, when it comes to salt sensitivity and HTN, Caribbean-origin Hispanics may have some similarities to non-Hispanic blacks that have been underappreciated and require further study. Understanding some of the genetic diversity within the Hispanic population can help to make sense of the limited and sometimes seemingly contradictory data on HTN and salt sensitivity in this group.

A study of antihypertensive medication efficacy in 117 subjects, 76% of whom were Caribbean Hispanic, found this group to respond similarly to AAs.[107] Subjects were randomized to receive placebo, beta blocker, ACEI, calcium channel blocker (CCB), hydrochlorothiazide (HCTZ) monotherapy, or a combination of HCTZ and ACEI for 8 to 12 weeks. Results showed BP reduction only by CCB, HCTZ, or the combination of ACEI and HCTZ to be significantly greater than placebo. These results suggest that Caribbean Hispanics, who have a greater proportion of African ancestry than Mexican-origin Hispanics, may exhibit a similar hypertensive phenotype to non-Hispanic blacks. In non-Hispanic blacks, a stronger response to diuretics than to renin–angiotensin–aldosterone system inhibiting drugs is thought to reflect an etiology of HTN that implicates sodium retention and volume overload, which can be measured as salt sensitivity, as causes of the observed decrease in renin–angiotensin–aldosterone system activity.[106]

The 2005 to 2008 NHANES study reports an age-adjusted HTN prevalence of 42.0% among non-Hispanic blacks, 28.8% among NHWs, and 28.8% among Mexicans. The NOMAS found HTN to be more common in non-Hispanic blacks and in a population of Hispanics that is largely Caribbean, compared with NHWs, with rates of 62%, 58%, and 43%, respectively.[108] The MESA study also revealed that, when looking at Hispanic subgroups, the prevalence of HTN among Hispanics of Caribbean origin approximated that of non-Hispanic blacks, whereas the prevalence in Mexican-origin Hispanics approximated that of NHWs.[109] Additionally, in a study of 438 non-Hispanic black, NHW, and Caribbean Hispanic hypertensives, the 24-hour average BP was similar in all racial groups; however, the absence of nocturnal dipping was more common in non-Hispanic black and Caribbean Hispanic men.[110]

In addition, there has been an association between salt sensitivity and obesity that was evaluated in a 12-month study of 20 otherwise healthy, salt-sensitive, obese Caribbean Hispanics. After obtaining baseline values including weight and BP on low- and high-salt diets, subjects were put on a lifestyle program with a goal of weight reduction, and prescribed metformin, titrated up to 500 mg 3 times a day.[111] This intervention achieved a significant reduction in subject's weight by 13%, reductions in systolic and diastolic BP, and, most notably, reduced the sensitivity of the participant's BP to salt intake by about 40%. Researchers also measured urinary excretion of nitrous oxide (NO) metabolites. At baseline, excretion of NO metabolites (suggestive of NO production) decreased on the high-sodium diet versus the low-sodium diet. After the weight loss and metformin intervention, NO metabolite excretion remained high regardless of whether the participant was on a low-salt or high-salt diet. This small study supports the notion that obesity acts as a contributor to the salt sensitivity phenotype via a mechanism that may involve blunted NO production in the obese state.

Treatment

Control of BP is a major intervention for reducing the burden of CVD, and the target for BP control in has been debated for several decades. Some argue that there are no clinical trial data at present to suggest that lower than usual BP targets should be set for high-risk demographic groups such as AAs, Hispanics, and AI/ANs.[112] Others have argued the minority populations should have lower BP targets than NHWs.[113] However, it is clear that treatment to control BP reduces CVD risks. In addition, ethnic minorities may demonstrate differences in treatment response and side effects to antihypertensive medications that impact BP control. Also, treatment resistant HTN is found more often in AA, but has not been shown in other ethnic minorities. In this study, AA women had the lowest BP control rate (59%) and non-AA men the highest (70%).[114]

Optimal antihypertensive treatment requires a comprehensive approach that encompasses multifactorial lifestyle modifications (eg, weight loss, salt and alcohol restriction, and increased physical activity) plus drug therapy. The most important initial step in the evaluation of patients with elevated BP is to appropriately risk stratify to determine their hypertensive status and BP goals. The primary means of prevention and early treatment of HTN in minorities is the use of lifestyle modification, including dietary sodium reduction and increased physical activity. Regarding pharmacotherapy for HTN, the responsiveness of AA to monotherapy with ACEIs, angiotensin receptor blockers, and beta blockers may be less than the responsiveness to diuretics and CCBs, but these differences are corrected when diuretics are added to these neurohormonal antagonists. Of note, AA patients with systolic BP of greater than 15 mm Hg or a diastolic BP of greater than 10 mm Hg above goal should be treated with first-line combination therapy.[112] Thus, the overwhelming majority of minority hypertensive patients will require combination antihypertensive drug therapy to maintain BP consistently below target levels. The emphasis is now appropriately on using the most effective drug combinations for the control of BP and protection of target organs in this high-risk population. The preferred combination is a calcium antagonist/ACEI or, alternatively, in edematous and/or volume overload states, a thiazide diuretic/ACEI.[113]

Single pill amlodipine/atorvastatin therapy was well-tolerated and effectively targeted HTN in a population of AAs who were at risk of CVD. In the CAPABLE trial (Clinical Utility of Caduet in Simultaneously Achieving Blood Pressure and Lipid End Points), 236 of 489 patients (48.3%) reached both their BP and LDL-C goals (vs 4

[0.8%] of 484 at baseline) and 280 (56.8%) of 493 reached BP goals (vs 7 [1.4%] of 494 at baseline).[115] The Hypertension in AA Working Group of the International Society of Hypertension in AAs recently developed a consensus document that presented a practical, evidence-based approach aimed at achieving better BP control. A new targeted approach was needed to achieve better BP control and enhance target tissue protection in AAs. Key elements include (1) an emphasis on the importance of therapeutic lifestyle modification such as weight loss, decreased sodium ingestion, increased potassium intake, exercise, and weight loss, to name a few, (2) the recommendation of combination antihypertensive agents because of the high prevalence of individuals with greater than 15 mm Hg above SBP goal and/or 10 mm Hg above DBP goal (140/90 unless there is also diabetes and/or kidney disease with >1 g proteinuria daily), and (3) that the recommendations do not differ from other racial/ethnic groups where specific or compelling indications for the use of specific classes of antihypertensive agents exist.[116]

As a single agent therapy, the diuretic chlorthalidone was associated with greater reductions in BP than ACEI and was also associated with a RR reduction in stroke.[115] Although the use of diuretics in AA patients may be a logical first-line choice for BP reduction, most patients will require combination therapy. As mentioned, AA patients with systolic BP of greater than or equal to 15 mm Hg above the target level or a diastolic BP of greater than or equal to 10 mm Hg above target should be considered for first-line combination therapy. Although certain combinations have been shown to be effective in non-AA patients, the choice of drugs for combination therapy in AA patients may be different.[51] Effective combinations include beta adrenoceptor antagonist/diuretic, ACEI/diuretic, ACEI/calcium channel antagonist, and angiotensin receptor antagonist/diuretic.

Despite these data on the effectiveness of ACEIs, other studies suggest that ACEIs were associated with a greater risk of cardiovascular events when compared with CCBs or thiazide diuretics.[117] ACEI-based therapy was superior to either a BB- or CCB-based regimen and a CCB-based regimen combined with strict BP control may be the next best choice to an ACEI-based regimen in this population.[118]

A study of antihypertensive medication efficacy in 117 subjects, 76% of whom were Caribbean Hispanic, found this group to respond similarly to non-Hispanic blacks.[107] Subjects were randomized to receive placebo, beta blocker, ACEI, CCB, HCTZ monotherapy, or a combination of HCTZ and ACEI for 8 to 12 weeks. Results showed that the BP reduction only by CCB, HCTZ, or the combination of ACEI and HCTZ to be significantly greater then placebo.

There are also nonpharmacologic approaches that are important considerations in the management of HTN in AAs. A peer and practice team intervention was used to reduce systolic BP and 4-year CHD risk in AAs. The reduction in risk favored the intervention, but was not significant. Among the 247 subjects, more intervention than control subjects achieved a greater than 5 mm Hg reduction (61% vs 45%, respectively; $P = .01$). After multiple imputation, the absolute reduction in systolic BP was also greater for the intervention group (difference of −6.47 mm Hg; 95% CI, -10.69 to −2.25; $P = .003$).[119] With regard to salt sensitivity, supported treatment avenues include diets high in potassium and soybean protein, the components of which stimulate nitric oxide production.

OTHER CARDIOVASCULAR DISEASE RISK FACTORS IN UNDERSERVED POPULATIONS

In addition to HTN, other major modifiable risk factors contribute to the high prevalence of CVD. These risk factors offer an opportunity for primary care interventions to alleviate the burden of CVD in UPs. Also, these factors are amenable to interprofessional team approaches and population management techniques. In fact, many are quality indications for primary care. Thus, incorporating techniques to address major cardiovascular risks such smoking cessation, hyperlipidemia, physical inactivity, obesity, and diabetes control not only improves the cardiovascular risk profile for UPs, but improves the overall quality of primary care practice.

Smoking Cessation

Tobacco abuse continues to be a problem in the US population, including UPs. In 2011, NHW high school students were more likely than Hispanic or AA students to report any current tobacco use, which includes cigarettes, cigars, or smokeless tobacco (26.5% compared with 20.5% for Hispanic students and 15.4% for non-Hispanic AA students). Among AA adults, 23.3% of males and 15.1% of females smoke cigarettes. Although the prevalence of tobacco use in similar between AAs and whites, AAs are less likely to be offered assistance with cessation and more likely to suffer higher rates of tobacco-related morbidity.[13]

Smoking cessation has substantial health benefits,[120] with a 50% reduction of the excess risk for a cardiovascular events within the first 2 years after stopping smoking. Despite reporting greater desires to quit and higher rates of attempted quits, AA smokers have lower rates of successful quit attempts when compared with the general population.[121–123] However, Ahluwalia and coworkers[121] found that the nicotine patch significantly improves short-term quit rates in inner-city AAs who are interested in trying to quit smoking. In a subsequent study in an AA population, bupropion sustained release was effective for smoking cessation and may be useful in reducing the health disparities associated with smoking with confirmed abstinence rates at the end of 7 weeks of treatment of 36.0% in the bupropion SR group and 19.0% in the placebo group (17.0% point difference; 95% CI, 9.7–24.4; $P<.001$).[122]

Overall, the prevalence of cigarette smoking is lower for US Hispanics than for NHWs and non-Hispanic blacks.[124,125] In 2012, among Hispanics aged 18 years or older, 16.6% of males and 7.5% of females smoked cigarettes. Although NHIS data from 2005 and 2010 showed significant declines in current smoking prevalence among Hispanic men and women (from 21.1% to 15.8% in men and from 11.8% to 9.0% in women),[126] smoking among Hispanic men and certain Hispanic subgroups approximates or exceeds the national average.[127,128]

Among MESA participants, Puerto Ricans had the highest rates of ever smoking.[20] In HCHS/SOL, the smoking prevalence was 25.7% for men, ranging from 11.1% among Dominicans to 34.7% among Puerto Ricans.[98] Although smoking prevalence was lower for women (15.2%), the ranges varied widely, from 8.7% for Central American women to 31.7% among Puerto Rican women.[98] The prevalence of smoking also increased with acculturation among women but not among men.[129] Central American women smoked significantly less than Puerto Rican or Cuban women.[130] Hispanic smokers were one-half as likely as NHW smokers to be advised on or offered assistance with smoking cessation.[4]

Guides such as *Pathways to Freedom* or videos such as *Kick It!*,[131,132] developed specifically for AA smokers were, for example, rated more favorably,[131] and perceived to be more useful (70% vs 65% for a nonadapted guide; $P = .14$).[132] One study reported greater satisfaction with the content of a culturally specific booklet compared with the content of a standard booklet, with an evaluation that the culturally specific booklet was better understood, felt to be more encouraging, and generated greater attention.[133] Interestingly, the same study reported that the standard booklet was perceived to be more credible/trustworthy.[133] One study reported greater use

(68.8% vs 59.6%; $P<.05$) of the targeted guide compared with a nonadapted guide, although it was not regarded as more salient by the participants. Interestingly, level of acculturation predicted how positively the adapted materials were evaluated: a culturally specific smoking cessation guide was rated as more useful, and enhanced readiness to quit in less acculturated AA smokers.[132,134]

High Blood Cholesterol and Other Lipids

Hyperlipidemia is a problem for individuals at risk for CVD, especially in AAs. Elevated cholesterol in the AAs may start as early as preadolescence. Among AAs age 20 and older, 38.6% of men and 40.7% of women have total blood cholesterol levels of 200 mg/dL or higher; 10.8% of men and 11.7% of women have levels of 240 mg/dL or higher; 33.1% of men and 31.2% of women have an LDL-C of 130 mg/dL or higher; and 20.3% of men and 10.2% of women have high-density lipoprotein cholesterol less than 40 mg/dL. Several familial and socioenvironmental factors lead to disparities in hyperlipidemia in AAs. The COMPASS showed that the 15q21.3 locus linked with elevated lipid levels in AAs. Social stressors and hypothalamic–pituitary–adrenal axis activation play a role in lipid dysregulation in AAs. Because of the high prevalence of hyperlipidemia, screening guidelines recommends beginning screening for hyper-lipidemia in AA at 40 years of age.

Treatment

The 2013 ACC/AHA guideline for cholesterol management recommend 4 groups for statin therapy. These new guidelines are important because many minority and female patients may need to be treated more aggressively to reduce their short-term risk for CVD. The new guidelines identify 4 categories of people who can benefit from treatment with a statin:

1. Patients with clinically evident atherosclerotic CVD;
2. Those with primary elevations of LDL-C of at least 4.9 mmol/L (190 mg/dL);
3. Middle-aged individuals (40–75 years) with diabetes and LDL-C levels of at least 1.8 mmol/L (70 mg/dL); and
4. Middle-aged people with an estimated 10-year risk for atherosclerotic CVD of at least 7.5% and with LDL-C levels of at least 1.8 mmol/L (70 mg/dL).

After lifestyle changes including low cholesterol diets and increase physical activity, statin therapy remains the mainstay of treatment of hyperlipidemia in CVD. In the ALL-HAT study (Antihypertensive and Lipid Lowering Treatment to Prevent Heart Attack Trial), AAs in the pravastatin group had a 29% lower risk of CHD (HR, 0.71; 95% CI, 0.57–0.90; $P = .005$) compared with those in the usual care group.[135] In a letter to the editor, Messerli and colleagues[135] indicate that the ALLHAT study showed pravastatin had no effect on all-cause mortality or CHD mortality but significantly reduced CHD mortality in AAs only. However, pravastatin also increased kidney disease mortality and (nonsignificantly) stroke mortality in AAs.

In other studies, single pill therapy containing atorvastatin was well-tolerated and effectively targeted dyslipidemia in AAs who were at risk of CVD.[136,137] Nonpharmacologic approaches also effective adjunct to cholesterol management. Church-based interventions showed improvement in management of cardiovascular risk including hyperlipidemia. One community based research program in AAs in Dallas, Texas, showed that intervention participants had higher rates of treatment and control of most cardiovascular risks with improvements in the treatment of hyperlipidemia (95% vs 64%; $P<.001$), controlling diabetes (95% vs 21%; $P<.001$), controlling HTN (70% vs 52%; $P = .003$), greater physically active (233 vs 177 metabolic equivalent units-min/week; $P<.0001$); and less of a likelihood to smoke (10% vs 30%; $P<.001$).[138]

Physical Inactivity

Physical inactivity is a key risk factors for CVD, especially for UPs. The prevalence of inactivity in children was highest among AA (26.7%) and Hispanic (21.3%) girls, followed by white girls (13.7%), black boys (12.3%), Hispanic boys (10.7%), and white boys (8.5%). In the National Health Interview Survey, AA adults had higher adjusted odds of physical inactivity compared with Whites in the national sample (OR, 1.40; 95% CI, 1.30–1.51).[139] A variety of factors explain the physical activity disparities in AAs. Physical activity barriers that exist in the AA community include the "built environment" (ie, the immediate exercise/walking environment). Lack of access to recreational or free exercise facilities, sidewalks, or age-appropriate physical activity programs are significant barriers to physical activity among AAs. Furthermore, oftentimes older AAs report they are less likely to exercise owing to family responsibilities or the lack of knowledge of the benefits of exercise.

In older AAs, like many other older adults, safety is a concern ranging from the fear of falls or concerns for personal safety in unsuitable neighborhoods. Suggested ways of reducing progression of chronic disease is to address and improve the built environment by developing safe sidewalks and attractive parks. In addition, AAs report that improved health, social support, and spirituality motivate physical activity. Although many AAs may have financial problems restraining them from being active, 1 solution is to develop low-cost physical activity venues and/or encourage home exercise with use of videos. In addition, other low-cost options are indoor malls and/or sites at work that are made available to employees at a reduced cost. Because safety from crime is an issue, this barrier can be attenuated by adjusting the time of day when exercising. Finally, public messages are needed that target the importance of exercise in populations such at risk for chronic diseases such as AAs.[138,139]

In 2010, only 14.4% of Hispanics aged 18 years or older met the 2008 Federal Physical Activity Guidelines.[51] Data from the NHIS showed that Hispanics were 2.09 times more likely to report inadequate levels of physical activity than NHWs.[140] Older Hispanic women were classified as among the least physically active groups in the country.[141,142] However, these prior studies did not account for the physical activity that occurs during normal working hours or for transportation-related physical activity. Occupational physical activity may be more important among Hispanics, because many more of them work in blue collar than white collar jobs, which tend to be more demanding physically.[143] When the BFRSS included occupation-related activity, the prevalence ratio for meeting physical activity guidelines increased from 0.85 to 0.97 of Hispanic men and from 0.88 to 0.93 for Hispanic women compared with NHW men and women, respectively.[144] Thus, previous studies that have only assessed leisure time physical activity may have underestimated levels of physical activity among Hispanic/Latino individuals. Acculturation may also play an important yet complex role. Previous research suggests that as immigrants become more acculturated, their lifestyle patterns approximate the pattern of US-born populations, experiencing a decline in physical activity, an increase in sedentary behavior, and greater consumption of calorie-rich foods.[145]

Overweight and Obesity

Obesity is a growing problem for US adults and an important cause of health disparities. An estimated 31.8% of children age 2 to 19 are overweight or obese. Among AA children, the rates are 36.9% of boys and 41.3% of girls. An estimated 68.2% of

Americans age 20 and older are overweight or obese with 68.7% of AA men and 79.9% of AA women are obese. Although obesity is similarly prevalent in AA and white men, it is twice as common in AA as in white women. From 1988 to 2000, the age-adjusted prevalence of obesity increased by 11.5% in AA women compared with 7.2% in white women.

The prevalence of obesity among Hispanic populations is generally higher than among NHW populations in the United States[146,147] and has increased from 1999 to 2002[148] (among Mexican participants in NHANES 2005–2008, 77.5% of men and 75.1% of women were overweight/obese [BMI $\geq$25 kg/m^2], and 31.4% of men and 43.4% of women were obese [BMI $\geq$30 kg/m^2]).[149] More recent NHANES 1999 to 2010 data show even higher rates of overweight/obesity and obesity among Mexicans (81.3% and 35.6% for men and 78.5% and 44.3% for women, respectively), with significant increases in overweight and obesity from 1999 through 2010.[150] Mexican HHANES participants had a higher mean BMI and higher age-adjusted prevalence of being overweight compared with Puerto Ricans and Cubans.[149] Contrary to what was seen in HHANES, the prevalence of obesity (BMI $\geq$30 kg/m^2) among HCHS/SOL participants was higher for Hispanic women (42.6%) than for men (36.5%), whereas the highest prevalence of obesity occurred among Puerto Rican men (40.9%) and women (51.4%) compared with the other Hispanic groups.[98] There is limited research regarding the efficacy of dietary and weight loss interventions in Hispanics. An important review by Lindberg and Stevens[151] discussed weight loss interventions that targeted Hispanics and concluded that most studies were limited in differentiation of Hispanic subgroups, level of acculturation, and socioeconomic status.[151]

Twelve articles compared rates of obesity among AI/AN communities versus other racial/ethnic groups. BRFSS survey data from 1997 through 2000 revealed higher rates of self-reported obesity for AI/AN respondents compared with respondents from all other racial/ethnic groups (23.9% vs 18.7%).[152] Aggregated BRFSS data from a later cohort (2000–2006) suggest that obesity is disproportionately increasing among AI/ANs compared with the NHW participants (29.6% compared with 20.9%).[153] Similarly, NHIS data between 2004 and 2008 found even higher rates of obesity among all racial/ethnic groups, but in particular among AI/AN populations in whom 39.4% were obese compared with 24.3% among NHW.[6] Higher rates of obesity are also observed among older AI/AN populations (>50 years of age) compared with NHWs (29.2% vs 22.7%; P = .05) based on BRFSS data between 2001 and 2004.[154] In the aforementioned study based on BRFSS data from 2000 to 2006, differences in obesity rates were slightly more pronounced for women (28.8% compared with 19.3%) compared with men (30.2% compared with 22.4%).[153] Amparo and colleagues[96] used BRFSS data from 2005 and 2007 to look at rates of obesity among AI/AN women of reproductive age and found that they were significantly more likely to report being obese than non-Hispanic women (25.8% vs 19.2%; P = .001). In terms of regional data, obesity rates across regions and communities are consistently higher among AI/AN populations compared with non-AI/ANs; however, the highest rates of obesity reported were among certain tribes of North Carolina.

Treatment

Faith-based interventions for obesity seem to be effective in AAs. Overall, 70% of interventions reported success in reducing weight, 60% reported increased fruit and vegetable intake, and 38% reported increased physical activity.[155] Several clinical interventions have shown success in obesity management in AAs. After 6 months, AA men had a mean 5.1% weight loss in the Weight Loss Maintenance trial's intensive intervention phase,[156] a mean 6.8% weight loss in the Look AHEAD trial (Action for Health in Diabetes),[157] and a 3% to 5% weight loss in PREMIER.[158] After 30 months, AA men maintained weight losses of 4.1, 6.1, and 3.7 kg across the weight loss maintenance trial's 3 arms (self-directed, interactive technology, and personal contact maintenance phases, respectively)[159] and maintained a significant 4.0% weight loss across the entire study.[160] A statistically significant weight loss (4.8 kg; 5.1% of weight) in the lifestyle component of the DPP was also noted after 30 months versus the placebo group ($P<.05$; West 2008). Hooker and colleagues[161] showed a statistically significant decrease in body weight (mean of 1.1 kg) across 8 weeks of intervention ($P<.05$). Treadwell and colleagues[162] showed a 2.5-kg weight loss after 6 weeks, and a 7% decrease in the percentage of individuals who were obese and overweight. A 6-month intervention showed a nonsignificant 2.0-kg difference between a weight loss/physical activity promotion intervention and a usual care group ($P = .26$). Kumanyika and colleagues[163] reported that weight loss for AA men in the weight loss intervention was 3.5 kg after 18 months in TOHP I (Trial of Hypertension Prevention I) and 0.7 kg after 36 months in the HPT (Hypertension Prevention Trial) weight loss intervention group. Mean net weight loss for AA men in the weight loss arm in TOHP II was 1.6 kg after 36 months.[164] Only 5% of men in the Cardiovascular Dietary Education System counseling intervention lost greater than 5% of their body weight.[165,166]

Ninety-one percent of Hispanics report some religious affiliation, with Roman Catholic affiliation being the most common (56%), although Protestant denominations are embraced by 23%. As such, Hispanics are often religious, and their way of expressing religious worship is often different from that of the US dominant culture.[167] Hispanics are more likely to see a link between body, mind, and spiritual health. A consequence of spirituality is a sense of fatalism or *destino*, in which life experiences, events, and adversities are inevitable and cannot be controlled or prevented. Such thinking leads to the fatalistic attitude that "whatever God wants, shall be" ("*lo que Dios quiera*"). Fatalistic beliefs have been correlated with a variety of negative health outcomes, including CVD,[168] as well as protective factors that reduce drug abuse among Hispanic youths.[167,169] Because religious networks and norms sometimes help to guide health behaviors, there is evidence that the deployment of interventions at Hispanic churches can serve as a motivating source of health education and fellowship, similar to what has occurred in the non-Hispanic black community.[170–172]

Diabetes Mellitus

In the total population age 20 and older, 8.3% have physician-diagnosed diabetes. Among AAs, the prevalence is 13.5% of men and 15.4% of women. Diabetes mellitus increases risk for CHD at least 2-fold to 4-fold. Furthermore, vascular complications in patients who have diabetes appear at a younger age, affect women as often as men, and are more often fatal than in patients who do not have diabetes. Atherosclerotic plaques in patients who have diabetes seem to be morphologically similar to those in patients who do not have diabetes and differ only by the extent and severity of atherosclerotic disease. AAs and other nonwhite minorities have a greater burden of diabetes, and its vascular complications are greater than in whites. The prevalence of type 2 diabetes mellitus in AAs is 2 to 3 times higher than in whites. In the United States, approximately 11.4% of AAs aged 20 years or older (2.7 million) have diabetes.

Glycemic control is worse in Hispanics than in NHWs, and Hispanics are more likely to have undiagnosed diabetes mellitus than non-Hispanic blacks and NHWs.[173] Although the prevalence of diabetes mellitus also varied by educational attainment among all Hispanic subgroups, it remained higher among Mexican participants compared with NHWs irrespective of their level of education.[174] Not only is the burden of diabetes mellitus higher for Hispanics, but the profile of diabetes mellitus-related complications in Hispanics (compared with NHWs) is variable: chronic kidney disease and retinopathy are more prevalent, whereas CVD morbidity and mortality are lower, although increasing acculturation leads to higher mortality.[175] The prevalence of type 2 diabetes mellitus is found to be consistently higher among Hispanics than among NHWs. Major surveys (NHANES, BRFSS) show that the prevalence of diabetes mellitus is twice as high among Hispanics as among NHWs.[176] Hispanics are also 1.5 times more likely to die of diabetes mellitus than NHWs.[175] People of Hispanic descent currently lead the epidemic of diabetes mellitus in the United States, particularly in areas of south Florida, Texas, and California.[177] The prevalence of physician-diagnosed diabetes mellitus was 11% in Mexican men and 12.7% in Mexican women; an additional 6.3% and 3.8% were estimated to have undiagnosed diabetes mellitus (fasting plasma glucose $\geq$126 mg/dL).[59] The higher incidence of diabetes mellitus among Mexicans is attributable to a large extent to a higher prevalence of insulin resistance.[178] Among HHANES participants, the age-standardized prevalence of diagnosed and undiagnosed diabetes was similar for Mexicans and Puerto Ricans (approximately 13%) but lower among Cubans (9.3%).[179] In the NHIS, rates of self-reported diabetes mellitus were higher among Puerto Ricans and Mexicans (11% and 10%), whereas Cubans, Dominicans, and Central/South Americans had a lower prevalence. Among MESA participants, Mexicans had the highest prevalence of diabetes mellitus[20] (HCHS/SOL documented a higher prevalence of diabetes mellitus among Hispanic women [17.2%] than among Hispanic men [16.7%]). The prevalence of diabetes mellitus was highest among Mexican men, Mexican women, and Puerto Rican women (19%); both South American men and women had the lowest prevalence of diabetes mellitus (10%).

Eighteen studies reported data on diabetes. One combined BRFSS data from 1997 through 2000 and showed that the prevalence for AI/AN was self-reported to be 9.7% (95% CI, 8.3–11.1) compared with a prevalence of 5.7% (95% CI, 5.6–5.8) for all other races.[152] Analyses of later BRFSS surveys reveal a marked increase in diabetes among AI/AN: the prevalence of diabetes among AI/ANs in 2000 to 2006 had increased to 12.4%, whereas the rate among NHWs remained relatively stable at 6.0%.[153] NHIS data between 2004 and 2008 corroborate this trend, revealing diabetes in 17.5% of AI/AN respondents compared with 6.6% of NHWs (17.5% vs 6.6%).[10] Rios Burrows and colleagues[180] also described this alarming increase in the rate of diabetes among AI/AN, using the Indian Health Service national outpatient database from 1990 through 1997. These investigators found that the rate (both crude and age adjusted) increased by 29% over this period. This trend varied by region, ranging from a 16% increase in the Northern Plains to 76% in the Alaska region. The authors compared these rates of increased prevalence to national increases of 14% in the general US population during this period.[180] The age-adjusted prevalence was found to be almost 3 times the prevalence among US NHWs. A report in *Morbidity and Mortality Weekly* also used the Indian Health Service national outpatient database to identify diabetes prevalence for each year between 1994 and 2002 and compared these rates to the prevalence of diabetes during the same time period based on BRFSS national results. The study revealed that the age-adjusted prevalence of diabetes increased by 33.2% (from 11.5% to 15.3%) for the AI/AN population, whereas the prevalence of diabetes in all US adults increased by 54.0% (4.8% to 7.3%).[181] Notably, the age-adjusted prevalence of diabetes in AI/AN adults was more than twice that of US adults for each year of the study.[181]

Risk Factor Clustering and the Metabolic Syndrome

UPs are more likely than whites to have multiple CHD risk factors. The presence of multiple risk factors increases CHD risk in an exponential fashion. Although the etiology of risk factor clustering is unknown, genetic and environmental factors have been implicated. The metabolic syndrome—also known as insulin resistance syndrome—refers to a specific clustering of cardiovascular risk factors in the same individual (abdominal obesity, atherogenic dyslipidemia, elevated BP, insulin resistance, a prothrombotic state, and a proinflammatory state). The AHA and the National Heart, Lung, and Blood Institute define the metabolic syndrome as a constellation of metabolic risk factors strongly associated with type 2 diabetes—atherogenic dyslipidemia (elevated triglycerides and apolipoprotein B, small LDL-C particles, and low levels of high-density lipoprotein cholesterol), elevated BP, elevated plasma glucose, a prothrombotic state, and a proinflammatory state. Patients with the metabolic syndrome are at increased risk for the development of diabetes and CVD. According to a recent analysis of data from the NHANES III, approximately 47 million Americans (23.7% of the population) have the metabolic syndrome. AA women and Hispanic men and women have the highest prevalences of the metabolic syndrome, which may be attributable to the disproportionate occurrence of elevated BP, obesity, and diabetes in AAs and the high prevalence of obesity in Hispanics. Management of the metabolic syndrome consists primarily of modification glucose intolerance and treatment of the risk factors. The first strategy involves weight reduction and increased physical activity, both of which can improve all components of the syndrome. The second strategy involves treatment of the individual risk factors to further improve BP, lipids, and glucose, thereby decreasing the risk of CVD. According to 1 recent analysis, aggressive management of elevated BP and dyslipidemia in individuals with the metabolic syndrome and control to optimal levels could result in the prevention of more than 80% of cardiovascular events.

Data from the 1999 to 2002 NHANES reports combined CVD risk profiles (BP, metabolic and inflammatory risk) and found that although foreign-born Mexicans and NHWs had similar combined risk profiles, US-born Mexicans were at higher risk.[182] HCHS/SOL recently examined the prevalence of combined adverse CVD risk factors (including hypercholesterolemia, HTN, diabetes mellitus, obesity, and smoking) and found that the prevalence was highest among Puerto Ricans, lower socioeconomic status Hispanics, and those with higher acculturation levels.[98] The prevalence of 3 or more major CVD risk factors was higher for Hispanic men (21.3%) than women (17.4%). Among Hispanic subgroups, both Puerto Rican men (24.9%) and women (25.0%) had the highest prevalence of having 3 or more major CVD risk factors. Similarly, ideal cardiovascular health (CVH) among Hispanics is low. Among Mexican NHANES participants, the prevalence of low CVD risk factor burden was only 7.5% in 1988 to 1994 and decreased to 5.3% in 1999 to 2004.[183] A Hispanic cohort of mostly Caribbean Hispanics also showed lower ideal CVH among Hispanics (3.2%) than NHWs (7.7%).[184,185] Although recent results from HCHS/SOL are better than what has been documented previously, only 20.2% of Hispanic men and 29.3% of Hispanic women met ideal CVH targets.[98]

Two studies provided data on comparative rates of the metabolic syndrome. Schumacher and colleagues[186] measured the prevalence of metabolic syndrome using a convenience sample of Alaska natives living in 26 villages as well as members of the Navajo Nation in Arizona and New Mexico. Sufficient data to determine presence of metabolic syndrome (including fasting blood sugar) was obtained for 3498 Alaskan natives and 4534 Navajos between 2004 and 2006. Because women were oversampled in the Alaska native population, data were presented stratified by gender. The authors found that 34.9% of AI/AN men and 40.0% of AI/AN women had metabolic syndrome, versus 24.8% and 22.8% among non-Hispanic men and women, respectively, based on NHANES data from 1988 to 1994.[186] Another cross-sectional study measured the prevalence of the metabolic syndrome between 2003 and 2006 among 4457 AI individuals living on or near reservations in the Northern Plains and Southwestern Unite States.[39] They found that the overall age-adjusted prevalence of the metabolic syndrome was 49.8% (95% CI, 47.8–50.7), compared with 34.0% in the general population based on NHANES data during the same period.[187] In subgroup analyses, they found that the prevalence of metabolic syndrome in nondiabetic AI men between the ages of 20 and 39 years was nearly twice the rate for similarly aged NHWs without diabetes (39.2% compared with 20%).[187] The differences in rates of metabolic syndrome were also striking among younger individuals, in which more than one-half of the AI population under 40 years of age had the metabolic syndrome compared with 20.3% of the younger NHANES population.

SUMMARY

AAs are at increased risk for HTN, hyperlipidemia, obesity, and diabetes, which contribute to the burden of CVD. The disparities of CVD in UPs require targeted attention from primary care clinicians to eliminate. Primary care can provide this targeted care for their patients by assessing cardiovascular risk, addressing BP control, and selecting appropriate intervention strategies. Using community resources is also effective for addressing CVD disparities in the UP.

REFERENCES

1. CDC High Blood Pressure Facts. Available at: http://www.cdc.gov/bloodpressure/facts.htm. Accessed December 6, 2015.
2. American Heart Association Statistical Fact Sheet 2013 Update. Available at: www.heart.org/idc/groups/heart public/@wcm/@sop/@smd/documents/downloadable/ucm_319568.pdf. Accessed December 6, 2015.
3. Rodriquez CJ, Allison M, Daviglus ML, et al. Status of cardiovascular disease and stoke in Hispanics/Latinos in the United States. Circulation 2014;130(7): 593–625.
4. National Alliance for Hispanic Health. Delivering health care to Hispanics: a manual for providers. Washington, DC: National Alliance for Hispanic Health; 2003.
5. Mosca L, Ferris A, Fabunmi R, et al. Tracking women's awareness of heart disease: an American Heart Association national study. Circulation 2004;109: 573–9.
6. Borrell LN, Lancet EA. Race/ethnicity and all-cause mortality in US adults: revisiting the Hispanic paradox. Am J Public Health 2012;102:836–43.
7. Abraído-Lanza AF, Dohrenwend BP, Ng-Mak DS, et al. The Latino mortality paradox: a test of the "salmon bias" and healthy migrant hypotheses. Am J Public Health 1999;89:1543–8.
8. Hummer RA. Adult mortality differentials among Hispanic subgroups and non-Hispanic whites. Soc Sci Q 2000;81:459–76.
9. Hajat A, Lucas JB, Kington R. Health outcomes among Hispanic subgroups: data from the National Health Interview Survey, 1992–95. Adv Data 2000;(310):1–14.

10. Barnes PM, Adams PF, Powell-Griner E. Health characteristics of the American Indian or Alaska Native adult population: United States, 2004–2008. Natl Health Stat Report 2010;20:1–22.

11. Jernigan VB, Duran B, Ahn D, et al. Changing patterns in health behaviors and risk factors related to cardiovascular disease among American Indians and Alaska Natives. Am J Public Health 2010;100:677–83.

12. Davis AM, Vinci LM, Okwuosa TM, et al. Cardiovascular health disparities: a systematic review of health care interventions. Med Care Res Rev 2007;64(5 Suppl):29S–100S.

13. Singh V, Deedwania P. Dyslipidemia in special populations: Asian Indians, African Americans, and Hispanics. Curr Atheroscler Rep 2006;8(1):32–40.

14. Mozaffarian D, Benjamin EJ, Go AS, et al, on behalf of the American Heart Association Statistics Committee and Stroke Statistics Subcommittee. Heart disease and stroke statistics—2015 update: a report from the American Heart Association. Circulation 2015;131(4):e535.

15. Giovannucci E, Liu Y, Hollis BW, et al. 25-hydroxyvitamin D and risk of myocardial infarction in men. Arch Intern Med 2008;168(11):1174–80.

16. Harris RA, Pedersen-White J, Guo DH, et al. Vitamin D3 supplementation for 16 weeks improves flow-mediated dilation in overweight African-American adults. Am J Hypertens 2011;24(5):557–62.

17. Pilz S, Gaksch M, Kienreich K, et al. Effects of vitamin D on blood pressure and cardiovascular risk factors: a randomized controlled trial. Hypertension 2015; 65(6):1195–201.

18. Donneyong MM, Hornung CA, Taylor KC, et al. Risk of heart failure among postmenopausal women: a secondary analysis of the randomized trial of vitamin D plus calcium of the women's health initiative. Circ Heart Fail 2015;8(1):49–56.

19. Bild DE, Detrano R, Peterson D, et al. Ethnic differences in coronary calcification: the Multi-Ethnic Study of Atherosclerosis (MESA). Circulation 2005;111: 1313–20.

20. Allison MA, Budoff MJ, Wong ND, et al. Prevalence of and risk factors for subclinical cardiovascular disease in selected US Hispanic ethnic groups: the Multi-Ethnic Study of Atherosclerosis. Am J Epidemiol 2008;167:962–9.

21. Diez Roux AV, Detrano R, Jackson S, et al. Acculturation and socioeconomic position as predictors of coronary calcification in a multiethnic sample. Circulation 2005;112:1557–65.

22. Gallo LC, de Los Monteros KE, Allison M, et al. Do socioeconomic gradients in subclinical atherosclerosis vary according to acculturation level? Analyses of Mexican-Americans in the Multi-Ethnic Study of Atherosclerosis. Psychosom Med 2009;71:756–62.

23. Detrano R, Guerci AD, Carr JJ, et al. Coronary calcium as a predictor of coronary events in four racial or ethnic groups. N Engl J Med 2008;358:1336–45.

24. McClelland RL, Jorgensen NW, Budoff M, et al. 10-Year Coronary Heart Disease Risk Prediction Using Coronary Artery Calcium and Traditional Risk Factors: Derivation in the MESA (Multi-Ethnic Study of Atherosclerosis) With Validation in the HNR (Heinz Nixdorf Recall) Study and the DHS (Dallas Heart Study). J Am Coll Cardiol 2015;66(15):1643–53.

25. Lackland DT, Elkind MS, D'Agostino R Sr, et al, American Heart Association Stroke Council, Council on Epidemiology and Prevention, Council on Cardiovascular Radiology and Intervention, Council on Cardiovascular Nursing, Council on Peripheral Vascular Disease, Council on Quality of Care and Outcomes Research. Inclusion of stroke in cardiovascular risk prediction instruments: a

statement for healthcare professionals from the American Heart Association/ American Stroke Association. Stroke 2012;43(7):1998–2027.

26. Raheem OA, Su JJ, Wilson JR, et al. The association of erectile dysfunction and cardiovascular disease: a systematic critical review. Am J Mens Health 2016. [Epub ahead of print].

27. Stone NJ, Robinson JG, Lichtenstein AH, et al, American College of Cardiology/ American Heart Association Task Force on Practice Guidelines. 2013 ACC/AHA guideline on the treatment of blood cholesterol to reduce atherosclerotic cardio-vascular risk in adults: a report of the American College of Cardiology/American Heart Association Task Force on Practice Guidelines. J Am Coll Cardiol 2014; 63(25 Pt B):2889–934.

28. Park SJ, Park DW. Percutaneous coronary intervention with stent implantation versus coronary artery bypass surgery for treatment of left main coronary artery disease: is it time to change guidelines? Circ Cardiovasc Interv 2009;2(1): 59–68.

29. Poludasu S, Cavusoglu E, Khan W, et al. All-cause mortality after drug-eluting stent implantation in African-Americans. Coron Artery Dis 2008;19(8):551–7.

30. McBean AM, Gornick M. Differences by Race in the Rates of Procedures Per-formed in Hospitals for Medicare Beneficiaries. Health Care Financ Rev 1994; 15(4):77–90.

31. Lillie-Blanton M, Maddox TM, Rushing O, et al. Disparities in cardiac care: rising to the challenge of Healthy People 2010. J Am Coll Cardiol 2004;44(3):503–8.

32. Hravnak M, Ibrahim S, Kaufer A, et al. Racial disparities in outcomes following coronary artery bypass grafting. J Cardiovasc Nurs 2006;21(5):367–78.

33. Yeo KK, Li Z, Amsterdam E. Clinical characteristics and 30-day mortality among Caucasians, Hispanics, Asians, And African-Americans in the 2003 California coronary artery bypass graft surgery outcomes reporting program. Am J Cardiol 2007;100(1):59–63.

34. Michael Smith J, Soneson EA, Woods SE, et al. Coronary artery bypass graft surgery outcomes among African-Americans and Caucasian patients. Int J Surg 2006;4(4):212–6.

35. Efird JT, Griffin WF, Sarpong DF, et al. Increased long-term mortality among black CABG patients receiving preoperative inotropic agents. Int J Environ Res Public Health 2015;12(7):7478–90.

36. Vandvik PO, Lincoff AM, Gore JM, et al, American College of Chest Physicians. Primary and secondary prevention of cardiovascular disease: antithrombotic therapy and prevention of thrombosis, 9th ed: American College of Chest Phy-sicians evidence-based clinical practice guidelines. Chest 2012;141(2 Suppl): e637S–68S.

37. Cruden NL, Din JN, Janssen C, et al. Prolonged clopidogrel use is associated with improved clinical outcomes following drug-eluting but not bare metal stent implantation. Am J Cardiovasc Drugs 2016;16(2):111–8.

38. Johnson D, Sacrinty M, Mehta H, et al. Cardiac rehabilitation in African Ameri-cans: evidence for poorer outcomes compared with whites, especially in women and diabetic participants. Am Heart J 2015;169(1):102–7.

39. Schneider RH, Grim CE, Rainforth MV, et al. Stress reduction in the secondary prevention of cardiovascular disease: randomized, controlled trial of transcen-dental meditation and health education in Blacks. Circ Cardiovasc Qual Out-comes 2012;5(6):750–8.

40. Shah S. Review: heart failure with preserved ejection fraction in African Ameri-cans. Ethn Dis 2012;22(4):432–8.

41. Ferdinand KC. African American heart failure trial: role of endothelial dysfunction and heart failure in African Americans. Am J Cardiol 2007;99(6B):3D–6D.

42. Baharami H, Kronmal R, Bluemke DA, et al. Differences in the incidence of congestive heart failure by ethnicity: the Multiethnic Study of Atherosclerosis. Arch Intern Med 2008;168:2138–45.

43. Cuyjet AB, Akinboboye O. Acute heart failure in the African American patient. J Card Fail 2014;20:533–40.

44. Yancy CW. Heart failure in African Americans. Am J Cardiol 2005;96(7B):3i–12i.

45. Mansour IN, Bress AP, Groo V, et al. Circulating procollagen type III N-terminal peptide and mortality risk in African Americans with heart failure. J Card Fail 2016;22(9):692–9.

46. El-Refai M, Hrobowski T, Peterson EL, et al. Race and association of angiotensin converting enzyme/angiotensin receptor blocker exposure with outcome in heart failure. J Cardiovasc Med (Hagerstown) 2015;16(9):591–6.

47. Anand IS, Win S, Rector TS, et al. Effect of fixed-dose combination of isosorbide dinitrate and hydralazine on all hospitalizations and on 30-day readmission rates in patients with heart failure: results from the African-American Heart Failure Trial. Circ Heart Fail 2014;7(5):759–65.

48. Ferdinand KC, Elkayam U, Mancini D, et al. Use of isosorbide dinitrate and hydralazine in African-Americans with heart failure 9 years after the African-American Heart Failure Trial. Am J Cardiol 2014;114(1):151–9.

49. Taylor JSW, Ellis GR. Racial Differences in Response to Drug Treatment: Implications for Pharmacotherapy of Heart Failure. Am J Cardiovasc Drugs 2002; 2(6):389–99.

50. Ziaeian B, Zhang Y, Albert NM, et al. Clinical effectiveness of CRT and ICD therapy in heart failure patients by racial/ethnic classification: insights from the IMPROVE HF registry. J Am Coll Cardiol 2014;64(8):797–807.

51. Go AS, Mozaffarian D, Roger VL, et al, on behalf of the American Heart Association Statistics Committee and Stroke Statistics Subcommittee. Heart disease and stroke statistics: 2014 update: a report from the American Heart Association. Circulation 2014;129:e28–292.

52. Vivo RP, Krim SR, Krim NR, et al. Care and outcomes of Hispanic patients admitted with heart failure with preserved or reduced ejection fraction: findings from Get With The Guidelines–Heart Failure. Circ Heart Fail 2012;5:167–75.

53. Aronow WS, Ahn C, Kronzon I. Comparison of incidences of congestive heart failure in older African-Americans, Hispanics, and whites. Am J Cardiol 1999; 84:611–2.

54. Bressler J, Franceschini N, Demerath EW, et al. Sequence variation in telomerase reverse transcriptase (TERT) as a determinant of risk of cardiovascular disease: the Atherosclerosis Risk in Communities (ARIC) study. BMC Med Genet 2015;16:52.

55. Carty CL, Keene KL, Cheng YC, et al, COMPASS and METASTROKE Consortia. Meta-Analysis of Genome-Wide Association Studies Identifies Genetic Risk Factors for Stroke in African Americans. Stroke 2015;46(8):2063–8.

56. Caughey MC, Loehr LR, Key NS, et al. Sickle cell trait and incident ischemic stroke in the Atherosclerosis Risk in Communities study. Stroke 2014;45(10): 2863–7.

57. Ruland S, Gorelick PB. Stroke in Black Americans. Curr Cardiol Rep 2005;7(1): 29–33.

58. Smith MA, Risser JM, Lisabeth LD, et al. Access to care, acculturation, and risk factors for stroke in Mexican Americans: the Brain Attack Surveillance in Corpus Christi (BASIC) project. Stroke 2003;34:2671–5.

59. Roger VL, Go AS, Lloyd-Jones DM, et al, on behalf of the American Heart Association Statistics Committee and Stroke Statistics Subcommittee. Heart disease and stroke statistics: 2012 update: a report from the American Heart Association. Circulation 2012;125:e2–220.

60. White H, Boden-Albala B, Wang C, et al. Ischemic stroke subtype incidence among whites, blacks, and Hispanics: the Northern Manhattan Study. Circulation 2005;111:1327–31.

61. Rodriguez CJ, Homma S, Sacco RL, et al, PICSS Investigators. Race-ethnic differences in patent foramen ovale, atrial septal aneurysm, and right atrial anatomy among ischemic stroke patients. Stroke 2003;34:2097–102.

62. Ayala C, Croft JB, Greenlund KJ, et al. Sex differences in US mortality rates for stroke and stroke subtypes by race/ethnicity and age, 1995–1998. Stroke 2002; 33:1197–201.

63. Rhoades DA. Racial misclassification and disparities in cardiovascular disease among American Indians and Alaska Natives. Circulation 2005;111:1250–6.

64. Howard BV, Lee ET, Cowan LD, et al. Rising tide of cardiovascular disease in American Indians. The Strong Heart Study. Circulation 1999;99:2389–95.

65. Zhang Y, Galloway JM, Welty TK, et al. Incidence and risk factors for stroke in American Indians: the Strong Heart Study. Circulation 2008;118:1577–84.

66. Liebson PR. Cardiovascular disease in special populations III: stoke. Prev Cardiol 2010;13(1):1–7.

67. Howard VJ. Reasons underlying racial differences in stroke incidence and mortality. Stroke 2013;44(601):S126–8.

68. Gorelick PB, Richardson D, Kelly M, et al, African American Antiplatelet Stroke Prevention Study Investigators. Aspirin and ticlopidine for prevention of recurrent stroke in black patients: a randomized trial. JAMA 2003;289(22):2947–57.

69. Ghidei W, Collins TC. African Americans and peripheral arterial disease: a review article. Vasc Med 2012;2012:9.

70. Collins TC, Johnson SL, Souchek J. Unsupervised walking therapy and atherosclerotic risk-factor management for patients with peripheral arterial disease: a pilot trial. Ann Behav Med 2007;33(3):318–24.

71. Selvin E, Erlinger TP. Prevalence of and risk factors for peripheral arterial disease in the United States: results from the National Health and Nutrition Examination Survey, 1999– 2000. Circulation 2004;110(6):738–43.

72. Hankey GJ, Norman PE, Eikelboom JW. Medical treatment of peripheral arterial disease. J Am Med Assoc 2006;295(5):547–53.

73. Morrissey J, Giacovelli J, Egorova N, et al. Disparities in the treatment and outcomes of vascular disease in Hispanic patients. J Vasc Surg 2007;46:971–8.

74. Lavery LA, Ashry HR, van Houtum W, et al. Variation in the incidence and proportion of diabetes-related amputations in minorities. Diabetes Care 1996;19: 48–52.

75. Collins TC, Petersen NJ, Suarez-Almazor M, et al. The prevalence of peripheral arterial disease in a racially diverse population. Arch Intern Med 2003;163: 1469–74.

76. Mendelson G, Aronow WS, Ahn C. Prevalence of coronary artery disease, atherothrombotic brain infarction, and peripheral arterial disease: associated risk factors in older Hispanics in an academic hospital-based geriatrics practice. J Am Geriatr Soc 1998;46:481–3.

77. Hirsch AT, Haskal ZJ, Hertzer NR, et al. ACC/AHA 2005 practice guidelines for the management of patients with peripheral arterial disease (lower extremity, renal, mesenteric, and abdominal aortic): a collaborative report from the American Association for Vascular Surgery/Society for Vascular Surgery, Society for Cardiovascular Angiography and Interventions, Society for Vascular Medicine and Biology, Society of Interventional Radiology, and the ACC/AHA Task Force on Practice Guidelines (Writing Committee to Develop Guidelines for the Management of Patients With Peripheral Arterial Disease. Circulation 2006;113: e463–654.

78. Allison MA, Peralta CA, Wassel CL, et al. Genetic ancestry and lower extremity peripheral artery disease in the Multi-Ethnic Study of Atherosclerosis. Vasc Med 2010;15:351–9.

79. Aronow WS. Office management of peripheral arterial disease. Am J Med 2010; 123(9):790–2.

80. Girolami B, Bernardi E, Prins MH, et al. Treatment of intermittent claudication with physical training, smoking cessation, pentoxifylline, or nafronyl: a meta-analysis. Arch Intern Med 1999;159(4):337–45.

81. Barone Gibbs B, Dobrosielske DA, Althouse AD, et al. The effect of exercise training on ankle-brachial index in type 2 diabetes. Atherosclerosis 2013; 230(1):125–30.

82. Ferdinand KC. Recommendations for the management of special populations: racial and ethnic populations. Am J Hypertens 2003;16(11 Pt 2):50S–4S.

83. Flack JM, Nasser SA, Levy PD. Therapy of hypertension in African Americans. Am J Cardiovasc Drugs 2011;11(2):83–92.

84. Kones R. Primary prevention of coronary heart disease: integration of new data, evolving views, revised goals, and role of rosuvastatin in management. A comprehensive survey. Drug Des Devel Ther 2011;5:325–80.

85. Do AN, Lynch AI, Claas SA, et al. The effects of genes implicated in cardiovascular disease on blood pressure response to treatment among treatment-naive hypertensive African Americans in the GenHAT study. J Hum Hypertens 2016; 30(9):549–54.

86. Dolezsar CM, McGrath JJ, Herzig AJ, et al. Perceived racial discrimination and hypertension: a comprehensive systematic review. Health Psychol 2014;33(1): 20–34.

87. Hajjar I, Kotchen TA. Trends in prevalence, awareness, treatment, and control of hypertension in the United States, 1988–2000. JAMA 2003;290:199–206.

88. Haffner SM, Mitchell BD, Stern MP, et al. Decreased prevalence of hypertension in Mexican-Americans. Hypertension 1990;16:225–32.

89. Go AS, Mozaffarian D, Roger VL, et al, on behalf of the American Heart Association Statistics Committee and Stroke Statistics Subcommittee. Heart disease and stroke statistics: 2013 update: a report from the American Heart Association. Circulation 2013;127:e6–245.

90. Qureshi AI, Suri MF, Kirmani JF, et al. Prevalence and trends of prehypertension and hypertension in United States: National Health and Nutrition Examination Surveys 1976 to 2000. Med Sci Monit 2005;11:CR403–9.

91. Ong KL, Cheung BM, Man YB, et al. Prevalence, awareness, treatment, and control of hypertension among United States adults 1999–2004. Hypertension 2007;49:69–75.

92. Burt VL, Whelton P, Roccella EJ, et al. Prevalence of hypertension in the US adult population: results from the Third National Health and Nutrition Examination Survey, 1988–1991. Hypertension 1995;25:305–13.

93. Egan BM, Zhao Y, Axon RN. US trends in prevalence, awareness, treatment, and control of hypertension, 1988–2008. JAMA 2010;303:2043–50.

94. Cutler JA, Sorlie PD, Wolz M, et al. Trends in hypertension prevalence, awareness, treatment, and control rates in United States adults between 1988–1994 and 1999–2004. Hypertension 2008;52:818–27.

95. Zhao G, Ford E, Mokdad A. Racial/ethnic variation in hypertension-related lifestyle behaviours among US women with self-reported hypertension. J Hum Hypertens 2008;22:608–16.

96. Amparo P, Farr SL, Dietz PM. Chronic disease risk factors among American Indian/Alaska Native women of reproductive age. Prev Chronic Dis 2011;8:A118.

97. Harwell TS, Gohdes D, Moore K, et al. Indians. Am J Prev Med 2001;20:196–201.

98. Daviglus ML, Talavera GA, Avilés-Santa ML, et al. Prevalence of major cardiovascular risk factors and cardiovascular diseases among Hispanic/Latino individuals of diverse backgrounds in the United States. JAMA 2012;308(17):1775–84.

99. Sorlie PD, Allison MA, Aviles-Santa ML, et al. Prevalence of hypertension, awareness, treatment, and control in the Hispanic community health study/study of Latinos. Am J Hypertens 2014;27(6):793–800.

100. Todorova IL, Falcon LM, Lincoln AK, et al. Perceived discrimination, psychological distress and health. Sociol Health Illn 2010;32:843–61.

101. Hakimzadeh S, Cohn D. English usage among Hispanics in the United States. Washington, DC: Pew Research Center; 2007. Pew Research Hispanic Trends Project.

102. Pérez DJ, Fortuna L, Alegria M. Prevalence and correlates of everyday discrimination among U.S. Latinos. J Community Psychol 2008;36:421–33.

103. Pew Hispanic Center. Between two worlds: how young Latinos come of age in America. Washington, DC: Pew Research Center; 2009. Pew Research Hispanic Trends Project.

104. Lee MA, Ferraro KF. Perceived discrimination and health among Puerto Rican and Mexican Americans: buffering effect of the Lazo matrimonial? Soc Sci Med 2009;68:1966–74.

105. Brondolo E, Hausmann LR, Jhalani J, et al. Dimensions of perceived racism and self-reported health: examination of racial/ethnic differences and potential mediators. Ann Behav Med 2011;42:14–28.

106. Richardson SI, Freedman BI, Ellison DH, et al. Salt sensitivity: a review with a focus on non-Hispanic blacks and Hispanics. J Am Soc Hypertens 2013;7(2):170–9.

107. Laffer CL, Elijovich F. Essential hypertension of Caribbean Hispanics: sodium, renin, and response to therapy. J Clin Hypertens (Greenwich) 2002;4:266–73.

108. Sacco RL, Boden-Albala B, Abel G, et al. Race-ethnic disparities in the impact of stroke risk factors. Stroke 2001;32:1725–31.

109. Rodriguez CJ, Diez-Roux AV, Moran A, et al. Left ventricular mass and ventricular remodeling among Hispanic subgroups compared with non-Hispanic blacks and whites: MESA (Multi-ethnic Study of Atherosclerosis). J Am Coll Cardiol 2010;55:234–42.

110. Hyman DJ, Ogbonnaya K, Taylor AA, et al. Ethnic differences in nocturnal blood pressure decline in treated hypertensives. Am J Hypertens 2000;13:884–91.

111. Hoffmann I, Alfieri A, Cubeddu L. Effects of lifestyle changes and metformin on salt sensitivity and nitric oxide metabolism in obese salt-sensitive Hispanics. J Hum Hypertens 2007;21:571–8.

112. Ferdinand KC, Armani AM. The management of hypertension in African Americans. Crit Pathw Cardiol 2007;6(2):67–71.

113. Flack JM, Okwuosa T, Sudhakar R, et al. Should African Americans have a lower blood pressure goal than other ethnic groups to prevent organ damage? Curr Cardiol Rep 2012;14(6):660–6.

114. Calhoun DA, Jones D, Textor S, et al. Resistant hypertension: diagnosis, evaluation, and treatment: a scientific statement from the American Heart Association Professional Education Committee of the Council for High Blood Pressure Research. Circulation 2008;117:e510–26.

115. Flack JM, Victor R, Watson K, et al. Improved attainment of blood pressure and cholesterol goals using single-pill amlodipine/atorvastatin in African Americans: the CAPABLE trial. Mayo Clin Proc 2008;83(1):35–45.

116. Douglas JG. Clinical guidelines for the treatment of hypertension in African Americans. Am J Cardiovasc Drugs 2005;5(1):1–6.

117. Bangalore S, Ogedegbe G, Gyamfi J, et al. Outcomes with Angiotensin-converting enzyme inhibitors vs other antihypertensive agents in hypertensive blacks. Am J Med 2015;128(11):1195–203.

118. Toto RD. Lessons from the African-American Study of Kidney Disease and Hypertension: an update. Curr Hypertens Rep 2006;8(5):409–12.

119. Turner BJ, Hollenbeak CS, Liang Y, et al. A randomized trial of peer coach and office staff support to reduce coronary heart disease risk in African-Americans with uncontrolled hypertension. J Gen Intern Med 2012;27(10):1258–64.

120. Bala M, Strzeszynski L, Cahill K. Mass media interventions for smoking cessation in adults. Cochrane database of systematic reviews. Chichester (United Kingdom): John Wiley & Sons, Ltd; 2008.

121. Ahluwalia JS, McNagny SE, Clark WS. Smoking cessation among inner-city African Americans using the nicotine transdermal patch. J Gen Intern Med 1998; 13:1–8.

122. Ahluwalia JS, Harris KJ, Catley D, et al. Sustained-release bupropion for smoking cessation in African Americans a randomized controlled trial. JAMA 2002; 288:468–74.

123. Giovino GA. Epidemiology of tobacco use in the United States. Oncogene 2002; 21:7326–40.

124. Chowdhury PP, Balluz L, Okoro C, et al. Leading health indicators: a of Hispanics with non-Hispanic whites and non-Hispanic blacks, United States 2003. Ethn Dis 2006;16:534–41.

125. Centers for Disease Control and Prevention (CDC). Cigarette smoking among adults and trends in smoking cessation: United States, 2008. MMWR Morb Mortal Wkly Rep 2009;58:1227–32.

126. Centers for Disease Control and Prevention (CDC). Vital signs: current cigarette smoking among adults aged $\geq$18 years: United States, 2005–2010. MMWR Morb Mortal Wkly Rep 2011;60:1207–12.

127. Pérez-Stable EJ, Ramirez A, Villareal R, et al. Cigarette smoking behavior among US Latino men and women from different countries of origin. Am J Public Health 2001;91:1424–30.

128. Centers for Disease Control and Prevention (CDC). Tobacco use among adults: United States, 2005. MMWR Morb Mortal Wkly Rep 2006;55:1145–8.

129. Bethel JW, Schenker MB. Acculturation and smoking patterns among Hispanics: a review. Am J Prev Med 2005;29:143–8.

130. Derby CA, Wildman RP, McGinn AP, et al. Cardiovascular risk factor variation within a Hispanic cohort: SWAN, the Study of Women's Health Across the Nation. Ethn Dis 2010;20:396–402.

131. Orleans CT, Boyd NR, Bingler R, et al. A self-help intervention for African American smokers: tailoring cancer information service counseling for a special population. Prev Med 1998;27:S61–70.

132. Ahluwalia JS, Okuyemi K, Nollen N, et al. The effects of nicotine gum and counseling among African American light smokers: a 2 × 2 factorial design. Addiction 2006;101:883–91.

133. Webb MS. Culturally specific interventions for African American smokers: an efficacy experiment. J Natl Med Assoc 2009;101:927–35.

134. Webb MS. Does one size fit all African American smokers? The moderating role of acculturation in culturally specific interventions. Psychol Addict Behav 2008; 22:592–6.

135. Messerli FH, Bangalore S, Agarwal V. Lipid-lowering in African Americans in ALLHAT-optimism bias? J Clin Hypertens (Greenwich) 2013;15(12):940.

136. Pearson TA, Denke MA, McBride PE, et al. Effectiveness of ezetimibe added to ongoing statin therapy in modifying lipid profiles and low-density lipoprotein cholesterol goal attainment in patients of different races and ethnicities: a substudy of the Ezetimibe add-on to statin for effectiveness trial. Mayo Clin Proc 2006;81(9):1177–85.

137. Rodney RA, Sugimoto D, Wagman B, et al. Efficacy and safety of coadministration of ezetimibe and simvastatin in African-American patients with primary hypercholesterolemia. J Natl Med Assoc 2006;98(5):772–8.

138. Powell-Wiley TM, Banks-Richard K, Williams-King E, et al. Churches as targets for cardiovascular disease prevention: comparison of genes, nutrition, exercise, wellness and spiritual growth (GoodNEWS) and Dallas County populations. J Public Health (Oxf) 2013;35(1):99–106.

139. Wilson-Frederick SM, Thorpe RJ Jr, Bell CN, et al. Examination of race disparities in physical inactivity among adults of similar social context. Ethn Dis 2014;24(3):363–9.

140. McGruder HF, Malarcher AM, Antoine TL, et al. Racial and ethnic disparities in cardiovascular risk factors among stroke survivors: United States 1999 to 2001. Stroke 2004;35:1557–61.

141. Brownson RC, Eyler AA, King AC, et al. Patterns and correlates of physical activity among US women 40 years and older. Am J Public Health 2000;90:264–70.

142. Dergance JM, Mouton CP, Lichtenstein MJ, et al. Potential mediators of ethnic differences in physical activity in older Mexican Americans and European Americans: results from the San Antonio Longitudinal Study of Aging. J Am Geriatr Soc 2005;53:1240–7.

143. Centers for Disease Control and Prevention (CDC). Contribution of occupational physical activity toward meeting recommended physical activity guidelines: United States, 2007. MMWR Morb Mortal Wkly Rep 2011;60:656–60.

144. Sussner KM, Lindsay AC, Greaney ML, et al. The influence of immigrant status and acculturation on the development of overweight in Latino families: a qualitative study. J Immigr Minor Health 2008;10:497–505.

145. Bowie JV, Juon HS, Cho J, et al. Factors associated with overweight and obesity among Mexican Americans and Central Americans: results from the 2001 California Health Interview Survey. Prev Chronic Dis 2007;4:A10.

146. Ogden CL, Carroll MD, Curtin LR, et al. Prevalence of overweight and obesity in the United States, 1999–2004. JAMA 2006;295:1549–55.

147. Nichaman MZ, Garcia G. Obesity in Hispanic Americans. Diabetes Care 1991; 14:691–4.
148. Flegal KM, Ogden CL, Carroll MD. Prevalence and trends in overweight in Mexican-American adults and children. Nutr Rev 2004;62(pt 2):S144–8.
149. Crespo C, Loria C, Burt V. Hypertension and other cardiovascular disease risk factors among Mexican Americans, Cuban Americans, and Puerto Ricans from the Hispanic Health and Nutrition Examination Survey. Public Health Rep 1996;111(Suppl 2):7–10.
150. Flegal KM, Carroll MD, Kit BK, et al. Prevalence of obesity and trends in the distribution of body mass index among US adults, 1999–2010. JAMA 2012;307: 491–7.
151. Lindberg NM, Stevens VJ, Halperin RO. Weight-loss interventions for Hispanic populations: the role of culture. J Obes 2013;1–5.
152. Denny CH, Holtzman D, Cobb N. Surveillance for health behaviors of American Indians and Alaska Natives. Findings from the Behavioral Risk Factor Surveillance System, 1997–2000. MMWR Surveill Summ 2003;52:1–13.
153. Steele CB, Cardinez CJ, Richardson LC, et al. Surveillance for Health Behaviors of American Indians and Alaska Natives –Findings from the Behavioral Risk Factor Surveillance System, 2000–2006. Cancer 2008;113:1131–41.
154. Balluz LS, Okoro CA, Mokdad A. Association between selected unhealthy lifestyle factors, body mass index, and chronic health conditions among individuals 50 years of age or older, by race/ethnicity. Ethn Dis 2008;18: 450–7.
155. Lancaster KJ, Carter-Edwards L, Grilo S, et al. Obesity interventions in African American faith-based organizations: a systematic review. Obes Rev 2014; 15(Suppl 4):159–76.
156. Hollis JF, Gullion CM, Stevens VJ, et al. Weight loss during the intensive intervention phase of the weight-loss maintenance trial. Am J Prev Med 2008;35: 118–26.
157. Wadden TA, West DS, Neiberg RH, et al. One-year weight losses in the Look AHEAD study: factors associated with success. Obesity (Silver Spring) 2009; 17:713–22.
158. Svetkey LP, Erlinger TP, Vollmer WM, et al. Effect of lifestyle modifications on blood pressure by race, sex, hypertension status, and age. J Hum Hypertens 2005;19:21–31.
159. Svetkey LP, Stevens VJ, Brantley PJ, et al. Comparison of strategies for sustaining weight loss: the weight loss maintenance randomized controlled trial. JAMA 2008;299:1139–48.
160. Svetkey LP, Ard JD, Stevens VJ, et al. Predictors of long-term weight loss in adults with modest initial weight loss, by sex and race. Obesity (Silver Spring) 2012;20:1820–8.
161. Hooker SP, Harmon B, Burroughs EL, et al. Exploring the feasibility of a physical activity intervention for midlife African–American men. Health Educ Res 2011; 26:732–8.
162. Treadwell H, Holden K, Hubbard R, et al. Addressing obesity and diabetes among African–American men: examination of a community-based model of prevention. J Natl Med Assoc 2010;102:794–802.
163. Kumanyika SK, Obarzanek E, Stevens VJ, et al. Weight-loss experience of black and white participants in NHLBI-sponsored clinical trials. Am J Clin Nutr 1991; 53:1631S–8S.

164. Stevens VJ, Obarzanek E, Cook NR, et al. Long-term weight loss and changes in blood pressure: results of the Trials of Hypertension Prevention, Phase II. Ann Intern Med 2001;134:1–11.

165. Kumanyika SK, Cook NR, Cutler JA, et al. Sodium reduction for hypertension prevention in overweight adults: further results from the Trials of Hypertension Prevention Phase II. J Hum Hypertens 2005;19:33–45.

166. Kumanyika SK, Adams-Campbell L, Van Horn B, et al. Outcomes of a cardiovascular nutrition counseling program in African–Americans with elevated blood pressure or cholesterol level. J Am Diet Assoc 1999;99:1380–91.

167. Torres V. La familia as locus theologicus and religious education in lo cotidiano [daily life]. Relig Educ 2010;105:444–61.

168. Urizar GG Jr, Sears SF Jr. Psychosocial and cultural influences on cardiovascular health and quality of life among Hispanic cardiac patients in South Florida. J Behav Med 2006;29:255–68.

169. Heathcote JD, West JH, Hall PC, et al. Religiosity and utilization of complementary and alternative medicine among foreign-born Hispanics in the United States. Hisp J Behav Sci 2011;33:398–408.

170. Hodge DR, Marsiglia FF, Nieri T. Religion and substance use among youths of Mexican heritage: a social capital perspective. Soc Work Res 2011;35:137–46.

171. Jurkowski JM, Kurlanska C, Ramos BM. Latino women's spiritual beliefs related to health. Am J Health Promot 2010;25:19–25.

172. Castro F, Elder J, Coe K, et al. Mobilizing churches for health promotion in Latino communities: Compañeros en la Salud. J Natl Cancer Inst Monogr 1995;1995:127–35.

173. Boltri JM, Okosun IS, Davis-Smith M, et al. Hemoglobin A1c levels in diagnosed and undiagnosed black, Hispanic, and white persons with diabetes: results from NHANES 1999–2000. Ethn Dis 2005;15:562–7.

174. Borrell LN, Crawford ND, Dallo FJ, et al. Self-reported diabetes in Hispanic subgroup, non-Hispanic black, and non-Hispanic white populations: National Health Interview Survey, 1997–2005. Public Health Rep 2009;124:702–10.

175. Diabetes and Hispanic Americans. US Department of Health & Human Services, Office of Minority Health; Web site. Available at: http://minorityhealth.hhs.gov/templates/content.aspx?ID=3324. Accessed June 19, 2015.

176. Caballero AE. Type 2 diabetes in the Hispanic or Latino population: challenges and opportunities. Curr Opin Endocrinol Diabetes Obes 2007;14:151–7.

177. Narayan KM, Boyle JP, Thompson TJ, et al. Lifetime risk for diabetes mellitus in the United States. JAMA 2003;290:1884–90.

178. Lorenzo C, Hazuda HP, Haffner SM. Insulin resistance and excess risk of diabetes in Mexican-Americans: the San Antonio Heart Study. J Clin Endocrinol Metab 2012;97:793–9.

179. Flegal K, Ezzati T, Harris M, et al. Prevalence of diabetes in Mexican Americans, Cubans, and Puerto Ricans from the Hispanic Health and Nutrition Examination Survey, 1982–1984. Diabetes Care 1991;14:628–38.

180. Burrows NR, Geiss LS, Engelgau MM, et al. Prevalence of diabetes among Native Americans and Alaska Natives, 1990–1997: an increasing burden. Diabetes Care 2000;23:1786–90.

181. Centers for Disease Control and Prevention (CDC).. Diabetes prevalence among American Indians and Alaska Natives and the overall population–United States, 1994–2002. MMWR Morb Mortal Wkly Rep 2003;52:702–4.

182. Crimmins E, Kim J, Alley D, et al. Hispanic paradox in biological risk profiles. Am J Public Health 2007;97:1305–10.

183. Ford ES, Li C, Zhao G, et al. Trends in the prevalence of low risk factor burden for cardiovascular disease among United States adults. Circulation 2009;120: 1181–8.

184. Dong C, Rundek T, Wright CB, et al. Ideal cardiovascular health predicts lower risks of myocardial infarction, stroke, and vascular death across whites, blacks, and Hispanics: the Northern Manhattan Study. Circulation 2012;125:2975–84.

185. Rodriguez CJ. Disparities in ideal cardiovascular health: a challenge or an opportunity? Circulation 2012;125:2963–4.

186. Schumacher C, Ferucci ED, Lanier AP, et al. Metabolic syndrome: prevalence among American Indian and Alaska native people living in the southwestern United States and in Alaska. Metab Syndr Relat Disord 2008;6:267–73.

187. Sinclair KA, Bogart A, Buchwald D, et al. The prevalence of metabolic syndrome and associated risk factors in Northern Plains and Southwest American Indians. Diabetes Care 2011;34:118–20.

FURTHER READINGS

Abraham PA, Kazman JB, Zeno SA, et al. Obesity and African Americans: physiologic and behavioral pathways. ISRN Obes 2013;2013:314295.

Artaza JN, Contreras S, Garcia LA, et al. Vitamin D and cardiovascular disease: potential role in health disparities. J Health Care Poor Underserved 2011;22(4 Suppl):23–38.

Clark LT, El-Atat F. Metabolic syndrome in African Americans: implications for preventing coronary heart disease. Clin Cardiol 2007;30(4):161–4.

Cox LS, Okuyemi K, Choi WS, et al. A review of tobacco use treatments in U.S. ethnic minority populations. Am J Health Promot 2011;25(5 Suppl):S11–30.

Flack JM, Sica DA. Therapeutic considerations in the African-American patient with hypertension: considerations with calcium channel blocker therapy. J Clin Hypertens (Greenwich) 2005;7(4 Suppl 1):9–14.

Gotto AM, Moon JE. Merits and potential downsides of the 2013 ACC/AHA cholesterol management guidelines. Nutr Metab Cardiovasc Dis 2014;24(6):573–6.

Gustat J, Srinivasan SR, Elkasabany A, et al. Relation of self-rated measures of physical activity to multiple risk factors of insulin resistance syndrome in young adults: the Bogalusa Heart Study. J Clin Epidemiol 2002;55(10):997–1006.

Kumanyika SK, Hebert PR, Cutler JA, et al. Feasibility and efficacy of sodium reduction in the trials of hypertension prevention, phase I. Trials of Hypertension Prevention Collaborative Research Group. Hypertension 1993;22:502–12.

Lopes AA, James SA, Port FK, et al. Meeting the challenge to improve the treatment of hypertension in blacks. J Clin Hypertens (Greenwich) 2003;5(6):393–401.

Mukamal KJ, Tremaglio J, Friedman DJ, et al. APOL1 genotype, kidney and cardiovascular disease, and death in older adults. Arterioscler Thromb Vasc Biol 2016;36(2):398–403.

Piamjariyakul U, Werkowitch M, Wick J, et al. Caregiver coaching program effect: reducing heart failure patient rehospitalizations and improving caregiver outcomes among African Americans. Heart Lung 2015;44(6):466–73.

Puckrein GA, Egan BM, Howard G. Social and medical determinants of cardiometabolic health: the big picture. Ethn Dis 2015;25(4):521–4.

Robles GI, Singh-Franco D, Ghin HL. A review of the efficacy of smoking-cessation pharmacotherapies in nonwhite populations. Clin Ther 2008;30(5):800–12.

Stephens T, Braithwaite H, Johnson L, et al. Cardiovascular risk reduction for African–American men through healthy empowerment and anger management. Health Educ J 2008;67:208–18.

Wassertheil-Smoller S, Langford HG, Blaufox MD, et al. Effective dietary intervention in hypertensives: sodium restriction and weight reduction. J Am Diet Assoc 1985; 85:423–30.

West DS, Elaine Prewitt T, Bursac Z, et al. Weight loss of black, white, and Hispanic men and women in the Diabetes Prevention Program. Obesity (Silver Spring) 2008;16:1413–20.

Whitt-Glover MC, Keith NR, Ceaser TG, et al. A systematic review of physical activity interventions among African American adults: evidence from 2009 to 2013. Obes Rev 2014;15(Suppl 4):125–45.

Cancer in the Medically Underserved Population

Oluwadamilola O. Olaku, MD, MPH[a,b,*], Emmanuel A. Taylor, MSc, DrPH[c]

KEYWORDS

- Cancer • Incidence • Mortality • Underserved • Screening • Prevention
- Health disparities • Global health

KEY POINTS

- In the United States, the lifetime risk of developing cancer is about 1 in 2 in men and 1 in 3 in women. Liver cancer is increasing among all population groups.
- The World Cancer Research Fund estimates that about 20% of all cancers diagnosed in the United States are related to body fatness, physical inactivity, excess alcohol consumption, and/or poor nutrition.
- There was a decline in breast and cervical cancer screening between 2008 and 2013. However, there was significant increase in colorectal cancer screening during the same period.
- Disparities in cancer incidence and mortality are not fully explained by correlations of race and lower socioeconomic status, or minority race and insurance status.
- The incidence and mortality of cancer is decreasing in Western countries through decreasing prevalence of known risk factors, early detection, and improved treatment.

INTRODUCTION

Cancer is a group of diseases characterized by uncontrolled growth and spread of abnormal cells. If the spread is not controlled it can result in death.[1] Cancer is the second most common cause of death in the United States. It accounts for nearly 1 in 4 deaths. In the United States, the lifetime risk of developing cancer is 1 in 2 in men (42%) and 1 in 3 in women (38%). According to the American Cancer Society (ACS), 1,685,210 new cases of cancer will be diagnosed in 2016 and an estimated 595,690 deaths will occur as a result of cancer. A significant proportion of cancer can be

This article originally appeared in Primary Care: Clinics in Office Practice, Volume 44, Issue 1, March 2017.

[a] Office of Cancer Complementary and Alternative Medicine, National Cancer Institute, 9609 Medical Center Drive, 5-W622, MSC 9743, Bethesda, MD 20892-9743, USA; [b] Kelly Services, Kelly Government Solutions, 6101 Executive Boulevard, Suite 392, Rockville, MD 20852, USA; [c] Center to Reduce Cancer Health Disparities, National Cancer Institute, 9609 Medical Center Drive, 6-W104, MSC 9746, Rockville, MD 20850-9746, USA

* Corresponding author. Office of Cancer Complementary and Alternative Medicine, National Cancer Institute, 9609 Medical Center Drive, 5-W622, MSC 9743, Bethesda, MD 20892-9743.
E-mail address: Olakuo@mail.nih.gov

prevented. In 2016, about 188,800 of the estimated 595,690 cancer deaths in the United States will be caused by cigarette smoking, according to a recent study by ACS epidemiologists. In addition, the World Cancer Research Fund (WCRF) estimates that about 20% of all cancers diagnosed in the United States are related to body fatness, physical inactivity, excess alcohol consumption, and/or poor nutrition, and thus could also be prevented.[2] Cancers that are related to infectious agents, such as human papillomavirus (HPV), hepatitis B virus (HBV), hepatitis C virus (HCV), human immunodeficiency virus (HIV), and *Helicobacter pylori* could be avoided by preventing these infections through behavioral changes or vaccination, or by treating the infection.[1]

An Institute of Medicine report titled "Unequal Treatment: Confronting Racial and Ethnic Disparities in Health Care" mentioned that one of the core aims of health care is the provision of care that does not vary in quality because of race, ethnicity, sex, socioeconomic status, and geographic considerations. This report showed compelling evidence of significant variation in the rates of medical procedures by race, even when insurance status, income, age, and severity of conditions are comparable.[3] This report revealed that underrepresented and underserved populations are less likely to receive routine medical procedures and experience a lower quality of health services. As defined by Vincent Morelli in the introduction of this issue, medically underserved areas and medically underserved populations are determined by the Health Resources and Services Administration by measuring 4 variables: (1) ratio of primary care physicians per 1000 population; (2) infant mortality; (3) percentage of the population below the poverty level; and (4) percentage of the population age 65 years or older. It has been estimated that more than 100 million Americans are medically underserved.[4]

Otis Brawley,[5] Chief Medical and Scientific Officer and Executive Vice President of the ACS, observed in his study on colorectal cancer that there were similar age-adjusted mortalities in black and white people in the 1970s. Significant disparities in mortality began in the early 1980s. This disparity coincided with the advent of large-scale screening programs and coverage for colonoscopies. Although overall mortalities have declined for all racial/ethnic populations and socioeconomic levels, the rate of decrease among white people was faster, thus exacerbating the disparity over time.[4,5]

There are 2 predominant hypotheses that have formed the basis for why inequities exist. Current data do not support or refute either one. Genomic sequencing has not supported a definite biological construct on which to base disparities. However, there is some evidence that raise questions about possible differences in treatment response, and the need to consider interaction of tumor and host biology.[6]

Others have attributed disparities solely to societal and health care system factors as they relate to unequal access to care. Observed disparities are not fully explained by the correlations between minority race and lower socioeconomic status, or minority race and insurance status (uninsured or publicly insured).[7] It seems that underserved patients with Medicaid or no insurance present with more advanced cancer and are less likely to receive definitive cancer-directed surgery and/or radiation therapy. In addition, these patients have far worse survival rates.[8]

There is growing evidence to support different outcomes as a result of inequities in the structure of the health care system.[9] Patients from disadvantaged populations tend to receive care in settings that differ in terms of quality. For example, patients with breast and colon cancer treated at hospitals with large minority populations had higher mortality regardless of race.[10] Patient preferences in treatment and other clinical management options should be considered by providers; however, providers must distinguish between deeply rooted values and transient beliefs that may be amenable to information and intervention.[4]

CAUSES OF CANCER

Factors associated with increased risk for cancer include:

1. Genetics: some types of cancer run in certain families, but most causes are not clearly linked to genes that people inherit from their parents.
2. Tobacco smoke: there are more than 70 carcinogens in tobacco smoke.
3. Diet and physical activity: poor diet and not being active are key factors that can increase a person's cancer risk. WCRF International guidelines for cancer prevention include being physically active for at least 30 minutes every day; limiting consumption of energy-dense foods; eating a variety of vegetables, fruits, and wholegrains; and limiting consumption of red and processed meats.[2]
4. Sun and ultraviolet (UV) ray exposure: exposure to UV light from the sun has been shown to have a carcinogenic effect. Low skin exposure to UVB radiation from the sun or caused by specific individual behavior may also have a negative effect.[11]
5. Radiation: exposure to ionizing radiation increases the risk of cancer throughout the lifespan. Cancer risk increases after exposure to moderate and high doses of radiation (0.1–0.2 Gy).[12] The largest number of radiotherapy-related second cancers are lung, esophageal, and female breast cancer. The highest percentages of second cancers related to radiotherapy are among survivors of Hodgkin disease and cancers of the oral cavity, pharynx, and cervix uteri.[13]
6. Other carcinogens (environmental [eg, asbestos] and infectious agents [eg, herpes simplex virus]): the global burden of cancer attributable to infectious agents is estimated to be about 18%. The main infectious agents responsible for the global cancer burden are H pylori, HPV, HBV, HIV, and human herpes virus.[14]

EPIDEMIOLOGY

Overall, the age-adjusted cancer incidence rate for all cancers combined decreased by 0.5% per year for both sexes from 2002 to 2011 (P<.001) **(Fig. 1)**. This finding is based on trend analysis of the surveillance epidemiology and end result (SEER)-13 data. Among men, cancer incidence rates decreased on average by 1.8% annually from 2007 to 2011 (P = .003). Overall cancer incidence rates among women increased 0.8% annually from 1992 to 1998 (P = .003), but were stable from 1998 to 2011. Among children aged 0 to 14 and 0 to 19 years, rates have increased by 0.8% per year over the past decade, continuing a trend dating from 1992 (P<.001).[15]

The observed rates of all cancers combined in all racial groups were lower among women than among men between 2007 and 2011 (412.8 vs 526.1 per 100,000). Black men had the overall highest incidence of cancer among men of any racial/ethnic group (587.7 per 100,000). Among women, white women had the overall highest incidence of cancer (418.6 per 100,000). In each of the racial/ethnic groups, prostate cancer remains the most common cancer among men, followed by lung and colorectal cancer among all racial/ethnic groups respectively. However, these ranks are reversed in Hispanic men. Among women, breast cancer is the most common cancer among all racial/ethnic groups. Lung and colorectal cancer are the second and third most common cancers among all racial/ethnic groups, except among Asian people and Pacific Islanders (API) and Hispanic people, among whom the ranks are reversed again.[15]

The cancer death rate for all cancer sites combined (2007–2011) was higher for men than for women (211.6 vs 147.4 deaths per 100,000). Of all racial or ethnic groups, black men had the highest cancer death rate (269.3 deaths per 100,000 men). Lung cancer was the leading cause of death in both men and women. Among men, lung, prostate, and colorectal cancers were the leading causes of cancer death in every

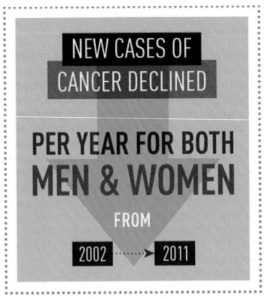

Fig. 1. Cancer incidence 2002 to 2011. (*From* National Cancer Institute. Cancer Incidence 2002 to 2011. Available at: https://www.cancer.gov/. Accessed February 17, 2016.)

racial and ethnic group except API men, for whom lung, liver, and colorectal cancers ranked highest. The leading causes of cancer death in women were lung, breast, and colorectal cancers, although the rank order of these top 3 cancers varied for American Indian/Alaska Native and Hispanic women.[15]

The 2015 report to the nation on the status of cancer used national data to determine the incidence of the 4 major molecular subtypes of breast cancer by age, race/ethnicity, poverty level, and other factors. The 4 molecular subtypes, which can be approximated by their hormone receptor (HR) status and expression of the HER2 gene are: luminal A (HR+/HER2−), Luminal B (HR+/HER2+), HER2-enriched (HR−/HER2+), and triple negative (HR−/HER2−). The 4 subtypes respond differently to treatment and have different survival rates. Non-Hispanic black people had the highest rates of late-stage disease and of poorly differentiated/undifferentiated disorder among all the subtypes. All of these factors are associated with lower survival among black people; resulting in the highest rates of breast cancer deaths[16] (**Fig. 2**).

SCREENING

The Healthy People (HP) initiative was initiated in 1979 as a Surgeon General's report. It tracks 10-year national objectives for improving the health of all Americans.[17] One of the goals of HP is a reduction in cancer deaths and a reduction in the incidence of late-stage cancers that may be reduced by screening (cervical, breast, colorectal, and prostate).[18] Brown and colleagues[18] observed marked disparities in cancer screening and provider counseling rates for certain population subgroups, including the uninsured and those with low income or no usual source of health care. The access to care of Hispanic people and those below the 200% federal poverty level were the most compromised as measured by not having health insurance and not having a usual source of care.[18]

BREAST CANCER IN WOMEN:
KNOW THE SUBTYPE

It's important for guiding treatment and predicting survival.

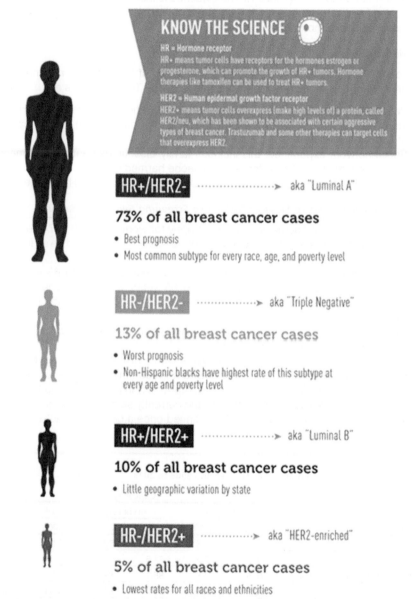

KNOW THE SCIENCE

HR = Hormone receptor
HR+ means tumor cells have receptors for the hormones estrogen or progesterone, which can promote the growth of HR+ tumors. Hormone therapies like tamoxifen can be used to treat HR+ tumors.

HER2 = Human epidermal growth factor receptor
HER2+ means tumor cells overexpress (make high levels of) a protein, called HER2/neu, which has been shown to be associated with certain aggressive types of breast cancer. Trastuzumab and some other therapies can target cells that overexpress HER2.

HR+/HER2- ··················> aka "Luminal A"

73% of all breast cancer cases

- Best prognosis
- Most common subtype for every race, age, and poverty level

HR-/HER2- ··············> aka "Triple Negative"

13% of all breast cancer cases

- Worst prognosis
- Non-Hispanic blacks have highest rate of this subtype at every age and poverty level

HR+/HER2+ ··················> aka "Luminal B"

10% of all breast cancer cases

- Little geographic variation by state

HR-/HER2+ ··············> aka "HER2-enriched"

5% of all breast cancer cases

- Lowest rates for all races and ethnicities

Fig. 2. Breast cancer subtypes. (*From* National Cancer Institute. Available at: https://www. cancer.gov/. Accessed February 17, 2016.)

From 2008 to 2013, self-reported cervical cancer screening overall declined by 3.8 percentage points, and breast cancer screening declined by 1.5 percentage points overall. The reason for the decrease is not certain. However, it could have been caused by the economic recession between 2008 and 2010. There is a link between economic recession and decreased health care coverage.[19] There was a significant increase of 6.1 percentage points for colorectal cancer screening in the overall population from 2008 to 2013 (**Table 1**). The evidence is insufficient to determine whether screening for prostate cancer with Prostate-specific antigen (PSA) or digital rectal examination reduces mortality from prostate cancer.[20]

Barriers to Screening

Ogedegbe and colleagues[21] identified 3 categories of barriers to screening in low-income minority women in community health centers. The categories are:

1. Patients' attitude and beliefs: examples are competing priorities, loss of privacy, lack of cancer screening knowledge, perception of good health, fear of pain and of cancer diagnosis.
2. Social network experience: this includes family discouragement, lack of medical recommendation, and knowledge of someone harmed by test.
3. Accessibility: this includes cost of test, lack of transportation, and language barrier.

United States Preventive Services Task Force Screening Recommendations

Breast cancer: biennial screening mammography for women age 50 to 74 years. The decision to start screening mammography before age 50 years should be an individual one.

Cervical cancer: screening recommended in women aged 21 to 65 years, with cytology every 3 years. Women aged 30 to 65 years who want to lengthen the screening interval are required to have a combination of cytology and HPV testing every 5 years.

Colorectal cancer: fecal occult blood testing, sigmoidoscopy, or colonoscopy in adults beginning at age 50 to 75 years.

Lung cancer: for adults aged 55 to 80 years with a history of smoking, the United States Preventive Services Task Force (USPSTF) recommends annual screening for lung cancer with low-dose computed tomography (CT) in adults aged 55 to 80 years who have a 30-pack-year smoking history and currently smoke or have quit within the past 15 years. Screening should be discontinued once a person has not smoked for

Table 1
Cervical, breast, and colorectal cancer screening 2008 to 2013

Race/Ethnicity	Cancer Type					
	Breast (%)		Cervix (%)		Colorectal (%)	
	2008	2013	2008	2013	2008	2013
Total	73.7	72.6	84.5	80.7	52.1	58.2
Asian	76.2	72.2	71.5	70.5	47.5	50.6
Black or African American	76.5	72.9	86.1	82.2	48.0	59.1
White	73.3	72.6	85.1	81.4	53.3	58.6
Hispanic or Latino	68.3	66.7	81.3	77.1	34.9	43.0

Data from National Health Interview Survey (NHIS), Centers for Disease Control and Prevention, National Center for Health Statistics (CDC/NCHS).

15 years or develops a health problem that substantially limits life expectancy or the ability or willingness to have curative lung surgery.

Prostate cancer: the USPSTF recommends against PSA-based screening for prostate cancer.[22]

PREVENTION

The second edition of *The Cancer Atlas* released by the ACS and the International Agency for Research on Cancer argues that many cancers are largely preventable and prevention is cost-effective.[23] There is evidence to suggest that a diagnosis or suspicion of cancer can be a financial stressor. In a population-based study in western Washington, 197,840 patients with cancer were matched with an equal number of controls by age, sex, and zip code. Patients with cancer were 2.6 times more likely to file for bankruptcy than cancer-free controls (*P*<.05).[24]

Observational epidemiologic studies have shown associations between the following modifiable lifestyle factors or environmental exposures and specific cancers.

Cigarette Smoking/Tobacco Use

Research has consistently shown the association between tobacco use and cancers of many sites. Specifically, cigarette smoking has been established as a cause of cancers of the lung, oral cavity, esophagus, bladder, kidney, pancreas, stomach, and cervix, and also acute myelogenous leukemia. It is estimated that cigarette smoking causes 30% of all cancer deaths in the United States. Smoking avoidance and cessation result in decreased incidence and mortality from cancer.[25] In addition, Andersen and colleagues[26] found that meeting ACS cancer prevention guidelines, especially regarding tobacco and alcohol consumption, was associated with a lower cancer risk in underserved populations.

Infections

Infectious agents have been estimated to cause 18% of all cancers globally.[14] The burden of cancers caused by infections is much greater in developing nations (26%) than in developed nations (8%). Infection with an oncogenic strain of HPV is considered a necessary event for subsequent cervical cancer. Immunity conferred by vaccines results in a marked decrease in precancerous lesions. Oncogenic strains of HPV are also linked with cancers of the penis, vagina, anus, and oropharynx. Other examples of infectious agents that cause cancer are HBV and HCV (liver cancer), and *H pylori* (gastric cancer).[14]

Radiation

Exposure to UV radiation and ionizing radiation are established causes of cancer. Nonmelanoma skin cancers are caused by exposure to solar UV radiation.[27] There is extensive epidemiologic and biological evidence that links exposure to ionizing radiation with the development of cancer, especially those that involve the hematological system, breast, lungs, and thyroid. The National Research Council of the National Academies, Committee to Assess the Health Risks from Exposure to Low Levels of Ionizing Radiation, the Biologic Effects of Ionizing Radiation VII report concluded that no dose of radiation should be considered completely safe.[28] The major sources of population exposure to ionizing radiation are medical radiation (including x-rays, CT, fluoroscopy) and naturally occurring radon gas in the basements of homes. There is a significant and negative correlation between income and radon levels.[29] Reducing radiation exposure and limiting unnecessary CT scans and other diagnostic studies are important prevention strategies.[30,31]

Diet

The WCRF/American Institute for Cancer Research (AICR) concluded that both fruits and nonstarchy vegetables were associated with probable decreased risk for cancers of the mouth, esophagus, and stomach. Fruits were also associated with probable decreased risk of lung cancer.[32,33]

Alcohol

The WCRF/AICR report judged the evidence to be convincing that drinking alcohol increased the risks of cancers of the mouth, esophagus, breast, and colorectum. Further, the evidence was judged to be probable that drinking alcohol increased the risk of liver cancer, and colorectal cancer in women.[32,33]

Physical Activity

In the WCRF/AICR report, the evidence was judged convincing that increased physical activity protects against colorectal cancer. The evidence was probable that physical activity was associated with lower risk of postmenopausal breast and endometrial cancer. As with dietary factors, physical activity seems to play a role in selected malignancies.[32,33]

Obesity

The WCRF/AICR report concluded that obesity is convincingly linked to postmenopausal breast cancer and cancers of the esophagus, pancreas, colorectum, endometrium, and kidney.

Chemoprevention

Chemoprevention refers to the use of natural or synthetic compounds to interfere with early stages of carcinogenesis before invasive cancer appears.[34] Daily use of selective estrogen receptor modulators (tamoxifen or raloxifene) for up to 5 years reduces the incidence of breast cancer by about 50% in high-risk women. Dutasteride (alpha-reductase inhibitor) has been shown to reduce the incidence of prostate cancer.[35] Other chemopreventive candidates include cyclooxygenase-2 inhibitors and aspirin. Secondary analyses from pooled data whose primary end points were vascular events showed that aspirin taken daily for 4 years was associated with an 18% reduction in overall cancer death.[36]

Vitamin and dietary supplement use

The evidence is insufficient to support the use of multivitamin and mineral supplements or single vitamins or minerals to prevent cancer.[37]

GLOBAL HEALTH

Cancer is a leading cause of death worldwide. The numbers of cases and deaths are expected to grow as populations grow, age, and adopt lifestyle behaviors that increase cancer risk.[38] In 2012, an estimated 14.1 million new cases and 8.2 million cancer deaths occurred worldwide.[39] The highest rates are in North America, Oceania, and Europe for both sexes. Prostate cancer is the most commonly diagnosed cancer among men in North and South America; northern, western, and southern Europe; and Oceania. In Eastern Europe, lung cancer is the most common. The leading cancers among men in Africa include prostate, lung, colorectum, liver, esophagus, Kaposi sarcoma, leukemia, stomach, and non-Hodgkin lymphoma. However, in Asia, they include lung, lip, oral cavity, liver, stomach, colorectal and prostate cancers.

Breast cancer is the most common cancer among women in North America, Europe, and Oceania. Breast and cervical cancers are the most frequently diagnosed cancers in Latin America and the Caribbean, Africa, and most of Asia. In addition, common female cancers in Asia include lung (China, Korea), liver (Mongolia), and thyroid (South Korea).[39]

Eight major cancers account for more than 60% of total global cases and deaths: lung and bronchus, colon and rectum, female breast, prostate, stomach, liver, esophagus, and cervix uteri.[39]

The incidence and mortality of cancer are decreasing in Western countries through decreasing prevalence of known risk factors, early detection, and improved treatment. However, rates of lung, breast, and colorectal cancers are increasing in low-income and middle-income countries. This increase is caused by increased risk of smoking, excess body weight, physical inactivity, and changing reproductive patterns. In addition, these countries also bear a disproportionate burden of infection-related cancers, such as cervix, liver, and stomach.[39]

SUMMARY

The incidence and mortality of cancer in the United States have been decreasing over the last few years, largely because of appropriate and timely screening, prevention, and better treatment. Despite this downward trend, disparities persist among the various ethnic and racial groups in the United States. The disparities can be minimized or eliminated by encouraging equitable distribution and use of resources. A sincere commitment by individual governments, international agencies, donors, and the private sector is required to reduce the burden of cancer globally.

REFERENCES

1. ACS. Cancer facts and figures 2016. Atlanta (GA): American Cancer Society; 2016.
2. WCRF, AIRC. Diet, nutrition, physical activity and prostate cancer. Washington, DC: AIRC; 2014.
3. Institute of Medicine. Unequal treatment confronting racial and ethnic disparities in health care. Washington, DC: National Academies Press; 2003.
4. Wong S. Medically underserved populations: disparities in quality and outcomes. J Oncol Pract 2015;11:193–4.
5. Brawley OW. Colorectal cancer control: providing adequate care to those who need it. J Natl Cancer Inst 2014;106:ju075.
6. Fine MJ, Ibrahim SA, Thomas SB. The role of race and genetics in health disparities research. Am J Public Health 2005;95:2125–8.
7. Haider AH, Scott VK, Rehman KA, et al. Racial disparities in surgical care and outcomes in the United States: a comprehensive review of the patient, provider, and systemic factors. J Am Coll Surg 2013;216:482–92.
8. Walker GV, Grant SR, Guadagnolo BA, et al. Disparities in stage at diagnosis, treatment and survival in non-elderly adult patients with cancer according to insurance status. J Clin Oncol 2014;27:3945–50.
9. Birkmayer NJ, Gu N, Baser O, et al. Socioeconomic status and surgical mortality in the elderly. Med Care 2008;46:893–9.
10. Breslin TM, Morris AM, Gu N, et al. Hospital factors and racial disparities in mortality after surgery for breast and colon cancer. J Clin Oncol 2009;27:3945–50.

11. Elwood JM, Jopson J. Melanoma and sun exposure: an overview of published studies. Int J Cancer 1997;73:198–203.
12. Kamiya K, Ozasa K, Akiba S, et al. Long term effects of radiation exposure on health. Lancet 2015;386:469–78.
13. Intidher Labidi-Galy S, Tassy L, Blay JY. Radiation induced soft tissue sarcoma. Available at: http://sarcomahelp.org/radiation-induced-sarcoma.html. Accessed February 8, 2016.
14. Parkin DM. The global health burden of infection-associated cancers in the year 2002. Int J Cancer 2006;118:3030–44.
15. Kohler BA, Sherman RL, Howlader N, et al. Annual report to the nation on the status of cancer, 1975-2011, featuring incidence of breast cancer subtypes by race/ethnicity, poverty and state. J Natl Cancer Inst 2015;107:djv048.
16. New analysis of breast cancer subtypes could lead to better risk stratifications; annual report to the nation shows that mortality and incidence for most cancers continue to decline. Available at: http://cancer.gov/news-events/press-releases/2015/report-nation-march-2015-press-release. Accessed February 17, 2016.
17. Department of Health, Education and Welfare, Public Health Service. Healthy People: the Surgeon General's report on health promotion and disease prevention. Washington, DC: Government Printing Office; 1979.
18. Brown ML, Klabunde CN, Cronin K, et al. Challenges in meeting Healthy People 2020 objective for cancer related preventive services, NHIS 2008 and 2010. Prev Chronic Dis 2014;11:E29.
19. William DR. Race, socioeconomic status and health. The added effect of racism and discrimination. Ann N Y Acad Sci 1999;896:173–88.
20. Prostate cancer screening for health professionals (PDQ). Available at: www.cancer.gov/types/prostate/hp/prostate-screening-pdq. Accessed February 29, 2016.
21. Ogedegbe G, Cassells AN, Robinson CM, et al. Perceptions of barriers and facilitators of cancer early development among low income minority women in community health centers. J Natl Med Assoc 2005;97:162–70.
22. US Preventive Services Task Force. Published recommendations. Available at: http://www.uspreventiveservicestaskforce.org/BrowseRec/Index/browse-recommendations. Accessed June 18, 2016.
23. Jemal A, Vineis P, Bray F, et al. The cancer atlas 2nd edition. Atlanta (GA): American Cancer Society; 2014.
24. Ramsey S, Blough D, Kirchhoff A, et al. Washington State cancer patients found to be at greater risk for bankruptcy than people without a cancer diagnosis. Health Aff (Millwood) 2013;32:1143–52.
25. National Cancer Institute. PDQ® Cancer Prevention overview. Bethesda (MD): National Cancer Institute; 2016. Available at: http://www.cancer.gov/about-cancer/causes-prevention/hp-prevention-overview-pdq. Accessed March 1, 2016.
26. Andersen SW, Blot WJ, Shu X, et al. Adherence to cancer prevention guidelines and cancer risk in low-income and African American populations. Cancer Epidemiol Biomarkers Prev 2016;25(5):846–53.
27. Scotto J, Fears TR, Fraumeni JF Jr. Solar radiation. In: Schottenfeld D, Fraumeni JF Jr, editors. Cancer epidemiology and prevention. 2nd edition. New York: Oxford University Press; 1996. p. 355–72.
28. National Research Council (US), Committee to Assess Health Risks from Exposure to Low Levels of Ionizing Radiation. Health risks from exposure to low levels

of ionizing radiation: BEIR VII phase 2. Washington, DC: National Academy Press; 2006.

29. National Council on Radiation Protection and Measurements. Ionizing radiation exposure of the population of the United States. Bethesda (MD): National Council on Radiation Protection and Measurement; 2009.
30. Reddy NK, Bhutani MS. Racial disparities in pancreatic cancer and radon exposure: a correlation study. Pancreas 2009;38:391–5.
31. Mettler FA Jr, Thomadsen BR, Bhargavan M, et al. Medical radiation exposure in the U.S. in 2006: preliminary results. Health Phys 2008;95:502–7.
32. World Cancer Research Fund/American Institute for Cancer Research, Food, Nutrition, Physical Activity, and Prevention of Cancer: a Global Perspective. Washington, DC: AICR; 2007.
33. Norat T, Aune D, Chan D, et al. Fruits and vegetables: updating the epidemiologic evidence for the WCRF/AICR lifestyle recommendations for cancer prevention. Cancer Treat Res 2014;159:35–50.
34. William WN Jr, Heymach JV, Kim ES, et al. Molecular targets for cancer chemoprevention. Nat Rev Drug Discov 2009;8:213–25.
35. Andriole GL, Bostwick DG, Brawley OW, et al. Effect of dutasteride on the risk of prostate cancer. N Engl J Med 2010;362:1192–202.
36. Rothwell PM, Fowkes FG, Belch JF, et al. Effect of daily aspirin on long term risk of death due to cancer: analysis of individual patient data from randomized trials. Lancet 2011;377:31–41.
37. Fortmann SP, Burda BU, Senger CA, et al. Vitamin and mineral supplements in the primary prevention of cardiovascular disease and cancer: an updated systematic evidence review for the US preventive services task force. Ann Intern Med 2013;159:824–34.
38. Torre LA, Siegel RL, Ward EM, et al. Global cancer incidence and mortality rates and trends. An update. Cancer Epidemiol Biomarkers Prev 2016;25(1):16–27.
39. Ferlay J, Soerjomataram I, Ervik M, et al. Cancer incidence and mortality worldwide: sources, methods and major patterns in GLOBOCAN 2012. Int J Cancer 2015;136:359–86.

International Comparisons in Underserved Health

Issues, Policies, Needs and Projections

Paul Hutchinson, PhD[a], Vincent Morelli, MD[b],*

KEYWORDS

- International health care • Global health care statistics • Health care spending
- Universal health care • Health care technology

KEY POINTS

- Primary care physicians/providers worldwide need to be aware of the issues and obstacles faced by the underserved patients they serve.
- Primary care physicians need to be aware of the changing issues involved with providing health care to underserved populations.
- Primary care physicians can participate in solving current and future challenges such as improving access to care, embracing new technologies, improving patient education, and being sensitive to the social/cultural prejudices.

Globally, there have been vast improvements in health over the past several decades, rapidly decreasing—but not eliminating—disparities between high-income and low-income countries. In the latter, the average life expectancy has increased rapidly—by 9 years in just the period from 1990 to 2012 (**Fig. 1**), and the difference in life expectancy between high-income countries and low-income countries has shrunk from 22 years to 17 years (**Fig. 2**). Excluding sub-Saharan Africa, the life expectancy gap is only 9 years.[1] Both infant mortality and mortality among those less than 5 years of age have decreased by nearly one-half, equivalent to a staggering 17,000 fewer child deaths each day.[1] Mothers are now more likely than ever to survive childbirth; the maternal mortality rate in low-income countries has decreased from 900 per 100,000 live births to 450 per 100,000 live births, largely owing to better prenatal care and increases in facility births. Similar proportional decreases have been evidenced in lower middle and upper middle income countries.[2]

This article originally appeared in Primary Care: Clinics in Office Practice, Volume 44, Issue 1, March 2017.

[a] Global Community Health Sciences, Tulane University School of Public Health and Tropical Medicine, 1440 Canal Street, Suite 2210, New Orleans, LA 70112, USA; [b] Department of Family and Community Medicine, Meharry Medical College, 1005 Dr D. B. Todd Boulevard, Nashville, TN 37208, USA
* Corresponding author.
E-mail address: morellivincent@yahoo.com

Physician Assist Clin 4 (2019) 287–304
https://doi.org/10.1016/j.cpha.2018.08.012
2405-7991/19/© 2018 Elsevier Inc. All rights reserved.

physicianassistant.theclinics.com

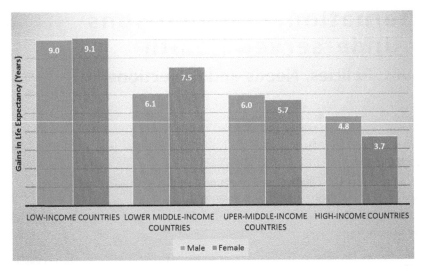

Fig. 1. Years gained in life expectancy 1990 to 2012, by sex and country income group. (*From* World Health Statistics 2014. A wealth of information on global public health. WHO. Available at: http://apps.who.int/iris/bitstream/10665/112739/1/WHO_HIS_HSI_14.1_eng.pdf? ua=1. Accessed June 10, 2016; with permission.)

Households in low-income countries, on average, are enjoying a higher quality of life than ever before. Currently, 90% of the world's population has access to safe drinking water and almost two-thirds have access to adequate sanitation.[1] Measles vaccination rates have reached 80% of children, and nearly three-quarters of births are

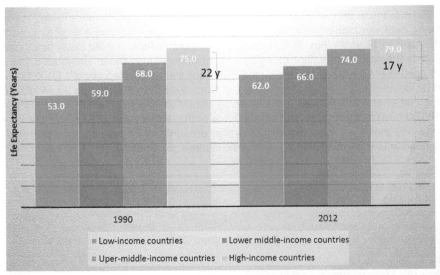

Fig. 2. Life expectancy (years) by level of income. (*From* World Health Statistics 2014. A wealth of information on global public health. WHO. Available at: http://apps.who.int/iris/bitstream/10665/112739/1/WHO_HIS_HSI_14.1_eng.pdf?ua=1. Accessed June 10, 2016; with permission.)

attended by skilled personnel. The percentage of those less than 5 years of age who are underweight decreased by 40%—from 25% in 1990% to 15% in 2009. The education gap between boys and girls has decreased dramatically, and now more than 90% of school-age girls are enrolled in primary school. Better access to family planning has given women more control over their fertility, allowing them to better time and limit births, with resultant decreases in infant and maternal mortality.[3]

In part, these improvements are owing to improved incomes globally. Poverty has decreased dramatically in much of the world. The percentage of people living in extreme poverty has decreased by more than one-half since 1990.[4] In 2015, less than 10% of the world's population was estimated to live on less than $1.90 per day, considered to be the benchmark for poverty. This represents 200 million fewer people living in poverty than in 2012.[5] In recent years, 7 of the 10 fastest growing economies of the past half-decade have been in Africa.[6]

These improvements are also owing to greater international focus, as evidenced by the United Nations Millennium Development Goals, which arose out of the Millennium Summit of the United Nations in 2000 and were intended to improve welfare in developing countries by 2015 through 8 subobjectives (eg, reducing poverty and hunger, improving education, reducing gender inequality, reducing child mortality, improving maternal health, and addressing human immunodeficiency virus (HIV) infection/AIDS, malaria, and other diseases). These objectives, many of which were met well before the 2015 deadline, are now being replaced by the broader and even more ambitious Sustainable Development Goals (available: https://sustainabledevelopment.un.org/post2015/transformingourworld), which also include ensuring prosperity for all and providing better protection for the planet.

In many low-income countries, an epidemiologic transition has begun, largely owing to population shifts, reflected in a change from a preponderance of mortality and morbidity owing to communicable diseases to an increase in the share attributable to noncommunicable diseases of older populations. "Where infectious disease and childhood illnesses related to malnutrition were once the primary causes of death, now children in many parts of the world—outside of sub-Saharan Africa—are more likely to live into an unhealthy adulthood and suffer from eating too much food rather than too little."[7] Over the past few decades, this shift has led to an increase in the importance of diseases such as diabetes, lung cancer, and chronic obstructive pulmonary disease, whereas the shares of other diseases, such as diarrhea, lower respiratory infections, and tuberculosis, have decreased.[7] This is apparent in composite measures of well-being—such as disability-adjusted life years (DALYs)—that combine both morbidity and mortality to give a more accurate picture of the burden of disease. For example, "in 1990, 47% of disability-adjusted life-years (DALYs) worldwide were from communicable, maternal, neonatal, and nutritional disorders, 43% from noncommunicable diseases, and 10% from injuries. By 2010, this had shifted to 35%, 54%, and 11%, respectively."[8]

First-world diseases are increasingly becoming problems globally. Currently, the top 5 causes of years of life lost globally are ischemic heart disease, lower respiratory infections, stroke, diarrheal diseases, and road injuries.[9] Again, although these patterns differ across low-income and high-income countries, convergence is apparent. The top 3 killers in low-income countries (heart disease, lower respiratory infections, stroke) are also in the top 10 in higher income countries. In terms of mortality, cancer now kills more people in low-income and middle-income countries than HIV, malaria, and tuberculosis combined,[10] although the latter diseases represent a larger loss of years of life lost. As a result, many low-income countries face a triple burden of disease: infections, noncommunicable diseases, and injuries. Early childhood conditions (eg, neonatal preterm complications, neonatal encephalitis, diarrheal diseases) and infectious diseases such as malaria and HIV/AIDS continue to afflict developing countries.

Although these gains have been widespread, they have not been shared by all. In sub-Saharan Africa, infectious diseases, childhood illnesses, and maternal causes of death still account for as much as 70% of the burden of disease. In other regions, such as south Asia and Oceania, these conditions account for only one-third of the burden, and less than 20% in all other regions. This discrepancy is readily apparent in mortality statistics. "While the average age of death throughout Latin America, Asia, and north Africa increased by more than 25 years between 1970 and 2010, it rose by less than 10 years in most of sub-Saharan Africa."[7]

DISEASE PATTERNS BY AGE
Under 5 Years of Age

In the past several decades, there have been major shifts in death rates and in the principal causes of death among those younger than 5 years. In 1990, 1 in 10 children died before their fifth birthday. Currently, that number is 1 in 20.[7] In 2000, the 5 major causes of death for those under 5 were acute respiratory infections (17%), diarrheal diseases (13%), prematurity (13%), intrapartum-related complications (11%), and malaria (8%). The top 5 causes of death are currently prematurity (17%), acute respiratory infections (15%), intrapartum-related complications (11%), diarrheal diseases (9%), and malaria (7%), but significant increases have been seen in neonatal sepsis (7%), congenital anomalies (7%), and injuries (6%).[1]

From 2000 to 2012, there were substantial decreases in measles deaths by 80%, HIV/AIDS deaths by 51%, diarrhea by 50%, pneumonia by 40% and malaria by 37% (**Fig. 3**).[1] These reductions have been achieved by multiple means. Countries have vastly improved their immunization rates for killers such as measles and pneumonia. Prevention and treatment for long-standing health issues such as malaria have

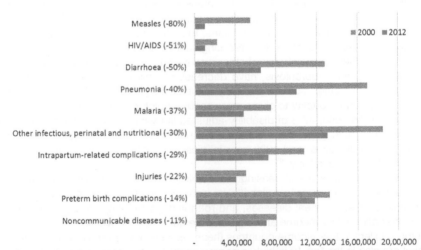

Fig. 3. Changes in major causes of deaths of those under 5 years of age globally, 2000 to 2012. HIV, human immunodeficiency virus. (*From* World Health Statistics 2014. A wealth of information on global public health. WHO. Available at: http://apps.who.int/iris/bitstream/10665/112739/1/WHO_HIS_HSI_14.1_eng.pdf?ua=1. Accessed June 10, 2016; with permission.)

improved, particularly through the development of new therapies and increased use of insecticide-treated nets. Improved sanitation and nutrition, most notably improved breastfeeding rates, have also contributed to improvements in diarrheal diseases.

However, positive trends with many diseases are being countered by negative trends in other areas. Obesity has become a global epidemic, including among children. In 1990, approximately 31 million (5%) children aged less than 5 years were overweight or obese. By 2012, that had increased to around 44 million (6.7%) of children. In Africa alone, the number of overweight children more than doubled, from 4 million to 10 million.[1] Further, "diseases such as diarrhea due to rotavirus and measles continue to kill more than 1 million children under the age of 5 every year, despite effective vaccines against those diseases."[7]

Pediatric/Adolescent

Adolescents, individuals aged 10 to 19 years, constitute 1.2 billion or roughly 17% of the world's population. In general, they are healthy; the vast majority of deaths in this age group are from preventable or treatable causes, such as road traffic injuries, which cause roughly 330 adolescents deaths each day. Although measles deaths are down for this age group, diarrhea, lower respiratory tract infections and meningitis remain among the top 10 causes of death.[11]

Nearly all adolescents become sexually active during this period, and approximately 11% of all births occur to girls aged 15 to 19 years. This marks a decline in recent years, which has translated to lower maternal mortality as well. However, there are more than 2 million adolescents who are HIV positive, and, although deaths have decreased, only 10% to 15% of adolescents in sub-Saharan Africa know their status, placing them at risk for perpetuating transmission and facing declining health themselves. In Sub-Saharan Africa, AIDS remains the number 1 killer among adolescents.[11]

Mental health is also a priority for this age group. Approximately 10% to 20% of children and adolescents worldwide face mental health problems.[12] Globally, "depression is the top cause of illness and disability among adolescents and suicide is the third cause of death."[11] Although approximately one-half of all adult mental health disorders appear by age 14, the majority of these cases are undetected and untreated.[11] Many adolescents face pervasive violence, and approximately 30% of girls aged 15 to 19 years experience intimate partner violence. In the low-income and middle-income countries of Latin America, approximately one-third of deaths among adolescent males are owing to violence.[11]

It is also at this age that many individuals develop harmful health habits. Smoking and its consequences (eg, cancer, heart disease, stroke, lung diseases, diabetes, and chronic obstructive pulmonary disease) is a leading cause of loss of life-years, and it is estimated that 1 in 5 boys aged 13 to 15 and 1 in 10 girls are smokers.[11] Consumption of alcohol can have multiple deleterious effects including increased risky behaviors, unsafe sex, traffic accidents and job related injuries.

Diet and exercise are primary concerns globally among this group, and are often tied to the environments in which adolescents live.[13] Obesity has been increasing in both low-income and high-income countries, and only 25% of adolescents meet the recommended requirements of 60 minutes of moderate activity per day. Lack of iron in diets leading to anemia is the third leading cause of loss of life-years among both girls and boys.[11]

Adults

The world is growing older. As child and other death rates have declined, the average age of the population has increased, leading to a higher proportion of deaths among

.

older populations.[9] Death rates from many diseases have been declining but others have been increasing, including HIV/AIDS, pancreatic cancer, atrial fibrillation and flutter, drug use disorders, diabetes, chronic kidney disease, and sickle cell anaemias.[9] In fact, the number of deaths among adults aged 15 to 49 increased by 44% between 1970 and 2010. Much of this can be attributed to HIV/AIDS, which kills 1.5 million people each year, and increased violence in many parts of the world.[7]

As with adolescents, poor diets and physical inactivity have led to increasing rates of obesity and other lifestyle-related risk factors, including high blood pressure, tobacco smoking, and harmful alcohol use. It is now estimated that fully one-third of adult males globally smoke, including nearly one-half of all males in upper middle income countries. Further, among all adults, dietary risk factors and physical inactivity collectively cause 10% of the disease burden.[7] In 2008, globally 10% of adult males and 14% of adult females were obese.[1] In summary, "we have gone from a world 20 years ago where people weren't getting enough to eat to a world now where too much food and unhealthy food—even in developing countries—is making us sick."[7] Paradoxically, some researchers have noted a double burden of overnutrition and undernutrition within the same households.[14,15] For example, in a 7-country study, Doak and colleagues[14] found that in 6 of the countries, 22% to 66% of households with an underweight person also had an overweight person.

Even with improvements in so many other areas, it is estimated that approximately 1 woman still dies in childbirth every 2 minutes and an additional 20 to 30 experience serious complications.[2] Over time, with increased access to family planning methods, women have gained greater control over their own fertility. In all regions except Sub-Saharan Africa, the total fertility rate is fewer than 3 births per woman. In East Asia and Pacific, Europe and Central Asia and high-income countries, the total fertility rate is less than the replacement level (**Fig. 4**).

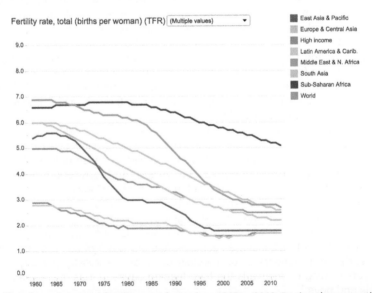

Fig. 4. Global trends in total fertility rates by region, 1960 to 2010. Regional aggregations are for all income levels. (*From* The World Bank. The Data Blog. Between 1960 and 2012, the world average fertility rate halved to 2.5 births per woman. © World Bank. Available at: http://blogs. worldbank.org/opendata/between960-and012-world-average-fertility-rate-halved5-births-woman. Accessed June 10, 2016. Creative Commons Attribution CC BY 3.0 IGO.)

Overall, there was a substantial increase of 37.6% from 1990 to 2010 in the burden of disease attributable to mental health and substance abuse disorders. In 2010, such disorders accounted for 7.4% (183.9 million DALYs) of all DALYs worldwide and were the leading cause of years lived with disability.[16] The problem is particularly acute in Africa, where "pain, anxiety, and depression—which erode quality of life and productivity—are ranked among the highest causes of years lived with disability throughout sub-Saharan Africa." As noted by one researcher, "African nations have not even begun to confront the consequences of exploding cases of mental illness, depression, pain, and the enormous burden of substance abuse that stem from those conditions."[7]

FUNDING

Health spending is a principal determinant of population health but global spending in health is far from equitable, with the preponderance of expenditures occurring in the wealthiest countries. In 2000, the ratio of health care spending per capita in high-income relative to low-income countries was 85 times, $2370 per capita versus $28 per capita. Since then, however, low-income and middle-income countries have renewed their focus on health as a priority area and have more than doubled their expenditures on health, by 129%, 114%, and 162% in low-income, lower middle-income, and upper middle-income countries, respectively. The gap between rich and poor, however, remains wide; in 2011, high-income countries still spent 68 times more per capita on health than low-income countries ($4319 vs $64).[17]

Even with the rapid increase in government spending, the majority of low-income countries fail to spend enough on care. It has been estimated that a minimum basic package of essential health services costs between $34 per capita[18] and $54 per capita.[19] Many low-income countries still currently fail to meet that target.[20]

The impact of spending on health is clear; countries that spend more have greater life expectancy and greater quality of life (**Fig. 5**). Further, "the returns on investing in health are impressive. Reductions in mortality account for about 11% of recent economic growth in low-income and middle-income countries."[21] In short, investing in health leads to a virtuous cycle, better health begets economic growth begets even more improvements in health.

International aid has contributed significantly to a changing global health environment. In 2013, global development assistance for health for low-income and middle-income countries reached an all-time high of $31.3 billion. Much of this increase was owing to increased assistance from the Global Fund to Fight AIDS,

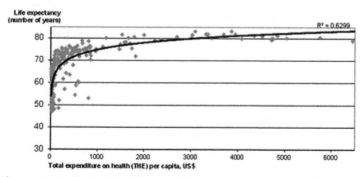

Fig. 5. Life expectancy by total health expenditure per capita. (*From* World Health Organization. Spending on health: a global overview. 2012. Available at: http://www.who.int/mediacentre/factsheets/fs319/en/; with permission.)

Tuberculosis, and Malaria; the GAVI (Global Alliance Vaccine Initiative) Alliance; and bilateral agencies in the United Kingdom. HIV/AIDS (25%) received the largest proportion of health assistance, followed by maternal, newborn, and child health (20%).[8]

Although the effectiveness of international aid has long been a question,[22,23] it is increasingly clear that global health initiatives have substantially improved the health situation in many countries. Since 2000, GAVI has funded vaccinations for 683 million children. Since 1988, the Global Polio Eradication Initiative has helped immunize 2.5 billion children, reducing the number of countries where polio is endemic from 125 to 3. To date, the Global Fund to Fight AIDS, Tuberculosis and Malaria has placed 6.1 million people on antiretroviral therapy, detected and treated 11.2 million cases of tuberculosis, and distributed 360 million insecticide-treated bed nets.[4]

THE WAY FORWARD

So what needs to be done to maintain these positive trends? And what can be done to ameliorate the remaining disparities? In short, what is the way forward? And how can primary care providers contribute?

Improve Access to Health Care

Limited access or complete absence of medical services clearly places many populations at risk for untoward health consequences. In Sub-Saharan Africa, it is estimated that 4 in 10 people do not have access to primary care.[24] Further, even when physical infrastructure is in place, access may be limited owing to scarcity of trained personnel. In low-income countries, for example, there are only 2.4 doctors per 10,000 population on average, far less than the 10 doctors per 10,000 population recommended by the World Health Organization (WHO).[25] The WHO estimates a current worldwide shortage of health workers of 7.2 million with trends indicating a 12.9 million person shortage by 2035.[25] This discrepancy is most evident in Sub-Saharan Africa, which has 25% of the global disease burden but only 3% of the world's health workforce. Within-country differences can be even more dramatic. In South Africa, for example, 43.6% of the population lives in rural areas but only 12% of the country's doctors are stationed in rural health facilities.[26]

Improving access to care can be accomplished even in low resource settings; some low-income and middle-income countries (eg, Sri Lanka, Costa Rica, Cuba) do quite well in ensuring access to care through a number of means, including prioritizing the health sector in public sector funding, establishing tiered referral networks starting at the village level, and innovative delivery systems.

An example of an innovative delivery system can be seen in Bangladesh, a poor country that historically had explosively high fertility rates and underuse of basic health services. Customs and norms in the highly conservative Muslim country restricted female mobility and women's ability to access services for themselves and their children. In 1977, researchers piloted a female-provided "doorstep delivery of care" program in 70 rural villages. After 18 months, contraceptive use had quadrupled and by just 24 months fertility rates had decreased by 25%. In addition, children were healthier, fewer women died of pregnancy-related causes, and child mortality decreased. All of these decreases persisted for more than 2 decades.[27]

Needed policy changes to address such access and shortage issues could include providing financial incentives to health workers to work in rural areas, providing ongoing professional development outside of urban areas, increasing the duration of the residency period during which health workers are given less flexibility with postings, and providing nonfinancial incentives such as free housing, better diagnostic facilities, and access to free or reduced price health care.[28]

Technology can also assist in health care delivery. For example, in many countries of Africa, where cellphone ownership is approaching 90% of adults, technology is already being used with great success. Mobisante, a startup company based in Redmond, Washington, has developed a cellphone-based ultrasound modality. Other companies have piloted mobile eye examinations, electronic medical record keeping, and smartphone microscopes. Still others help patients with medical compliance or assist health care providers with clinical decision making (Health Market Innovations 2016). All told, the WHO has identified 14 ways that cellphones can be used to promote population health.[29]

It is incumbent on the primary care physician working in underserved areas to be aware of these and other technologies to optimize access and health care delivery in their particular local. For example, in the United States, access to specialty care in underserved communities is a significant problem. The 25% of patients from Federally Qualified Health Centers needing specialist consultation often have to wait up to a year for an appointment[30,31] and these long waits have been shown to result in higher rates of chronic disease complications, disability, and death.[32] Such disparities are being addressed by asynchronous electronic consultation between primary care physicians and specialists using a secure Health Insurance Portability and Accountability Act of 1996 (HIPAA)-complaint platform. With specialist assistance, primary care physicians are then able to handle less common/more complex medical conditions. One study[33] showed that 70% of referrals could be handled in this manner, obviating the need for patient specialist appointments and long referral wait times. The average wait time for electronic consultations between physicians in this study was 5 days. Such electronic consultations have proven to be particularly effective in rural and sparsely populated areas.[34] Other studies have noted that telemedicine saves travel time and money for patients, provides better disease management, and increases rapport between specialists and primary care providers, providing education to primary care physicians and enhancing overall collaboration.[35] Technologies such as these will have to be embraced by primary care physicians working in underserved communities if they are to serve their constituents optimally.

Move Toward Universal Health Care Coverage

In many parts of the world, health services are unaffordable to vast numbers of people, and as a consequence individuals may seek care from informal or low-quality providers, forego necessary care, or, perhaps worst of all, suffer impoverishment from debilitating medical expenses, leading to further ill health and a downward cycle deeper into poverty. Carrin and colleagues,[36] looking at household expenditure surveys in 89 countries, found that the costs of accessing health services caused severe financial hardships for 44 million people annually, and an additional 25 million people were thrust into poverty because of such expenditures. Although the global average for household out-of-pocket medical expenditures as a percentage of total expenditures is 19%, in poorer countries it accounts for more than 50% of the total, meaning that poorer households are at greater risk of experiencing catastrophic health expenditures. In short, those least able to afford health care are the ones that must use a higher percentage of their wealth to access that health care.

As a result, the majority of countries have endorsed the idea that health is a fundamental human right, regardless of a person's income,[37] and in recent decades a movement has begun to ensure universal health coverage globally.[38] This means having a health care system that provides health care and financial protection to all citizens.[39] In 2012, the United Nations passed a resolution endorsing universal health coverage as a "pillar of sustainable development and global security." In 2014, a Global Coalition of more than 500 organizations launched a campaign to "Accelerate Access to Universal Health Coverage." According to the coalition, "Each year, 100 million people fall into poverty because they or a family member becomes seriously ill and they have to pay for care out of their own pockets. Around one billion people worldwide can't even access the health care they need, paving the way for disease outbreaks to become catastrophic epidemics."[38]

There is no one way to achieve universal health coverage. "Whether a nation chooses a mixed economy model of coverage, single-payer mode, donor-issued voucher mechanism, or other innovative models of universal financing is not the issue; provision of universal health coverage is the issue facing the entire global health construct."[37] The Lancet Commission on Global Health 2035 proposed 2 pathways toward achieving universal health coverage within the next 20 years: (1) a publicly financed health insurance that covers essential health care interventions or (2) a health insurance program, financed through a range of mechanisms, which covers a broader range of health services from which the poor would be exempt from payment.

Any plan to expand health coverage must tackle a number of fundamental issues. As noted by Marten,[40] the implementation of universal health coverage requires political support for the concept, the government resources to achieve it, and strong oversight to "design, implement, measure and manage complex technical challenges." One of the key challenges involves creating risk pools that promote subsidies from the rich to the poor, from lower risk to higher risk individuals, and from younger, healthier individuals to older ones. Health care providers also need to be incentivized to allocate resources in the most efficient way; health care providers who are expected to take a financial loss from providing care for the poor are apt to reduce the quality of that care or even to stop offering services used by the poor.

A second key challenge is providing coverage to informal workers, who make up 40% to 90% of the population in low-income and middle-income countries. "Most health system stewards employ some mixture of three discrete approaches: (a) using a tax-based system to offer health coverage to all people within a country; (b) enrolling informal workers by "building out" from covering the formal sector through contributory schemes; or (c) employing a combination of tax-based subsidies and contributions to enroll informal workers."[40]

Because of these efforts, approximately 58 countries globally have achieved universal health coverage, including 9 in Africa. Rwanda, for example, uses a mutual insurance scheme paid for by a combination of government and individual contributions of approximately $2 per year. Households that cannot afford to pay the $2 have their copay subsidized by the Global Fund to Fight AIDS, Tuberculosis and Malaria, which funds roughly 1.5 million Rwandans.[37]

Although the role of primary care physicians in policy design and implementation is often limited, it is important for them to be aware of the issues involved and the effects of shortcomings so that they may best advocate for optimal patient care when the opportunity arises.

Reduce Stigma and Prejudice Against Women and Marginalized Populations to Ensure a Safe, Supportive Environment in Which These Underserved Populations Can Fulfill Their Health Care Needs

Stigma—against women, the disabled, the mentally ill, minorities, men who have sex with men, commercial sex workers, injection drug users, among others—can be a huge barrier to care. Certain diseases, such as HIV/AIDS, have long carried devastating stigma—about sexual orientation, about promiscuity, and about divine retribution. Discrimination against people living with HIV and AIDS can prevent infected individuals from getting tested, from seeking treatment, and even from changing risky behaviors.[41] At the extreme, legislation—such as laws against homosexuality—can criminalize behavior, further marginalizing stigmatized populations. Currently, 79 countries have made homosexuality illegal, placing individuals at risk of incarceration if their sexual orientation is revealed through accessing health services.

Power differentials between men and women can determine whether or not women use necessary contraception, become victims of violence, fail to space births appropriately, or even access basic prenatal care or delivery care in a heath facility. A study of 23 low-income countries, for example, found that in none of them did a majority of women have decision making ability alone about their own health care.[42]

The poor also face stigma and discrimination. In the United States, for example, the Affordable Care Act expanded Medicaid coverage to many low-income individuals. However, qualitative interviews have indicated that perceptions of being treated poorly or unfairly because of Medicaid status inhibit many low-income individuals from using the health services to which they are entitled. Allen and colleagues,[43] for example, found

That stigma was most often the result of a provider-patient interaction that felt demeaning, rather than an internalized sense of shame related to receiving public insurance or charity care. An experience of stigma was associated with unmet health needs, poorer perceptions of quality of care, and worse health across several self-reported measures.

The effects of stigma and discrimination on the use of mental health services is perhaps even more pronounced. The WHO estimates that roughly 1 in 4 people will experience a mental or neurologic disorder in their lifetime and that approximately 350 million people worldwide suffer from depression.[44] They further estimate that 76% of people with mental disorders in low-income countries and 85% of people in middle-income countries receive no treatment for their disorder, largely because of stigma and absence of services. High-income countries are not immune either; roughly 35% to 50% of people with mental disorders also do not receive treatment.[44]

Health communication programs can work to reduce stigma against marginalized populations and to shift norms. Ongoing behavior change communication programs still have not reached many populations and are necessary to continue to shift norms and attitudes. In the case of HIV/AIDS, these efforts can include community interactions, such as focus group discussions with people living with HIV, the use of media to educate through entertaining nonstigmatizing "edutainment" messages, engagement with religious and community leaders and celebrities, inclusion of nondiscrimination in institutional and workplace policies, and peer mobilization and support for and by people living with HIV.[41]

To help combat stigma and discrimination, primary care physicians have key responsibilities as role models, advocates of policy change, and protectors of their clients. In Kenya, for example, 15% of HIV-positive individuals reported that a health care worker disclosed their HIV status without their consent.[45] In Lesotho, nearly 23% of people living with HIV stated that it was clear that their HIV records were not kept confidential.[45] Ensuring basic privacy of clients' health and treatment should be a minimal standard for care.

A key responsibility of primary care physicians is to familiarize themselves with human rights and ethics training. This serves 2 purposes. First, it enables primary care physicians to become familiar with their own health rights, including HIV prevention and treatment, universal precautions, and compensation for work-related infection. Second, such training can help to "reduce stigmatizing attitudes in health care settings and to provide health care providers with the skills and tools necessary to ensure patients' rights to informed consent, confidentiality, treatment and non-discrimination."[41]

Improve Surveillance Systems to Detect Threats More Quickly

We live in an increasingly connected world. Airline passengers can move from 1 continent to another in a matter of hours. New and emerging diseases have shown the potential to spread quickly: Ebola, Marburg, Chikungunya, H1N1 influenza, dengue, and most recently Zika. Even places where diseases have been eliminated can experience outbreaks. In 2015, a measles-infected international traveler visiting a theme park in the United States, where measles has been eliminated, is believed to have come into contact with unvaccinated individuals, leading to 147 measles cases across multiple states.

As noted by Bill Gates, the world has been "lucky" with recent outbreaks. The Ebola outbreak in 2014 in western Africa led to approximately 10,000 deaths. The toll, however, could have been far worse if it had not been for the diligent work of dedicated medical professionals, if the disease had been easier to transmit—Ebola is transmitted through bodily fluids—or if the disease had reached a major urban population center. According to Dr Tom Frieden, head of the Centers for Disease Control and Prevention, "With patterns of global travel and trade, disease can spread nearly anywhere within 24 hours. That's why the ability to detect, fight, and prevent these diseases must be developed and strengthened overseas, and not just here in the United States."[46]

Similarly, the influenza outbreak of 2009 also highlighted shortcomings in epidemiologic surveillance and outbreak control. "Shortcomings included the lack of standards for reporting illness, risk factor and mortality data and a mechanism for systematic reporting of epidemiologic data. Such measures would have facilitated direct comparison of data between countries and improved timely understanding of the characteristics and impact of the pandemic."[47]

Currently, only 1 in 5 countries can rapidly detect, respond to, or prevent global health threats caused by emerging infections. Improvements overseas, such as strengthening disease surveillance and laboratory systems for identifying threats, training disease detectives, and building facilities to investigate disease outbreaks make the world—and the United States—more secure.[48]

Achieving better systems to rapidly detect and handle global health threats requires a multifaceted solution. First, health systems need to be strengthened. This goes hand in hand with ensuring universal health coverage, so that disease may be reported quickly without financial concern. Second, there needs to be an abundant supply of health care professionals, most notably a medical reserve corps with training and expertise in epidemics who can respond quickly to threats. Bill Gates advocates pairing such a corps with military forces, who have the logistical capabilities to respond quickly and secure areas. Further, according to Gates, there is a "need to do simulations, germ games, not war games, so that we see where the holes are. The last time a germ game was done in the United States was back in 2001, and it didn't go so well. So far the score is germs: 1, people: 0." Finally, there is an ongoing need for research and development of vaccines and rapid diagnostic tests.[49] Already, research and development seems to have developed a rapid diagnostic test for the Zika virus, which may serve as a model for other new and emerging infectious diseases.[50]

Once again, technology and eHealth can help in dealing with potential outbreaks. For example, *eHealth Africa* developed an Android-based app to help caseworkers trace people who had had contact with Ebola patients. According to Justin Lorenzon, head of software development, "that's a huge deal in controlling an outbreak—making sure that if there's a new case, that it's followed up on and that person is isolated as quickly as possible, so you don't have just a continuation of transmission."[51] The app is an example of how epidemics can lead to innovations that address a current public health crisis. Originally designed to track and prevent polio, eHealth Africa's Ebola contact-tracing app helped to cut reporting times for new Ebola cases by 75%. Lane Goodman of the Center for Health Market Innovations noted that many analysts believe contact tracing was instrumental in helping Nigeria to eradicate the disease.

Primary care physicians are often the front line in detecting outbreaks. A key responsibility in preventing outbreaks is enhanced vigilance to unusual cases and familiarity with the symptoms of emerging diseases. Physicians working in endemic areas have a duty to maintain surveillance systems—reporting all unusual cases as rapidly as possible—so that larger patterns can be detected by surveillance agencies.

Governments Play a Large Role in the Health of Their Populations

Functioning governments are a requisite for good population health. The greatest decrements in health occur in places where governments and nations are failing (eg, Syria, Somalia). Armed conflict can quickly take advanced societies back generations, destroying vital health infrastructure, displacing populations, increasing the risk of disease transmission, and wreaking havoc on morbidity and mortality.[52] Violence can have both direct effects (eg, the loss of life and morbidity from conflict) and indirect effects (eg, the health repercussions of a depleted health care infrastructure).

Governments also play a role in prioritizing health within their public sector budgets. On average, the share of health in aggregate government expenditure is approximately 12%. However, considerable variation exists. Costa Rica spends approximately 28% of the government budget on health; Myanmar spends less than 1%.[20]

Finally, governments, by enforcing contracts, weeding out corruption and abiding by the rule of law, can ensure the maximal effects of public and private spending on health by insisting that limited resources are not leaked from the health system. Transparency International has defined corruption "as the abuse of entrusted power for private gain, which in health care encompasses bribery of regulators and medical professionals, manipulation of information on drug trials, diversion of medicines and supplies, corruption in procurement, and overbilling of insurance companies."[53] In India, unofficial bribes for spots in medical schools can cost up to US$200,000. Kickbacks from clinics and drug companies to physicians for prescribed tests and drugs have led to a climate of distrust between patients and physicians, who are generally not believed to have the well-being of their patients at heart.[54]

Primary care physicians can play an important role by refusing to engage in unethical behaviors, to prioritize patient health over financial gain, and by reporting instances of inappropriate medical conduct. Primary care physicians are encouraged to follow standard ethical of conduct such as the AMA's published code of ethics (available: http://www.ama-assn.org/ama/pub/physician-resources/medical-ethics/code-medical-ethics.page) in their governed areas. Such adherence will foster patient trust and promote "human values" over political expediency or self interest.

Behavioral Economics Is a New Frontier in Changing Healthy Behaviors

One area that has recently emerged for achieving the types of behavior change that can substantially improve health is the field of behavioral economics. Popularized in books such as *Nudge*,[55] *Predictably Irrational*,[56] and *Thinking Fast and Slow*,[57] behavioral economics marries psychology and economics to "nudge" people to change behaviors. This can include gentle nudges—such as reframing choices, getting people to view the future differently, using defaults (eg, automatic refilling of prescriptions or default health insurance plan options) to ensure that people do not succumb to status quo bias, and identity priming (eg, "a lot of people like yourself have started trying medicine *X*, treatment *Y*, or therapy *Z* to deal with problem *Q*") can have huge impacts. To date, these approaches have been small in scale, but promising. Some examples include providing vouchers to keep adolescents in school and avoid early pregnancy/disease, using routine child immunization visits as opportunities to present family planning options to women, making reenrollment in health insurance programs the default, and providing financial incentives to encourage health workers to work with underserved or remote populations.

An ongoing study in Kenya is examining why women fail to adequately plan for delivering in a health facility. This is important because 1 key means of reducing maternal and neonatal mortality is ensuring that women have access to safe, high-quality delivery services at health facilities. During pregnancy, women may express a desire to deliver in a facility but at the time of delivery they may find themselves faced with unexpected barriers that could have been foreseen through better planning. The study is using a key behavioral economics tool—a commitment device—in which women receive cash transfers—both conditional and unrestricted—that encourage them to deliver in a health facility.[58]

Another study examined the issue of early child marriage in Ethiopia, where early marriage is the norm, leading to early childbearing and subsequent increases in maternal and infant mortality. Surveys have found that 19% of girls are married by age 15 and the mean age of marriage is 16 years. Changing the social pressure to marry earlier presented an enormous challenge. The program paired adolescent girls with older female mentors, provided financial incentives for girls to stay in school, enrolled out-of-school girls in livelihood training (eg, basic literacy and numeracy), and engaged communities in problem solving conversations about early marriage. By the endline of the study, girls aged 10 to 14 years were more likely to still be in school and less likely to have gotten married.[59]

As health care technologies and delivery methods continue to evolve, it is vital that primary care physicians express their practical perspective to policy makers so that behavioral economics and other best practices may be used to inform policy creation and revision.

THE ROLE OF THE PRIMARY CARE PHYSICIAN IN ADDRESSING THE CHALLENGES

Primary care physicians in underserved areas are faced with a rapidly changing health environment. As the global epidemiologic transition continues, they will be faced with an increasing diversity of health issues. No longer are noncommunicable diseases the sole purview of first-world countries. Obesity is now a global problem and in many places coexists with undernutrition and more traditional patterns of communicable diseases. Primary care physicians need to be vigilant about addressing this double burden of disease, while also being aware of new and emerging diseases, such as Zika and chikungunya.

Primary care physicians will also have to embrace new technology, which will be essential to both disease surveillance and persistent shortages of health personnel globally. Despite movements toward universal health coverage, both physical and financial access to health care will continue to be a problem. New technology will allow for a greater dependence on telemedicine, which may serve to alleviate the short-term pressure on scarce health services.

As mentioned, primary care physicians working in underserved communities will have to be prepared to enhance access to care, to embrace technology, to be aware of health care policy and WHO universal coverage recommendations, to embrace patient education and the reduction of stigmatization and prejudice, to be aware of and ready to respond to activated disease surveillance systems and to be aware of governmental policy as it relates to health of their populations. To this end, the Centers for Disease Control and Prevention and other agencies have noted the need to enhance training for primary care physicians working in these areas. Education in public and population health,[60] leadership, community engagement, community collaboration and data analysis are all needed.[61,62] Such skills are vital to optimally addressing the chronic medical conditions that account for more than 75% of US health care costs and are disproportionately present in underserved communities. This type of primary care physician training may be even more important in the developing world.

REFERENCES

1. World Health Statistics 2014. A wealth of information on global public health. WHO. Available at: http://apps.who.int/iris/bitstream/10665/112739/1/WHO_HIS_HSI_14.1_eng.pdf?ua=1). Accessed June 10, 2016.
2. UNFPA. United Nations Population Fund. Maternal Health. Available at: http://www.unfpa.org/maternal-health. Accessed March 5, 2016.
3. Cleland J, Bernstein S, Ezeh A, et al. Family planning: the unfinished agenda. Lancet 2006;368:1820–7.
4. Gates B, Gate M. 2015 Gates annual letter: three myths that block progress for the poor. Available at: http://www.gatesfoundation.org/Who-We-Are/Resources-and-Media/Annual-Letters-List/Annual-Letter-2014. Accessed February 29, 2016.
5. World Bank. 2015. Global Monitoring Report: development goals in an era of demographic change. Available at: http://www.worldbank.org/en/publication/global-monitoring-report. Accessed June 10, 2016.
6. The Economist, 2011. Daily chart: Africa's impressive growth. Available at: http://www.economist.com/blogs/dailychart/2011/01/daily_chart. Accessed February 1, 2016.
7. Institute for Health Metrics and Evaluation. 2012. Global burden of disease: massive shifts reshape the health landscape worldwide. Available at: http://www.healthdata.org/news-release/global-burden-disease-massive-shifts-reshape-health-landscape-worldwide. Accessed February 17, 2016.
8. Dieleman JL, Graves CM, Templin T, et al. Global health development assistance remained steady in 2013 but did not align with recipients' disease burden. Health Aff 2013;33:878–86.
9. GBD 2013 Mortality and Causes of Death Collaborators. Global, regional, and national age-sex specific all-cause and cause-specific mortality for 240 causes of death, 1990-2013: a systematic analysis for the Global Burden of Disease Study 2013. Lancet 2015;385:117–71.
10. Allemani C, Weir HK, Carrera H, et al. Global surveillance of cancer survival 1995–2009: analysis of individual data for 25,676,887 patients from 279 population-based registries in 67 countries (CONCORD-2). Lancet 2015;385:977–1010.

11. World Health Organization. Adolescents: health risks and solutions, WHO Fact Sheet No. 345. Available at: http://www.who.int/mediacentre/factsheets/fs345/en/. Accessed February 18, 2016.

12. Kieling C, Baker-Henningham H, Belfer M, et al. Child and adolescent mental health worldwide: evidence for action. Lancet 2011;378:1515–25.

13. Gordon-Larsen P, McMurray RG, Popkin BM. Determinants of adolescent physical activity and inactivity patterns. Pediatrics 2000;105:E83.

14. Doak CM, Adair LS, Bentley M, et al. The dual burden household and the nutrition transition paradox. Int J Obes (Lond) 2005;29:129–36.

15. Megan J, Brewis A. Paradoxical malnutrition in mother–child pairs: untangling the phenomenon of over- and under-nutrition in underdeveloped economies. Econ Hum Biol 2009;7:28–35.

16. Whiteford HA, Degenhardt L, Rehm J, et al. Global burden of disease attributable to mental and substance use disorders: findings from the Global Burden of Disease Study 2010. Lancet 2013;382:1575–86.

17. The World Bank. Data. Health expenditure per capita. Available at: http://data.worldbank.org/indicator/SH.XPD.PCAP. Accessed on June 10, 2016.

18. World Health Organization. Macroeconomics and Health (CMH). Available at: http://www.who.int/macrohealth/en/. Accessed June 10, 2016.

19. World Health Organization. Constraints to Scaling up the Health Millennium Development Goals: costing and financial analysis gap, The taskforce for innovative international financing for health systems. 2010. Geneva.

20. Tandon A, Fleisher L, Li R, et al. Reprioritizing government spending on health: pushing an elephant up the stairs. Washington, DC: World Bank; 2014. HNP Discussion Paper 85773.

21. Jamison DT, Summers LH, Alleyne G, et al. Global health 2035: a world converging within a generation. Lancet 2013;382:1898–955.

22. Easterly W. The white Man's burden: why the West's efforts to aid the rest have done so much ill and so little good. New York: Penguin Press; 2006.

23. Kaufmann D. Aid effectiveness and governance. World Bank. Available at: https://openknowledge.worldbank.org/handle/10986/4571. Accessed May 14, 2016.

24. Knapp T, Richardson B, Viranna S. Three practical steps to better health for Africans. Available at: http://www.mckinsey.com/industries/healthcare-systems-and-services/our-insights/three-practical-steps-to-better-health-for-africans. Accessed January 13, 2016.

25. World Health Organization. Global Health Observatory (GHO) data. Density of physicians (total number per 1000 population, latest available year). Available at: http://www.who.int/gho/health_workforce/physicians_density/en/. Accessed June 10, 2016.

26. AHP. Africa Health Placements. The Need: No People = No Healthcare. Available at: http://ahp.org.za/the-need/. Accessed June 10, 2016.

27. Joshi S, Schultz TP. Family planning and women's and children's health: long-term consequences of an outreach program in Matlab, Bangladesh. Demography 2015;50:149–80.

28. World Health Organization. Global health workforce alliance. A universal truth: no health without a workforce. Third Global Forum on Human Resources for Health Report. Available at: http://www.who.int/workforcealliance/knowledge/resources/hrhreport2013/en/. Accessed on June 10, 2016.

29. World Health Organization. Health: new horizons for health through mobile technologies, 2011. Available at: http://www.who.int/goe/publications/goe_mhealth_web.pdf. Accessed June 10, 2016.

30. Kim Y, Chen AH, Keith E, et al. Not perfect, but better: primary care providers' experiences with electronic referrals in a safety net health system. J Gen Intern Med 2009;24:614–9.

31. Kim-Hwang JE, Chen AH, Bell DS, et al. Evaluating electronic referrals for specialty care at a public hospital. J Gen Intern Med 2010;25:1123–8.

32. Cook NL, Hicks LS, O'Malley AJ, et al. Access to specialty care and medical services in community health centers. Health Aff (Millwood) 2007;26:1459–68.

33. Olayiwola JN, Anderson D, Jepeal N. Electronic consultations to improve the primary care- specialty care interface for cardiology in the medically underserved: a cluster-randomized controlled trial. Ann Fam Med 2016;14:133–40.

34. O'Gorman LD, Hogenbirk JC, Warry W. Clinical telemedicine utilization in Ontario over the Ontario Telemedicine Network. Telemed J E Health 2016;22:473–9.

35. Meyers L, Gibbs D. Building a telehealth network through collaboration: the story of the Nebraska statewide telehealth network. Crit Care Nurs Q 2012;35:346–52.

36. Carrin G, Mathauer I, Xu K, et al. Universal coverage of health services: tailoring its implementation. Bull World Health Organ 2008;86:857–63.

37. Garrett LA, Chowdhury MR, Pablos-Méndez A. All for universal health coverage. Lancet 2009;374:1294–9.

38. Rockefeller Foundation. Universal health coverage: a commitment to close the gap. 2013. Available at: https://www.rockefellerfoundation.org/report/universal-health-coverage-a-commitment-to-close-the-gap/. Accessed June 10, 2016.

39. World Health Organization. What is universal health coverage? Available at: http://www.who.int/features/qa/universal_health_coverage/en/. Accessed March 19, 2016.

40. The World Bank. Marten R. Investing in health. Ten (Plus One) things to think about when planning and implementing universal health coverage. Available at: http://blogs.worldbank.org/health/ten-plus-one-things-think-about-when-planning-and-implementing-universal-health-coverage. Accessed June 10, 2016.

41. UNAIDS. May 15, 2012. Key programmes to reduce stigma and discrimination and increase access to justice in national HIV responses. Available at: http://www.unaids.org/en/resources/documents/2012/Key_Human_Rights_Programmes. Accessed June 10, 2016.

42. Kishor S, Subaiya L. 2008. 2008. Understanding women's empowerment: a comparative analysis of Demographic and Health Surveys (DHS) data. DHS Comparative Reports No. 20. Calverton, Maryland, USA: Macro International. Available at: http://dhsprogram.com/publications/publication-cr20-comparative-reports.cfm#sthash.NtUHytt2.dpuf. Accessed June 10, 2016.

43. Allen H, Wright BJ, Harding K, et al. The role of stigma in access to health care for the poor. Milbank Q 2014;92:289–318.

44. World Health Organization. Mental disorders. Fact sheet number 396; 2015. Available at: http://www.who.int/mediacentre/factsheets/fs396/en/. Accessed January 15, 2016.

45. The people living with HIV Stigma index: Kenya. 2009. Available at: http://www.stigmaindex.org/sites/default/files/reports/Kenya%20People%20Living%20with%20HIV%20Stigma%20Index%20Report%202009.pdf. Accessed March 3, 2016.

46. Centers for Disease Control and Prevention. 2013. Measles Still Threatens Security. Available at: http://www.cdc.gov/media/releases/2013/p1205-meales-threat.html. Accessed February 14, 2016.
47. Briand S, Mounts A, Chamberland M. Challenges of global surveillance during an influenza pandemic. Public Health 2011;125:247–56.
48. Centers for Disease Control and Prevention. Press Release, December 16, 2013. CDC looks back at 2013 health challenges, ahead to 2014 health worries. Available at: https://www.cdc.gov/media/releases/2013/p1216-eoy2013.html. Accessed June 10, 2016.
49. Gates, B. 2015. Ted Talks: the next outbreak: we're not ready. Available at: https://www.ted.com/talks/bill_gates_the_next_disaster_we_re_not_ready/transcript?language=en. Accessed June 10, 2016.
50. Biocan. 2016. Zika virus rapid test. Available at: http://www.zikatest.com/?page_id=24. Accessed March 3, 2016.
51. Center for Health market innovations, 2016. Available at: http://healthmarketinnovations.org/blog/developing-countries-lead-way-mobile-health-technologies. Accessed March 8, 2016.
52. Murray CJ, King G, Lopez AD, et al. Armed conflict as a public health problem. BMJ 2002;324:346–9.
53. Jain A, Nundy S, Abbasi K. Corruption: medicine's dirty open secret. BMJ 2014; 348:g4184.
54. Berger D. Corruption ruins the doctor-patient relationship. BMJ 2014;348:g3169.
55. Thaler RH, Sunstein C. Nudge: improving decisions about health, wealth, and happiness. New Haven (CT): Yale University Press; 2008.
56. Ariely D. Predictably irrational: the hidden forces that shape our decisions. Harper Perennial; 2007.
57. Kahneman D. Thinking, Fast and Slow. New York: Farrar, Straus and Giroux; 2011.
58. Cohen J, McConnell M. Behavioral economics in reproductive health initiative. 2016. Impact of pre-commitment to delivery facilities on the quality of maternal and neonatal care. Available at: http://www.beri-research.org/research/sub-saharan-africa/kenya-quality-delivery-facilities/. Accessed March 5, 2016.
59. Erulkar A, Muthengi E. Evaluation of Berhane Hewan: a program to delay child marriage in rural Ethiopia. Int Perspect Sex Reprod Health 2009;35:6–14.
60. Maeshiro R, Koo D, Keck CW. Integration of public health into medical education: an introduction to the supplement. Am J Prev Med 2011;41:S145–8.
61. Elliott L, McBride TD. Health care system collaboration to address chronic diseases: a nationwide snapshot from state public health practitioners. Prev Chronic Dis 2014;11:E152.
62. Institute of Medicine. Primary care and public health: exploring integration to improve population health. Released March 28, 2012. Available at: http://www.nationalacademies.org/hmd/Reports/2012/Primary-Care-and-Public-Health.aspx. Accessed March 30, 2016.

Printed and bound by CPI Group (UK) Ltd, Croydon, CR0 4YY

03/10/2024

01040475-0004